Mother Becoming

Empowering You in Pregnancy, Birthing and Early Mothering

WENDY JACKSON

MB PRESS

Acknowledgment of Country

I wish to acknowledge the traditional custodians of the land, the Whadjuk people of the Noongar nation, where this work has been created. I pay my respects to Elders past, present and emerging, especially to the matriarchal Elders of many nations currently working together to bring back Grandmother's Law and birthing wisdom to the forefront of Birthing on Country. I acknowledge that sovereignty of this land has never been ceded.

Published by MB Press
Website: www.motherbecoming.com.au

ISBN: 978-0-646-70791-4

Also available as an ebook. ISBN: 978-1-7642073-0-0

Cover illustration by Wendy Jackson
Illustrations by Wendy Jackson

Disclaimer

The information and materials in this book is provided "as is"; no representations are made that the content is error-free. While the author has made every effort to ensure the accuracy and completeness of the information, the book does not warrant or guarantee the accurateness. The author has made every effort to provide resources that are free. The choice to explore a resource further, such as buying a product or educational course, is the reader's own. The information in this book does not and is not intended to constitute medical or legal advice. This book does not guarantee results and is not a substitute for medical attention, treatment of existing conditions or diagnosis. It is not intended to provide a clinical diagnosis nor take the place of proper personalised, fully informed medical advice from a qualified midwife or medical practitioner.

The author has made every effort to contact copyright holders and gain permission to use quotations from other published works.

It takes a village ...

I was supported through the journey of writing this book by seven mothers who have written about their stories in the form of letters to you. Each chapter is in their name.

Liesja, Samantha, Ashleigh, Ally, Katie, Alysia and Clémentine are integral to this book because they care as deeply about supporting women becoming mothers as I do. Their journeys into mothering are as unique as yours will be. Their generosity of spirit will take your breath away. They kindly gave me photos for inspiration for the illustrations to help express the stories we wish to tell.

Have a box of tissues ready when you read their letters.

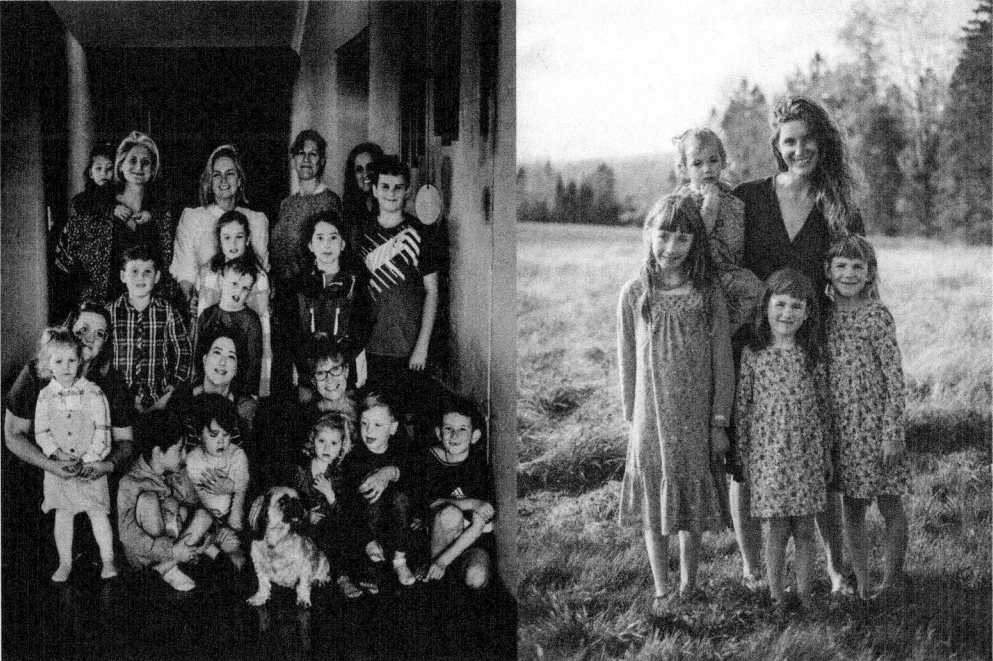

From top left: Charlie, Clémentine, Liesja, Alysia, Katie, Jake
Middle row: Casey, Freyja, Lachy, Bonnie
Bottom row: Layla, Samantha, Octavius, Ashleigh, Rafael, Wendy, Alizée, Mochi dog, Nicholas, Mason

From top left: Vance, Ally, Audrey, Edith, Norah

About the author

Wendy Jackson is a retired midwife after 30 years' practice. She has worked in all areas of clinical care, including neonatal intensive care, as a research midwife and health professional educator. Wendy is published in the British Journal of Midwifery on 'Breastfeeding and Type 1 diabetes mellitus.' She retired unhappily due to ill-health.

A yoga practitioner since the birth of her daughter, Wendy found the practice calming when suffering postpartum depression and post-traumatic stress disorder (PTSD) after a traumatic birth. She became an instructor in later life, and specialised in pregnancy, birthing and postpartum yoga. A graduate of the Make Birth Better birth trauma training, Wendy is also a matrescence coach and passionate matricentric feminist. She harnesses these to bring them into the pregnancy, birthing and early mothering space.

Wendy is totally nutty about mothers' wellbeing and passionate about empowering women and mothers in their pregnancy, birthing and early mothering journey towards emotional and physical wellness. She supports women to advocate for themselves and cultivate self-trust, so they can realise their own immense power and worth. She also creates connection and community so that mothers feel seen, honoured and supported in a safe environment.

Born in England to a Dutch mum and English dad, Wendy spent her childhood and early teens moving around overseas and feels a part of the global village. She migrated to Western Australia in 2006 with her husband and 2 children. Wendy lives beside a national park with her dogs, husband and plenty of wildlife. (Notice the order? Dogs first!) She is an artist who uses graphite, watercolour, acrylic and oils to express her love of nature and the power of women. Her happiest moments are when the house is filled with friends, family, mums, babies and children's laughter. With plenty of mess left behind as evidence of a joyful time.

Author's note on language usage

'Mother' is powerfully feminine; an archetypal noun used globally, representative of life-giving, nurturing and divinity. With utmost respect to diverse gender identities, I choose to use the terms 'woman', 'mother', 'matriarchal', 'matrescence' and 'matricentric' in the context of this piece of work.

With regard to 'postpartum' and 'postnatal', what's the difference? The word 'partum' refers to the one giving birth, so all about the mother, whereas 'natal' indicates the one who is born, so all about the baby. As this work is all about 'mother becoming' from a matricentric viewpoint, I use 'postpartum' here. Where other works use the term 'postnatal' to mean 'postpartum', I shall respectfully do so when referencing those works.

Praise for this book

This book is a poetic gift, full of wisdom. Through the power of storytelling, you can find yourself. Discovering what your journey can be, and determining what is right for you. *Mother Becoming* helps us to understand matrescence and the importance of honouring and supporting the immensity of this transition. This is the core of our humanity. Wendy draws strength from resources which enrich the journey of self-discovery. The resources are evidence based and centred around an understanding that women are the decision makers.

Dr Catherine Bell
Doula, author, birth cartographer and director of Maternity Choices Australia

Bringing new life into the world is one of the most transformative journeys a woman can embark upon. It is a path woven with anticipation, joy, and, at times, uncertainty. In a world where maternity care is constantly evolving, where choices can feel overwhelming, and where the voices of expectant parents are sometimes drowned out by institutional norms, there is an ever-growing need for resources that educate, support and give the power back to the woman. Wendy Jackson's book is one such resource – a guiding light for those navigating the sacred experience of pre-pregnancy, fertility, pregnancy, birth, and the postpartum period.

From the moment I began reading, I was captivated by the depth of knowledge, the clarity of thought, and the compassionate tone that underpins every chapter. This book is more than a manual; it is an invitation to embark on a deeply personal journey – one that honours the mind, body, emotions, and spirit. With evidence-based research, historical context, and a wealth of resources, Wendy has created a beautiful book that not only informs but also inspires.

What sets this book apart is its ability to bridge the gap between information and action. Each chapter offers a thoughtful "wish list," enabling readers to continue their exploration through books, podcasts, and research links that align with their own values and needs. It is a resource that meets people where they are and encourages them to go deeper, ask more questions, and become active participants in their maternity care, not passive bystanders. Additionally, the book includes the voices of women who share their varied lived experiences. These real and raw stories serve as powerful tools for education, reminding us of the diverse paths that birth and motherhood can take, and reinforcing the importance of sharing these journeys.

Wendy's words serve as a gentle but firm reminder that birth is not a one-size-fits-all experience. Instead, it is a deeply personal rite of passage —one that deserves thoughtful preparation, meaningful conversations, and a birth team that truly honours the woman's wishes.

This book is a gift for couples to read together, encouraging discussions that may not have otherwise arisen. It highlights the importance of negotiation with care providers, the creation of a birth map that acknowledges all potential pathways, and the integration of relaxation techniques, yoga traditions, pain relief options, and comfort measures. It is a book that nurtures confidence and encourages a proactive approach to perinatal care as a whole, not just birth.

Vicki Hobbs
Back to Basics Birthing Educator and Doula
Doula Trainer with Doula Training Academy Australia

I can well imagine loving something like this when I was pregnant with my first baby - I devoured everything I could find on being mentally and spiritually prepared for birthing, as many first time mums do, and I would have valued it when I was a midwifery student as well for the practice suggestions, evidence summations, and references.

Dr Sara Bayes PhD RN RM FACM
Vice Chancellor's Professorial Research Fellow
Edith Cowan University

I am certain Mother Becoming is the most profoundly empowering and supportive book an expecting mother could read in preparation for 'matrescence' - the journey to motherhood. Written by an experienced midwife, birthing educator and yoga teacher, this book is a trove of facts, insights, personal stories, helpful resources, and yoga methods all of which help women remain at the centre of their own birthing and motherhood experience. Birthing a baby is a profound rite of passage for women, yet for many the experience is unnecessarily reduced to a medicalised and sometimes dehumanising procedure. Wendy takes us back in time to when mothers, grandmothers and midwives were central and revered, and traces the history of birthing to modern times. She brings forward the insights and knowledge we collectively need to centralise the birthing mother's needs and perspectives - regardless of the place of birth. Mother Becoming is interwoven with fierce wisdom and gentle guidance. Wendy shares beautiful, powerfully effective yet simple yoga, breathing and mindfulness practices which can help a mother to manage her state of mind and body through pregnancy, birthing and the early months of intense mothering.

On reading this book I felt sadness that this information wasn't available to me when I brought my own babies into this world, and also happiness that it now exists for women now and onwards. *Mother Becoming* is a powerful handbook to help women reclaim birthing as the profound rite of passage it is.

Mandy Becker Knox
Creator, Hatha Yoga Method
Director, Kookaburra Yoga
www.kookaburrayoga.com

In Memory of Thomas Michael Treanor
Birth and Passing 13.2.2013

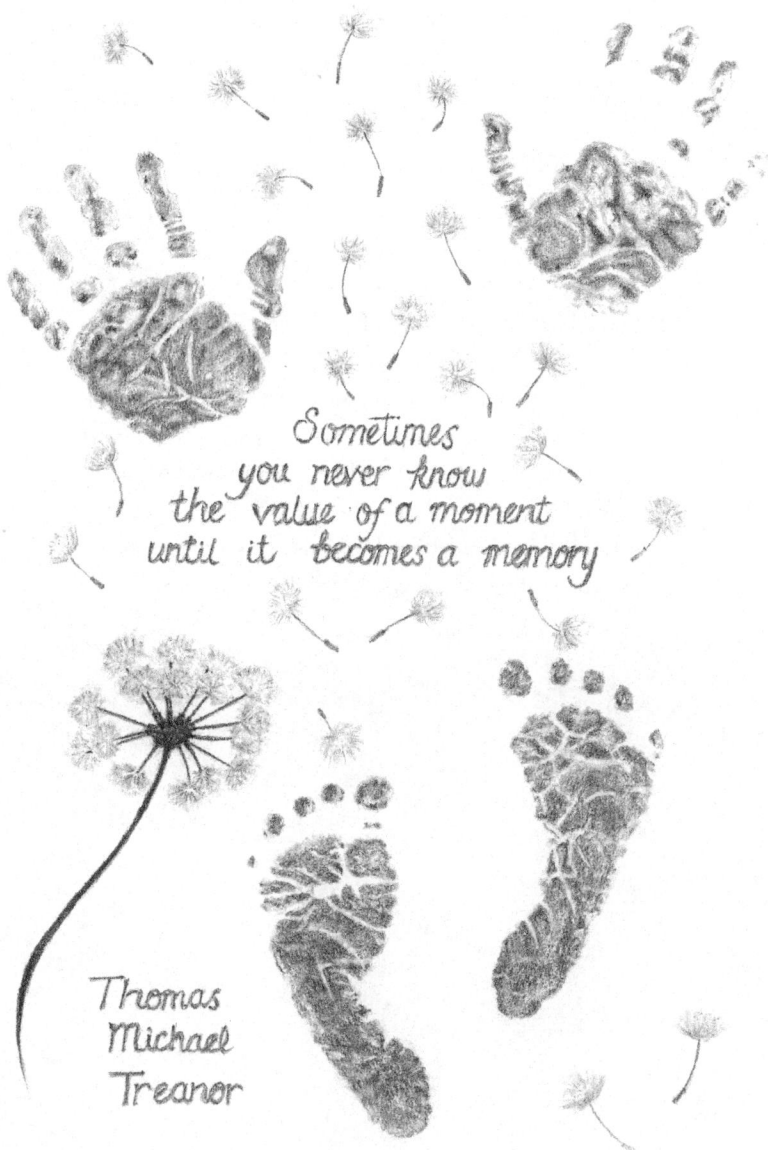

Sometimes
you never know
the value of a moment
until it becomes a memory

Thomas
Michael
Treanor

Dedication

Liesja, Samantha, Ashleigh, Ally, Katie, Alysia and Clémentine,
this book would not have been possible without you. Thank you for your vulnerability and
belief in this work to bring birthing and early mothering to the forefront of conversation.

For all mothers past, present and future.

And for Mum.

You gave birth to me at home. Dad had to pick up the midwife
because it was too snowy for her to cycle.
He told me he wanted to be there and said it was an "interesting scene". He
felt no anxiety, and held Mum's hand. The midwife sat beside the fire reading
War and Peace, with sage words like, "a bit of a way to go yet".

In the experience of labour, birth and the very new hours of
parenthood, they forgot it was New Year's Eve.

Contents

Chapter 2
The Middle Months with Samantha 53

Chapter 3
Ashleigh With You in Late Pregnancy   89

Chapter 7
Early Mothering and the Fourth Trimester with Clémentine

Abbreviations

ABA	Australian Breastfeeding Association
ABE	Antenatal breast expressing
ABTA	Australasian Birth Trauma Association
ACM	Australian College of Midwifery
ACOG	American College of Obstetricians and Gynaecologists
AHPRA	Australian Health Practitioner Regulation Agency
ARM	Artificial rupture of membranes
BASIS	Baby Sleep Information Source
BMI	Body mass index
BTA	Birth Trauma Association
CALD	Culturally and linguistically diverse
CMP	Community Midwifery Program
COC	Continuity of carer
COPE	Centre of Perinatal Excellence
CS	Caesarean section
CTG	Cardiotocography
CVS	Chorionic villus sampling
DMER	Dysphoric milk ejection reflex
DNA	Deoxyribonucleic acid
DRA	Diastasis rectus abdominis
ECV	External cephalic version
EDA	Epidural analgesia
EDD	Estimated due date
EFM	External fetal heart monitoring
FIGO	Federation of International Gynaecologists and Obstetricians
FNT	Fetal nuchal translucency
GA	General anaesthetic
GBS	Group B streptococcus
GD	Gestational diabetes
GP	General practitioner
HRiC	Human Rights in Childbirth
ICM	International Confederation of Midwives
KICO	Knees in, calves out
LHS	Learning Health System
MBB	Make Birth Better
MCA	Maternity Choices Australia
MCN	Maternity Consumer Network
MGP	Midwifery Group Practice
MHC	Midwifery Homebirth Care
MHM	Maternal Health Matters
MRI	Magnetic resonance image

MTFHR	Methylenetetrahydrofolate reductase
NICE	National Institute for Health and Care Excellence
NICU	Neonatal intensive care units
NIPT	Non-invasive prenatal test
PND	Postnatal depression
PPL	Paid parental leave
PTSD	Post-traumatic stress disorder
PTSS	Post-traumatic stress syndrome
RANZCOG	Royal Australian and New Zealand College of Obstetrics and Gynaecology
SANDS	Stillbirth and Neonatal Death Society
SIDS	Sudden infant death syndrome
SUDI	Sudden unexpected death of an infant
TMCC	Transforming Maternity Care Collaborative
TOLAC	Trial of labour after caesarean
USS	Ultrasound scan
VBAC	Vaginal birth after caesarean
WGEA	Workplace Gender Equality Agency
WHO	World Health Organization

Foreword

As an obstetrician, I have walked beside many women as they journey through pregnancy, birth, and the early days of motherhood. I've witnessed the intensity of that transition—physically, emotionally, and spiritually. Yet, no matter how many times I observe it, I remain in awe of the strength, vulnerability, self-discovery and transformation that motherhood brings. That transformation—or matrescence—deserves more than clinical observation; it deserves reverence, compassion, and guidance. That is exactly what this book offers.

Mother Becoming is a call to reframe how we view motherhood. It centres the woman—her voice, her story, her autonomy. In a world that too often medicalises, politicises, or commercialises birth, this book invites us to return to the heart of it all: the woman becoming a mother.

Wendy brings to this work the wisdom of decades in midwifery, her lived experience, and her unrelenting passion for women's holistic wellbeing. She writes with the kind of care only a mother, midwife, and advocate can bring. Her grounding in evidence-based knowledge, combined with the power of lived stories and her profound respect for the sacred nature of birth, make this an invaluable resource for every woman—whether she is preparing to conceive, currently pregnant, birthing, grieving, or navigating the fourth trimester.

Wendy paints the physiological and hormonal changes of pregnancy and birth not as isolated biological events, but as a magnificent orchestration—where every hormone and physiological change is like a different instrument playing in concert. Sometimes in harmony, sometimes in discord, but always moving towards the birth of not just a child, but of a new mother. This understanding allows women to feel the innate intelligence of their bodies, to trust the music within them even when the journey takes unexpected turns.

Wendy and I have shared many conversations—sometimes from different starting points, but always with the shared goal of respectful, woman-centred care. I believe deeply in shared decision-making, in informed choice, and in care that is free from coercion or bias. Wendy's voice echoes these values in every chapter. She invites women to reclaim ownership of their journey, to honour their beliefs and intuition, and to find strength even in unexpected outcomes.

The unique structure of this book—framed around the roots of matrescence—allows for an exploration of the physical, cultural, social, and spiritual influences on the mothering journey. This is not about prescribing a "right" way to birth or parent. It is about inviting reflection, offering practical tools, and helping each reader find what is right for her.

For those of us who work in maternity care, this book is also a mirror. It asks us to consider the impact of our systems, our language, and our presence. It reminds us that empowerment and safety are not mutually exclusive. It challenges us as Doctors and Midwives to co-create a space where women are informed, respected, and deeply supported during one of the most challenging metamorphosis of their lives.

Thank you, Wendy, for pouring your soul into providing this formidable guide to matrescence.

Dr Liza Fowler
Obstetrician, Perth, Western Australia

Introduction

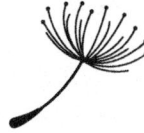

Dear Mother Becoming,

Hello, and a heartfelt, warm, embracing welcome.

Women enter pregnancy and motherhood with certain aspirations, imagining how the future for themselves and their children will be. They anticipate challenges and hurdles, but do not fully comprehend the lived experience because the truth is rarely told. Australian women are among the greatest consumers of private antenatal education. Yet many come out the other side of our current system of maternity care shocked, scarred, confused, bewildered, frustrated and angry. They are unprepared for the differences between anticipation of birthing and mothering, and the intensity of the reality.

Currently, one in 5 women experiences postnatal depression (PND) in Australia and our leading cause of maternal death is suicide. In the UK, Canada, the USA and NZ, the picture is similar. One in 3 mothers experiences birth trauma in Australia. One in 10 of these mums goes on to develop PTSD and others post-traumatic stress syndrome (PTSS). Our system of birthing and (lack of) postpartum care is failing women, and this needs to change. Some work has begun. The 2024 New South Wales Legislative Council Select Committee on Birth Trauma report made 43 recommendations to reduce birth trauma and provide care for women who have birth trauma. Some of the recommendations are emphasised in this book. It is important to note that recommendations are not legally binding, and the government or institutions do not have to act on them.

The suffering of mothers is so often invisible because we expect them to have it all under control, to not complain. There is a wall of silence about mental health and problems 'down there'. The shame and stigma associated with feelings of self-blame for not coping, having 'failed at birth' and not living up to others' expectations cause suffering and depression. By the time these mothers ask for help, they are broken. There is also the reality of boredom, repetitiveness, fatigue beyond words, overwhelm, invisibility, and not enjoying being a mother. These are not spoken about for fear of judgement, so mothers are isolated in their suffering and silence themselves.

How about we turn our birthing and early mothering world upside-down? And place you, the woman and mother, at the centre. A focus that nurtures you in mind, body and spirit on your pregnancy, birthing and early mothering journey. A place that cheers you on, believes in you, empowers you and puts your autonomy in your hands. A home for you to come and find community, respect, trustworthy information and love. Where you can become informed and empowered, and able to adjust to unexpected changes, while still being a part of the process.

In this book are letters gifted from 7 women, who have courageously shared their experiences with you. They begin each chapter of this journey we are embarking on. Liesja, Samantha, Ashleigh, Ally, Katie, Alysia and Clémentine are integral to this book because they care as deeply about supporting women becoming mothers as I do. Their journeys into mothering are as unique as yours will be. Their generosity of spirit takes my breath away. They kindly gave me photos for inspiration for the illustrations to help express the stories we wish to tell. Have a box of tissues ready when you read their letters. You will share in their utter joy, anguish, laughter, grief, crippling fatigue – the entire spectrum of emotions – and come away with a sense of awe at their fortitude. They will inspire you and encourage you to believe that you have that same strength within yourself too. You will be reassured that you are not alone in your experiences.

Mother Becoming is not a textbook that talks *at* you. This is not a book that makes you feel you have failed if you don't achieve what is suggested to be 'the best way' to be pregnant, to birth and to parent. Take away what you will. There is no judgement here about how to be pregnant, how to birth or how to mother your baby. I don't care if you are purple or green, what you believe in, your sexual orientation, shape or nation. This is for all women, no matter your heritage, culture or beliefs, because the practices and philosophy expressed in this book transcend our differing qualities.

This is an interactive journey together. There is a **wishlist** 🌾 of 7 resources in each chapter that I hope you are happy to read, watch and listen to, but the choice is entirely yours. Choice – your choice – is of utmost importance and is always supported here. To strengthen your mind and body during this enormous transition in your life, there are practice offerings of yoga, mindfulness, meditation and breathwork in each chapter. They will all support your experiences, helping you be fully present and autonomous in a mindful way during pregnancy, birth and postpartum. This is especially useful if unexpected complications occur. Nothing ever goes exactly to plan. We know this. It's essential to know how to navigate unexpected experiences, and how to find more information or support, or acceptance so you can adjust to changes while still feeling part of the process.

In addition to the **wishlist** 🌾, there are other resources throughout, placed in a goody box of information – podcasts, blogs, videos, books, e-books, PDFs, websites, apps, research references, news articles and links to professional bodies. They are to be used as tools, evidence, support and further information to empower and enrich you. This is one way of sharing and discussing a condensed version of the latest available knowledge, which is easy to understand, useful, reliable and illuminating. These are fabulous free resources, cherry-picked for their reliability and transparency, so you don't have to do the legwork. It's important to state that I do not endorse any of the advertisers in these podcasts, videos, blogs and websites. It is your choice to explore a resource further at cost.

Resources do change over time, so please refer to www.motherbecoming.com.au, the Mother Becoming website, for updated **wishlist** 🌾 resources and the latest research.

Together, we will identify themes, attitudes and beliefs that have led to the development of our current maternal care pathways. It is important to understand the ingrained attitudes within the culture of birthing and mothering in westernised societies today. This book will explain why we have our current maternity care choices, how they developed and why some women are increasingly opting out of the available care. The book will help you become confident and proactive in your choices. It will inform you about your right to choice and respect. It will support you in preparing for the reality of 'mother becoming'.

This is going to be real and raw, to prepare you for the real world of mothering. No flim-flam. No rose-tinted glasses. The reality of modern experiences of pregnancy, birthing and early parenthood will be aired and shared. This reality check will empower change. You will become proud, accepting and confident in the changes and capacity of your body. Enjoy this expression of your femininity because you are extraordinary.

Most importantly, no matter what your experiences are, you have not 'failed' in any way. There is no 'right way' to do any of this, because we and our babies are all so unique.

The Why of *Mother Becoming*

It is my dearest wish to provide awareness, thoughts and strategies that will lead to a much-needed return to mothering the mother – to nourish the mother physically and emotionally, to prepare her for the mother she is becoming. I aim to support mothers to speak up when they need help and to accept support with grace – without guilt or shame, or fear of being perceived as failing when they can't cope. I wish to highlight how to recognise postnatal depression early and help you find out where to go for help. We'll talk about the importance of creating a village to support you in this process. And we'll start that support from the beginning of pregnancy, as a natural thing to do. *Mother Becoming* is about developing a you-centred network.

As a culture, we tend to become absorbed in preparing for birth, but what about preparing for our experiences of mothering? Our birthing experience is deeply embedded, forever remembered like yesterday, incredibly important. Birthing, though, is a few days of our lives, and we prepare for it to the nth degree. Mothering is for the rest of our lives, yet we don't prepare for it enough.

Enter matrescence. If society understood the essence of what becoming a mother involves, by supporting that incredible process, we may reduce experiences of isolation, lack of self-worth and self-esteem, overwhelm, anxiety and stress. This insight would help reduce depression and depletion, and release mothers from the unhappiness of unattainable, unrealistic expectations. Universal understanding of matrescence could lead to the re-emergence of matricentric care, where mothering is respected as a foundational pillar of society.

Matricentric (woman- and mother-focused) feminism needs to be drawn into the early stages of fertility, pregnancy, birthing and early mothering. It isn't strident or scary. It recognises the significance of emotional nurturing and caregiving as a source of strength and knowledge. The skills of mothering need to be recognised, valued and respected in all aspects of life. We need matricentric feminism in the birthing space, because feminism very much left birthing and early mothering behind. Understanding matrescence strengthens matricentric feminism; both are seeking to bring mothers to the forefront of attention. Mothers are not broken in their abilities to mother and don't need fixing, but they do need understanding and support.

We will be debunking a few myths along the way too, such as the unrealistic 'perfect mother' and 'good mother' myths – the supposed ability to 'do and have it all', being fulfilled by motherhood, all while 'looking good'. We will talk about the notion of the so-called 'perfect birth'. The mental and physical load of childcare has become associated with the chores of home, garden, school runs, extracurricular activities, social secretary, taxi, homework, yadda, yadda, yadda. It is taken for granted that these are the roles of the woman in mothering. And it's rubbish. Dear Mother Becoming, you will come to know it is enough to be a 'good enough mother'. This understanding will grow with each page you turn.

We will also explore unrealistic body expectations and the myth of 'bouncebackability' after birth. We will look at the perception that motherhood is 'a blissful experience' … hmmmmmmm … and how the myth of 'baby brain' makes mothers out to seem less capable, when the opposite is true!

This is a journey of discovering your physical and emotional capacity for reconnecting mind and body by understanding the physiological effects of hormones in pregnancy, labour, birthing and early mothering. You will use this wisdom wherever you choose to birth, whether at home, a birthing unit or in a hospital birthing room – especially when medical care is needed to assist your labour and birth. You can harness your intrinsic capacity and feel that your birthing experience is your own.

We will talk about building partnerships with your care providers, with reciprocal respect for each other's knowledge. Ultimately this will empower you to feel confident and take responsibility for your body and growing baby. Thank goodness for modern-day medicine and access to excellent care if complications arise. We are incredibly lucky to have that. However, it is a fact that health professionals in maternity and obstetric care are working in a climate of understaffed midwifery services, institutional financial pressures, time constraints, non-matricentric policies, and unfortunately, convenience.

Health professionals should never use their status to influence you for their own convenience. They sometimes use biased language or withhold information to pressure you into non-evidence-based care or something that you know just isn't right. Over-medicalisation of obstetric care is very real in Australia. We will explore that more and come up with approaches for resolving this issue. Making available mother-centric care shouldn't be governed by efficiency, politics, and economic and time constraints in an institutionalised hospital environment. We expect evidence-based care, implemented in a timely manner. We deserve care that is not harmful and is respectful to all, no matter ethnicity, beliefs or culture. Working towards improving these maternal experiences enhances bonding, maternal satisfaction and the transition to mothering.

We will have some difficult conversations, discussed in a balanced but subjective way, to deepen your understanding about them. This book is not an anti-men manifesto, nor a bashing of the medical profession. It isn't about complaining and negativity. Rather, this book is full of ideas, information and action that can create positive experiences and inspire change. It's about learning how to reclaim what we have lost in caring for mothers in westernised culture.

Mother Becoming is also an invitation to claim ways to prepare, celebrate, acknowledge and work with your emotional, psychological and physical strengths in pregnancy, birthing and mothering. And for some mothers, to heal. There will be moments when you feel angry, frustrated, saddened and outraged as the pages turn. I'm not going to leave you high and dry with that, because it's toxic to remain in those emotions. The supportive practices are there if you need them to aid you through such deep feeling.

Birthing partners are not forgotten throughout this experience, and there are resources for them too. Although this book is titled *Mother Becoming*, it is in fact a journey for 2. After all, it isn't just a new mother who is being born here, but a new father or parent-partner too. Support is vitally important and the more your partner is involved, the easier it will be to transition into parenthood.

A matricentric view nurtures the change and evolution that happens each time a mother becomes. It is a philosophy where you and all women feel respected, supported, visible, informed, listened to, empowered and autonomous. It's time to reframe the internal and external narrative so you, the birthing woman and mother, are front and centre. This book provides guidance, advocates for you, and is a touchstone of a new kind of village where you are the beating heart. A matricentric village.

There are some big thought-provoking discussion points at the end of each chapter, so have a pen ready to write down what pops into your mind. If you are reading the eBook version, you will definitely need a note book! Scribble down comments, questions, doodles and ideas. Brainstorm with your partner.

Matrescence explained

Long ago, we were a matricentric society, where the mother and child were respected, and childrearing was a responsibility shared by the community. In their research, anthropologists Holly Dunsworth and Leah Eccleston highlight how we evolved to alloparent (share the care of children), which was the norm for millennia.[1] We didn't evolve to birth and mother in isolation. Joint parenting happened among family and friends, with shared responsibility and care. There was support for the mother through wisdom handed down through the ages. Anthropologically, the time since the Industrial Revolution and the beginning of the nuclear family 250 years ago is but a blink in our evolution and we haven't had time to adjust.

In our modern world, the state of heightened anxiety, fear around birth, occurrence of birth trauma, PND, depletion and burnout that mothers experience serves no one, least of all the mother. It's unsustainable. Add in how birthing has become medicalised and institutionalised over the past 100 years. Currently 97% of births in Australia are in hospital and there is little postpartum support. When one in 3 women has been traumatised and one in 5 is depressed, this is unhealthy for our continued existence. The fallout from our current system of maternity care is isolated, bewildered, frustrated, resentful, anxious and depleted mothers. We have lost the ways of knowing, explaining and supporting the myriad of changes we undergo as we become a mother. We have lost the respect for, connection to and support of this profound life transition. Much of this book is about regaining what has been lost and supporting a mother when she needs it most.

Technological change, advances in sciences and medicine, and historical and social change have combined to give rise to our neoliberal, patriarchal, westernised society. Sadly, our modern culture has little reverence or respect for pregnancy, birthing and, especially, early mothering. We live with the ideals of individualism, competition and material gain, and are raised to believe we can be, do and have it all. We are expected to mother as if we don't work and work as though we are not mothers. We are expected to be uncomplaining about our role as a mother. Fulfilled, loving it —with a clean home, fresh meals, well-behaved children, and being sexy and looking good as we do it all. Woe betide you if you are frustrated, angry, snappy, resentful, unfulfilled or unhappy. Bad mother, they say.

Westernised culture has forgotten ancient practices and the knowledge of 'matrescence'. This needs to change in a deeply fundamental way. We can change by learning from other cultures, from history and from research.

Dr Alexandra Sacks, a reproductive psychiatrist, has noted that many mothers experience an emotional tug of war on becoming a mother. Women came to her concerned that something was wrong with them because they couldn't measure up to how they thought a mother should be. They were not enjoying it, were overwhelmed, and felt like they were failing. Falling short of their own expectations and what they believed society expected of them. They felt betrayed by society's portrayal of mothering as blissful, and asked why nobody told them it would be like this. Some women were shocked by the ambivalence they felt towards their baby, and were confused by their reaction. They felt broken, abnormal and unable to tell anyone. Ultimately, women were ashamed of themselves.

Yet when Sacks informed them that they didn't have PND, that they weren't sick, it didn't help them. She wanted to find a way for mothers to understand and normalise their experiences of the transition to motherhood, and the discomfort that becoming a mother can bring. Sacks discovered the 1973 work of medical anthropologist Dr Dana Raphael. Raphael described the all-encompassing emotional, physical, psychological and cultural changes that affect a woman as she transitions to motherhood: "The critical period which has been missed is matrescence: the time of mother becoming ..."[2]

In 2008 Dr Aurélie Athan, a clinical psychologist, revived the term 'matrescence' from Raphael's work. Athan studies and teaches matrescence from a holistic perspective, offering a 'strengths of the mother' approach towards normalising women's experiences. One of her students suggested that matrescence is like adolescence. Understanding that becoming a mother is like the transition of adolescence has made many women weep with relief. The acknowledgment that what they are experiencing is real, has a name and can be described is powerful.

Athan's definition of the matrescence experience is "a developmental passage where the woman transitions through pre-conception, pregnancy, and birth, surrogacy or adoption, to the postnatal period and beyond. The exact length of matrescence is individual, recurs with each child, and may arguably last a lifetime! The scope of the changes encompasses multiple domains ... bio-psycho-social-political-spiritual ... and can be likened to the developmental push of adolescence. Increased attention to mothers has spurred new findings, from neuroscience to economics, and supports the rationale for a new field of study known as matrescence. Such an arena would allow the roundtable of specialists to come together and advance our understanding of this life passage."[3]

The neuroplastic changes that rewire a mother's brain is evidence of this amazing process. What a relief to have a word to explain and understand what happens to a woman as she becomes a mother! Owning the term helps us advocate for ourselves. We now understand that hormonal changes, bodily adjustment, identity and relational changes remake a woman as a mother with each birth, including surrogacy and adoption. These changes also encompass how the social, political, economic and spiritual effects of culture and society influence a mother. All this has an integral role to play in how the new mother sees herself, and is seen, valued and cared for. Matrescence can now be found in the Oxford English Dictionary.

So, let's bring this word and its knowledge, value and awareness into our everyday language so it is embedded into our social psyche as normality.

- **Wishlist** 🌿 **Dr Sacks TED Talk**, YouTube.
  https://www.ted.com/talks/alexandra_sacks_a_new_way_to_think_about_the_transition_to_motherhood?subtitle=en&trigger=0s
- *Seasons of Matrescence* S1 #10. 'Matrescence, the developmental experience and spiritual awakening of motherhood' Apple 🎙 Spotify
- *Happy Mama Movement* #67. 'Matrescence and the Transition to Mother' Apple 🎙 Spotify

---

When matrescence is supported by matricentric feminism, a term first used by Professor Andrea O'Reilly, and founded in motherhood studies, something special can happen. Both these concepts enable us to make changes in our experiences of becoming and being a mother. They make pregnancy, birthing and early mothering visible, acknowledged, valued and supported.

Matricentric feminism explained

This is a feminist perspective that places motherhood and the experiences of mothering at the centre of study. It emphasises the importance of recognising and valuing the work and contribution of mothers. Matricentric feminism provides a foundation for activism that challenges patriarchal structures, which inherently devalue mothering. It advocates for policies and practices to support, empower and liberate mothers and their families. It redresses gender inequalities that limit women's choices and opportunities in work. It supports mothers in accessing paid maternity leave, affordable childcare, flexible work, health care and education. It values emotional, nurturing and caregiving labour as skills, and a source of strength and knowledge. It argues that these skills and experiences are valuable and should be recognised and respected in all aspects of life.

Matricentric feminism doesn't seek to exclude women who are not mothers. It seeks to recognise the unique challenges of mothering and the contributions matricentric feminism can bring to the feminist movement as a whole. It comes from a place of care.

O'Reilly writes: "The category of mother is distinct from the category of woman and that many of the problems mothers face – socially, politically, culturally and psychologically – are specific to women's work and identity as mothers. Indeed, mothers, arguably more so than women in general, remain disempowered despite forty years of feminism. Mothers need a feminism of their own, one that positions mothers' concerns as the starting point for a theory and politics of empowerment."[4] Vanessa Olorenshaw, a lawyer, so rightly says in her book *Liberating Motherhood: Birthing the Purple Stocking Movement*: "If feminism ignores the birthing room, focusing only on the boardroom, we fail women. We must push for greater respect for women's bodies, our being, and our births. A feminism which ignores birth is a feminism that has forgotten its heritage: remember, we are all born of our mothers."[5] Bringing matricentric feminism into the pregnancy, birth and early mothering space is important because change is desperately needed. The next wave of feminism needs to be matricentric.

This is a potent combination, powerfully expressed in the multi-award-winning documentary *Birthtime*, which blew the lid off the current culture of birthing in Australia. It exploded in 2021, demonstrating that our current system of maternity care is damaging to women. The film shows the raw power of undisturbed birthing. It aired interviews with women of many cultures whose birth experiences in the hospital system left them traumatised. There is commentary from multidisciplinary professionals who believe women should be at the centre of care. The result is an exposé of our current maternity system that is eye-opening, emotive and challenging.

The overwhelming conclusion is that women need continuity of midwifery care to improve birthing outcomes for themselves, their babies and their families, and to reduce birth trauma, PTSD and PND in our country. The current Medicare fee-for-service system increases interventions, particularly in private practice. The evidence is all there.

In *Birthtime*, author Milli Hill states: "Being a feminist, and having read feminist stuff, and thinking a lot about feminism from lots of different angles, and seeing progress being made, and then coming into birth as a woman, I felt like feminism hadn't really reached birth."[6]

The *Mother Becoming* Matricentric Framework

This book provides ways for you to rethink how you see and value yourself, with awareness and understanding of what's happening to you as you become a mother. It prepares you for the values you wish to embody during pregnancy, birth and as a parent. Your new knowledge will help you to negotiate autonomous choice and invoke change. You will relearn ways of navigating mothering in our modern world. There is so much emphasis on birthing, and rightly so. But there is so little preparation or recognition of the importance and value of supporting a new mother. Throughout *Mother Becoming*, I hope to start to redress this imbalance.

Through understanding and using matrescence as a framework of discovery, we acknowledge that preparing for mothering, and optimising our mother-wellbeing, is essential. We start to embody it, really live it.

At this point, many books will tell you all about what is happening in your body week by week and what to expect. I'm not going to. It is perfectly written and presented by others, and available in the resources and inspirational, informative quotes in each chapter. We are going to explore all that matrescence and positive matricentric feminism encompass. They form a framework that will help you rewrite internal narratives and beliefs about pregnancy, birthing and mothering.

You will notice that I talk to you in 2 voices. The voice of compassion and love, and the voice of a gentle teacher.

This book challenges outdated research, modes of maternity care and myths, helping you navigate your education, self-discovery, values, strengths and confident choices during your maternity care. It prepares you for the transition into, and realities of, mothering. It provides you with knowledge and strength to navigate through so much that is hidden, unsaid and has been subliminally impressed. And it places the power of knowledge in your hands to make choices and changes that work for you.

The *Mother Becoming* Tree of Matrescence

The Tree of Matrescence provides a structure that will help you to navigate and understand each chapter. All parts of the tree are interwoven because everything works together to provide holistic information and practices to nourish your mind, body and soul.

The 4 tree roots represent all the aspects of becoming a mother. They provide a strong foundation of knowledge, drawing from the past and present. Some roots are going to be weightier with information than others and differ in intensity in each chapter. Bear with me. It will all come together in the end!

The tree trunk. A strong pregnant woman and mother who is nourished by the roots of information. By understanding the knowledge provided by the roots, you can find your voice to achieve empowerment and autonomy in your present and future.

The leaves of mindfulness, meditations and yoga unfurl to strengthen and prepare your body and mind. With the leaves of kindness, gentleness, compassion, self-worth, love and trust we will create something beautiful together – while building a village with a you-centred focus and network. A matricentric village.

The tree icons in each chapter will remind you where you are on your information gathering journey.

Physical, Hormonal, Emotional Influences
Practice offerings of mindfulness, breathing, meditation and yoga

Cultural, Herstorical (not His-torical), Political Influences

Social, Economic, Media Influences

Self-identity, Beliefs/Values, Spiritual Influences
Practice offerings of breathing and further meditation

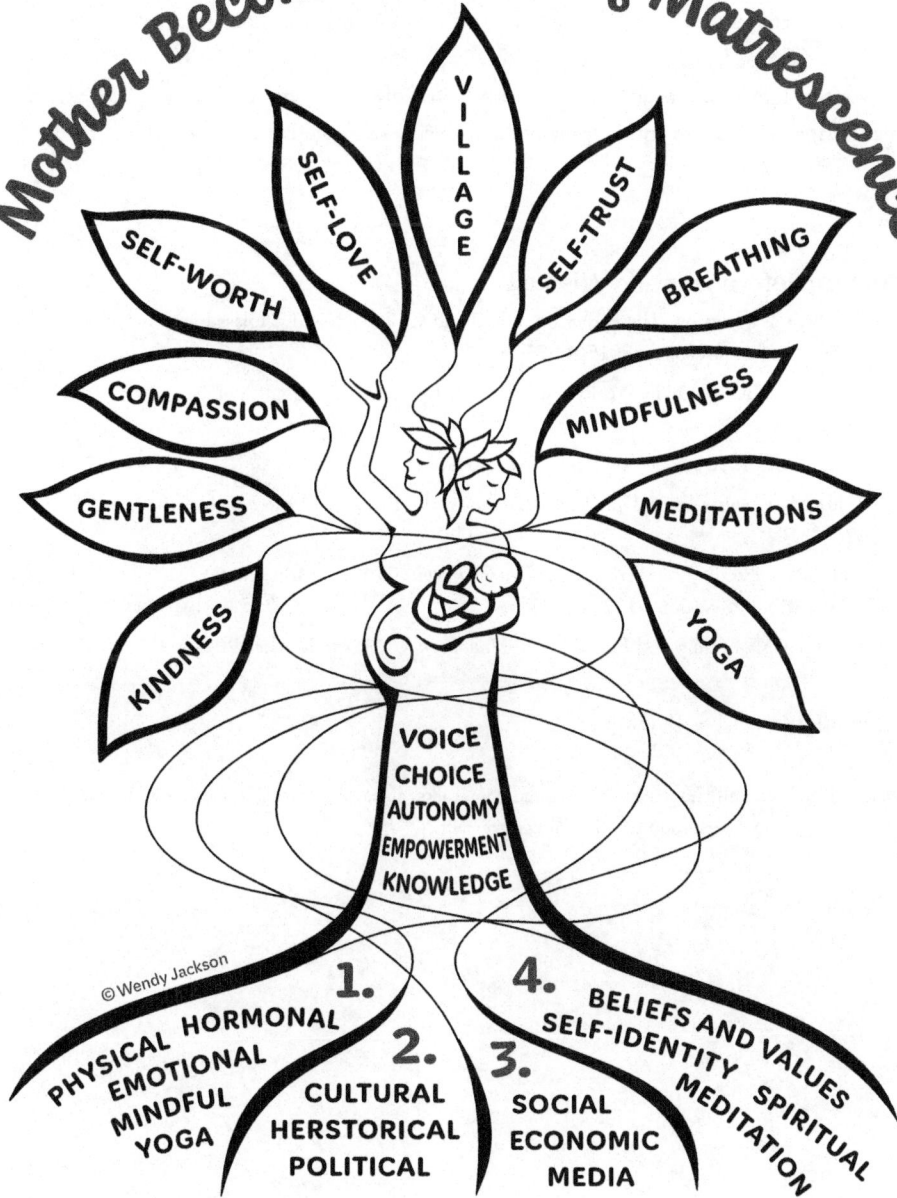

Mother Becoming Tree of Matrescence

VILLAGE

SELF-LOVE

SELF-WORTH

SELF-TRUST

BREATHING

COMPASSION

MINDFULNESS

GENTLENESS

MEDITATIONS

KINDNESS

YOGA

VOICE
CHOICE
AUTONOMY
EMPOWERMENT
KNOWLEDGE

© Wendy Jackson

1.
PHYSICAL HORMONAL
EMOTIONAL
MINDFUL
YOGA

2.
CULTURAL
HERSTORICAL
POLITICAL

3.
SOCIAL
ECONOMIC
MEDIA

4.
BELIEFS AND VALUES
SELF-IDENTITY SPIRITUAL
MEDITATION

Please don't feel you have to read this book in order. There is a lot of information. The detailed contents page is there for you to pick and choose what you want to know about and do. You can read the letters and information, do the practices of Tree Roots 1 and 4 of each chapter if you wish. Then read Tree Roots 2 and 3. Do whatever combination works for you.

At the end of each chapter is a 'How might it be for you if?' list that provokes thoughts about how you may wish to navigate your journey. It also prompts insight for change.

Through these pages Liesja, Samantha, Ashleigh, Ally, Katie, Alysia, Clémentine and I will cheer you on and support you in spirit. We know that you are more than enough. That you are to be valued, respected, acknowledged, appreciated and are totally awesome.

Put on your imaginary boots and carry a backpack full of nourishing snacks, chocolate, a thermos of tea, pen and paper. Let's begin this journey of empowering you together …

Introduction References and Wishlist

1   H Dunsworth, L Eccleston, 'The Evolution of Difficult Childbirth and helpless Hominin Infants' *The Annual Review of Anthropology*. 2015, 44:55–69

2   D Raphael PhD, Being female. World Anthropology, De Gruyer. Mouten Publishers, 1975, p66. ISBN 90-279-7599

3   Dr A Athan PhD. Matrescence. https://www.matrescence.com/

4   A O'Reilly, Matricentric Feminism: Theory, Activism and Practice, Demeter Press, 2021, p42. ISBN 9781772583762

5   V Olorenshaw. *Liberating Motherhood: birthing the Purple Stocking Movement*, Womancraft Publishing, 2016, p76. ISBN 978-910559-192

6   *Birthtime The Documentary* and *Birthtime The Handbook*, Clark and Mackay, 2021, p92.

Wishlist

1. Dr Sacks TED Talk, YouTube. https://www.ted.com/talks/alexandra_sacks_a_new_way_to_think_about_the_transition_to_motherhood?subtitle=en&trigger=0s

Chapter 1

Liesja with you in Early Pregnancy

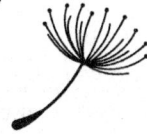

Meeting Liesja

Liesja and I met when we did our Hatha Vinyasa yoga teacher training (together with Ashleigh and Ally, whom you will meet later). Liesja has the most beautiful smile, introduced me to strawberry chia seed pudding, is mum to Freyja and Lachlan, and works in the corporate world. During that time, she blended the practices and philosophy of yoga into her career and home life. We connected over our deep passion for supporting mothers, while on an 8-day immersive program on pregnancy, birthing and postpartum yoga.

While there, after an emotional day for all of us, Liesja told me, "I'm not done yet." As she tells her story in her letter about struggling with fertility and loss, this tear-filled "I'm not done yet" statement will become clear. Her journey to becoming the mother of Freyja and Lachy illustrates her strength, tenacity and capacity of mother love to bring life to the world.

Mama of Frejya and Lachy, here is Liesja's letter to you

"To return home to my heart"

Dear Mama,

Wherever you are in your motherhood journey, just beginning, struggling with fertility, recently birthed a sleeping baby, just became a mum for the first time or perhaps awaiting the arrival of number 2 or 3, know that you are enough, and you are so supported and loved. You will find a way. That's our super strength as women. That is what we do as mums. We find a way, so you just do you!

Of all the names you can be called as a mother, mama has always been my favourite. Maybe it's because it was the first name both of my children, when they were small, called me. For a long time, nearly 4 years, I thought I may never get the chance to hear those words from beautiful babies.

When I met my future husband at 29, I had not long returned to my hometown after 4 years of living and working in the UK. The instant I met him, I knew he was someone I wanted to have children with. I felt this pull towards becoming a mother and wanting a family with my partner. We had been together for 2 years when we casually started talking about having children after a long walk along our local beach.

Once we'd made that decision, it felt like the most natural thing in the world. As we embarked on an amazing 6-week trip to Europe, I came off the pill and thought: *Let's just see what happens.* I imagined it would take some time to fall pregnant, but returning home from that holiday, much to my surprise, my period didn't arrive. A test confirmed we were pregnant. It was a shock, but a happy kind.

Instantly, I noticed how different I felt in my body: swollen tender breasts, crying at the drop of a hat. I had this niggling feeling that my life as I knew it was about to become completely different. If I'm really honest, I wasn't sure I was ready to surrender to it all just yet. I wasn't ready to give up my running, rein in my yoga practice, perhaps pause my career. These were all the thoughts running through my head that I hadn't really considered, even though I knew deep in my bones I wanted to be a mum. I just wasn't sure if I was ready to make the sacrifices and share my body.

As women, we may spend a lot of time trying not to fall pregnant. So, when it happens, even when it is planned, you can never be fully prepared for the changes occurring from the early stages of pregnancy. I felt an internal shift happening, like I could no longer selfishly think just about me, but about this little human I was growing. It is hard to not skip ahead of the pregnancy part and build a story of what it will be like holding your little baby, imagining all the things you want for them.

About a week later, while at work, I went to the toilet, wiped and saw pink spotting on the toilet paper. My heart sank. While I tried not to panic, deep down I felt perhaps I didn't want this baby enough and it was rejecting me. I tried not to look up symptoms on the internet or get ahead of myself, but it was a challenge to stop myself spiralling into considering the worst possible outcomes. I cycled between maybe this was normal – some women do have bleeding early on in their pregnancy and are able to carry to full-term – to this is the start of losing my baby.

A few days later, a scan confirmed there was no heartbeat. For the first time, I cried for all the things that were not going to be. My baby had decided I wasn't ready. I know this is an irrational thought. For lots of reasons, miscarriages occur. Yet that didn't stop my brain from going into a spin of over-analysis. Perhaps I had overdone it going for a run in the early weeks. Maybe my baby had felt my fear and doubt that I didn't really want it, or picked up on my innermost thoughts and emotions.

"This happens to one in 3," the doctor said. "You are healthy. Give yourself some time to heal and give it another go. I am sure next time will be different." I remember feeling fearful of trying for a baby again. I was working in a fairly senior human resources role, which often involved dealing with a lot of other people's emotions. I felt a responsibility to always deliver at a high level. I would never want to let down the team or have others think I wasn't doing a good enough job. After all, I had worked my whole life for this career. At this point, I wanted to continue working, regardless of whether I had children or not. I did a lot of soul-searching over the month to see if this was what I truly wanted.

When I felt ready to try again a few months later, I thought my body was set. After all, I'd been able to fall pregnant once; that must be a good sign. Again, I fell pregnant after trying for a month and as before I reached the seven-week mark. I booked to see a GP after a positive home pregnancy test and had a blood test to confirm. A couple of days later, the spotting started. The blood test confirmed my hCG levels were not where they were expected to be. It would likely lead to the loss of my baby. Another one. I had failed again. Not just failed myself, but failed my partner and family who so desperately wanted a baby and grandchild.

I was always the type A personality, always achieving, mostly doing what I was told, good at following the rules, reaching my goals … I didn't understand why my body could not do this one thing I wanted it to do.

Other than my partner, I had told only my mum about the losses … and after the second one came her story of loss: a baby boy at 20 weeks, fully formed, blond hair, peacefully curled up in a kidney dish. After some investigation, the doctor had confirmed her loss was from a rare bacterium. Mum had had a spa at a friend's place a few days previously, not realising the risks to her unborn baby. I have a rainbow brother; he would be 2 years younger than me. Dad left her at the hospital all alone to deal with it. He couldn't face it. A similar story surfaced of my nana losing a baby at nearly full-term. It is something the women in my bloodline have faced for generations.

I found some comfort in knowing that women do experience a whole range of challenges when bringing life into this world. I felt the strength of all the women who had come before me. I witnessed them finding an inner strength to heal and eventually thrive, just as my mother and grandmother had shown me.

I don't know why society doesn't talk about miscarriage or why we don't share our grief. I know I felt a shame attached to mine, that I was somehow less because of it, that I had let my partner down. I also felt that my grief wasn't warranted given I had lost my baby so early on; we never heard a heartbeat so did I really have the right to publicly grieve for my baby?

When my partner and I tried for the third time, it took a little longer to fall pregnant, but once I saw that positive test, I was quick to book an appointment with my GP. I shared my fears and reservations with the doctor. After suffering 2 miscarriages previously, I wanted some facts and was looking for a confirmation that this pregnancy would be different.

While my GP couldn't guarantee this pregnancy would be successful to full-term, they did confirm that they would investigate further if it wasn't, given I would have had 3 miscarriages in a row, or 12 months of trying to fall pregnant. If I was to lose this one, I wanted to know why this was happening to me.

A few days later, my bloods confirmed that my hCG levels were low and my GP wanted to monitor them for a few days to see what was happening. After 5 blood tests, the doctor suspected I had an ectopic pregnancy. I wasn't overly sure what this meant, but I was referred to the womens hospital for further investigations.

My mum came with me, not fully comprehending what was going on. It took 2 specialists via an ultrasound to find the egg stuck in my fallopian tube. They diagnosed an ectopic pregnancy; because they had caught it early, I was given the option of having the methotrexate injection and it being dissolved over a few weeks or having my tube removed.

At that time, I chose to dissolve it and save my tube. I guess I chose the less invasive option that I felt comfortable with. The procedure was fairly simple: having an injection and then being sent home to recover. What I perhaps didn't consider was that having a methotrexate injection required me to continue being monitored each week to ensure the egg was dissolving and my hCG levels were going down. I also had to wait 3 months before I could try for another baby to ensure the methotrexate was fully out of my system. At the time, we never knew what the right option was, but we listened to the advice and chose what felt right for us.

Once I had recovered from my ectopic pregnancy, I booked another appointment with my GP. I also asked for a referral to a fertility specialist. I wanted answers, but I needed to heal and find the fighter within as I could feel myself slipping. This was becoming all-consuming. I was losing my sense of self. When I looked in the mirror, I just saw failure and sorrow.

Not sharing all these losses with my wider family, friends and work colleagues, I felt like I was always hiding something, putting on a mask. Underneath, my sadness was so close to the surface. I worked hard every day to keep a lid on it, to stop it spilling over, to keep up the façade that everything was okay. It took a lot of energy not being able to be completely honest as to what I was dealing with.

Eventually, I met with the fertility specialist and went through a series of tests, completed the list of things asked of me. I ticked them off, like a shopping list, thinking that if I did all of this, I would get some answers and hopefully a baby. This included giving 17 vials of blood and having an endoscopy.

The surgery found I had severe endometriosis on my bowel, intestines and around my right fallopian tube where I'd had the ectopic pregnancy. I was kept on the same ward as those who were having babies. Then the morning after my surgery, a nurse announced they needed the bed and I needed to go and wait in the outpatient area to be collected. I was discharged without seeing a doctor or being given any after care.

I was left tender from the surgery. It took weeks to recover. The gas that they use in keyhole surgery to inflate the area so they can see all your organs was still surging around my body. I felt winded every time I moved, walked or sat. After 2 weeks, I still didn't understand the health implications. I had no real symptoms of endometriosis, no painful periods and my periods were fairly regular. I was shocked to receive this information and it took me time to process the diagnosis.

My partner and I were getting married in the February of the following year, so I parked the follow-up appointment for a few months and just focused on healing from surgery and getting our renovation complete in time for our backyard wedding.

When I did see the fertility specialist for a follow-up some months later, he was appalled by the treatment at the hospital and said he would make a complaint on my behalf. He then told me, "We couldn't really find any reason why you have infertility. Yes, some endometriosis, but it shouldn't affect your ability to carry a baby to term. However, we did find you have the MTFHR gene mutation. We advise patients with MTFHR to take vitamin B supplements and a high dose of folate while trying to conceive and during pregnancy. That should resolve the matter."

This was almost a passing comment at the end of the consultation as we were ushered out the door. I had no proper information about this gene mutation and felt a lack of empathy for the journey my partner and I had been on. Now I felt bereft, treated like a number and left to navigate this alone once again. At the time, I was seeking answers and information; when that was absent, it led me to a lot of online searching and misinformation.

I decided to complete a tracking cycle on advice from the consultant. This involved blood tests first thing every other morning at the clinic and being told the optimum time for conception during the month. I joined over 40 other women in the fertility clinic getting blood tests every 48 hours. I was surprised at how many women were there for support with their fertility journey.

"Today, go home and have sex with your husband, because you'll be ovulating in the next 12 hours." Not at all how I romanticised conceiving a baby! However, after our journey, I had long ago let go of romance. On the last day of the cycle tracking test, I got a positive pregnancy signal, only for it to end in a chemical pregnancy. I was heartbroken. I had done it all, everything that was asked of me, and still I did not have what I really wanted. Four potential babies lost. Four different due dates to remind me of what could have been.

I still had told very few people about my losses. I put on a brave face, fronted up to work, did a good job. I cleaned, cooked, put on a shiny, smiling exterior as I tried to hold on to something in my life that I could control. I researched all the reasons this was happening to me, but I can tell you there is a lot of crap out there on the internet.

I started to restrict all the things that were keeping me mentally sane. I stopped running, stopped doing any vigorous exercise, stopped drinking alcohol, stopped planning holidays, stopped drinking coffee, reduced any processed foods. I became a shell of my former self. It was all I thought about and the factor on which I based all my decisions around whether to participate in something. I didn't want to let anyone know how much of a failure I was. I congratulated all my friends who were becoming pregnant – and there were a lot – and I hid the deepest parts of myself. I pushed it all down. I couldn't open the grief. I was scared it would swallow me whole, that my fiancé would leave me if I couldn't have a baby.

In the meantime, life happened. We embarked on a massive renovation, got engaged, got married and decided to take a break from trying to grow our family. We needed time to regroup, find our way back to ourselves, add some light, joy and celebration back into our lives. We did not want this to break us. We recommitted to one another. We pushed away our sadness and our grief.

On a beautiful second honeymoon in Vietnam, sitting in a bath, we reopened the conception conversation. While I still wanted to be mother, I was reconciled with the idea that it may not happen for us. On that holiday, we agreed we would try to find a way through.

As a woman battling with infertility, with the physical side happening in my body, I don't think I had realised the toll that grief had taken on my husband. I am not sure men feel they have the right to be sad. Perhaps they are focused on getting their partner better after a loss and don't want to communicate their feelings as if it may make us feel bad about the situation. Not talking about it can be worse, though. I felt quiet alone at times, shouldering the burden of not being able to give my family a baby.

This holiday allowed us the space to talk through all of this and find a way to move forward. When you are in your routine, living day to day, it can be hard to find time to be present in such conversations. At the time of the miscarriages, I didn't have the space to hold anyone else's grief. I carried the weight of it with me. My brain was full of all the shoulda-coulda-wouldas and keeping up appearances. Sifting through all this were my lowest days.

As a way to cope and show I could handle the situation, I voiced that I was okay about a baby not being in my future. I allowed myself to think about all the things we would do, if we didn't have children of our own. I thought I could travel as much as I wanted and be a dog mum. I don't know if I really believed it and I am not sure my husband did either, but we entertained the idea. I needed this time to regroup, to let go of what was holding me tightly to this sad place, to find myself again.

After some time away from trying to fall pregnant, just living life, I found I was ready to give it another shot. I asked for all my notes to be reviewed by a senior consultant. I sought out a friend who was a midwife, told her my story and asked her who to go to for a second opinion. Who would she speak to if she were in my shoes? My friend put me in touch with a beautiful man, an obstetrician who dealt with all the tricky fertility cases and high-risk pregnancies. We met him, he gave me the odds, talked through my results, ordered a few more tests, suggested that I up my B vitamins, keep taking the higher folate dose, and introduce vitamin D as my levels were too low to sustain a pregnancy. He advised giving it another 6 months. "I think you just need all the stars to align. When you fall pregnant, give me a call and let's get you straight on progesterone suppositories to support the pregnancy through the first term."

That doctor gave us hope.

When I did fall pregnant again about 5 months later, we had a plan. I was put straight on progesterone supplements following a six-week scan that confirmed a heartbeat. I will never forget the joy my husband and I felt that day seeing our baby with a little heartbeat. We were both still feeling anxious about this pregnancy, given our history of loss, but we were so excited in this moment. It felt different to the others right from the start.

Morning sickness arrived around week 7. Well, it was afternoon sickness for me. I was unable to eat from lunchtime onwards, aside from an arrowroot biscuit. I would get home and lie in bed, maybe eat a bowl of cornflakes and sleep. I was so tired that first trimester and still quite anxious. I remember thinking I couldn't get too excited; we had a long way to go and I wasn't sure how either of us would deal with another loss of a baby. We were fairly fragile and I didn't want to share it with anyone outside of my family so we waited till about 16 weeks when I couldn't hide my growing belly. Every time I saw a scan of my baby, every week we made together, I just kept praying they would make it safely earthside. That this time would be different.

The funny thing was I was 4 months into a new job at a workplace I had been in for 6 years when I fell pregnant. I was in the middle of one of the most stressful projects of my life and yet it happened. Against all the odds, I got pregnant not when I was pulling back, but when I was at the height of life. The lesson there? When life is tough, we try to control everything to gain a sense of security. I will never know what helped. Maybe it was the combination of everything I had done to that point. Perhaps it was just fate. The stars aligning.

Aside from my own worries and anxieties of losing this baby, I had a relatively straightforward pregnancy. The morning sickness ceased around 14 weeks and I had no complications or scares. When I got to 26 weeks, I let myself believe it was really happening. *Okay*, I thought, *we are having a baby, and if it comes tomorrow, I know it can survive.*

At 33 weeks, the obstetrician confirmed my baby was in breech position, though there was still time and space for the baby to turn. The Spinning Babies website had some good tips, but my very first lesson in motherhood was: *surrender to what will be*. We can have all these ideas about how we think the birth will play out. We can put together a plan and consider the environment of how we want the baby to enter the world. Yet the reality is there are many factors. Ultimately, we have no control.

When I found out my baby was in breech position, I did everything within my control to turn that baby. I badly wanted a natural vaginal birth and was scared I would have to have a c-section if my baby didn't turn. After 3 weeks of swimming, handstands in the pool, lying on an ironing board against the couch, frozen peas at the top of my baby bump, inversions off the couch, sitting on an exercise ball – trying to get the baby's head to shift down to my cervix – nothing changed. At my 36-week check-up, they confirmed baby was still in the breech position. From that time, it was likely the baby wouldn't turn so we talked options.

I was lucky, although I didn't know how lucky. My obstetrician and his second-in-charge were trained in breech birth delivery and gave me the option to consider a vaginal breech delivery. My other option was a scheduled caesarean section, which I now know is the only option a lot of mothers are given if they are having a hospitalised birth.

I was practising antenatal yoga, going to class each week during my pregnancy. I didn't feel like sharing my journey or my anxieties, but I remember I kept showing up as I felt the need for a community. I was always less anxious after those antenatal yoga sessions. I do remember one teaching that really stuck with me: "This is the time to surround yourselves with positive birth stories. Don't let other women pass their trauma and fear on to you. Educate yourself and be informed about your options."

As I got closer to the due date, I didn't want to know anything about birthing. I needed to distance myself. I couldn't let myself go there. I was afraid and just wanted that part over. I wanted to be holding my baby. On reflection, with some distance and hindsight, I was protecting myself in case of any further pregnancy loss.

After lots of looking inwards and chatting to my mum about attempting a breech birth or opting for a c-section, I decided to try a breech vaginal birth. I went into it knowing that it could end in an emergency c-section and I was okay with that. My obstetrician was very encouraging, saying, "I think you can do this. Baby is a good size and I wouldn't suggest it if I didn't have confidence that we can deliver this baby safely."

Perhaps I was naive. I hadn't even watched or researched breech birth. However, I felt supported in my decision and my obstetrician knew how long we had waited for our baby.

I opted for a stretch and sweep at 38 weeks. In my mind, if I could go into spontaneous labour, I would know the baby was meant to arrive. Perhaps that would give me the best chance of a successful breech birth. (There is no research behind this – just my own rationalisation and attempt to control.) When the midwife did the internal examination, she said, "Your membranes are bulging. I think you are going to have this baby in the next 24 hours."

I left the clinic thinking: *Whatever. I am sure it won't be that quick.* I went home and started cooking spaghetti bolognaise to freeze so we had some supplies for when baby arrived. That afternoon, I had some lower back pain, but I ignored it. I lay down and had a sleep. Most likely, I was in labour then, but you don't know what to expect in your first experience so you can second guess yourself. I was also probably in denial that it would happen so fast. After all, I was still 2 weeks from my due date.

Before I went to bed, the back pain had gone, but I thought to put a towel under me to sleep on, just in case my waters broke. Luckily, I listened to that intuition, because at around midnight I woke to the sensation of wetting the bed. I quickly realised what was happening, woke my husband and called the hospital. They suggested I come in, though I had no contractions yet. "Take your time," they said, "It's your first baby."

By the time I was dressed and had finished packing the last-minute things into my hospital bag, the contractions started as I got in the car. I was watching the clock and feeling a contraction about every 2 minutes. What? I thought. Where are the 10-minute-apart ones? I was anxious now, because we had a half-hour drive to the hospital and I didn't know if the contractions would speed up or slow down.

By the time I got into the hospital, I could hardly walk. The contractions were coming one after the other, a little one followed by a long intense one. I tried to remember my breathing, but I was a deer in the headlights! "Wow!" said the midwife, "You are about 8 centimetres, but I don't think this baby is breech." I told her it had been breech all along, hadn't turned and that I needed some pain relief. "We just had a beautiful natural breech birth a couple of days ago," she replied. "You can do it too."

Having done no research on birthing, optimal positions, or movement in labour, I lay flat on my back on the bed, wanting the pain to go away. I didn't want gas; I wanted an epidural! My obstetrician was on holiday that week, so when his 2IC waltzed in and said, "Are you ready?" I said, "No way!"

As far as breech births go, I suppose it was fairly uneventful, albeit a little quick. I couldn't get off the bed. I wasn't good at relaxing between contractions. I struggled to focus and breathe. At one point, the bottom of the bed was dropped down and I was helped to sit up and get into a sort-of squat position. I pushed for some time. I don't think I'm doing this right, I thought, because it felt like forever.

Next thing I know, the obstetrician said, "Oh your baby is coming out pooing and weeing everywhere!" This is completely normal as you squeeze the abdomen and they come out bottom first. "Do you want to touch your baby?" he asked. "Errrm, no thank you!" I replied.

I remember the moment when my beautiful baby girl was put on my chest. There was this feeling of coming full circle, being so proud of myself, like a superwoman. There was also a real understanding of what my parents had felt when they breathed me into this world.

My daughter truly looked like an angel.

It was a very emotional first few minutes. My heart swelled with love. We finally had our baby earthside with us. Our beautiful girl had been sent to help heal us in all the ways we didn't know how to heal ourselves, to teach us the richness and challenges of being parents. I would learn to drop my guard, give up pretences, soften, be compassionate. She cracked me open and allowed me to lead from the heart. I hadn't realised how life had hardened me until I held her.

In hindsight, I wish I'd shared more of my journey at the time and even since. One of my biggest regrets is not communicating what I was going through as I was going through it. Even since then, I have been reluctant to open the door on my trauma of loss. I had a happy ending though. I have 2 beautiful babies from 9 pregnancies. I realise this isn't always the outcome for many women who struggle with fertility. Taking a pause can sometimes give you time and space to sift through all the emotions, trauma and grief, but no one tells you when to give up on your dream of holding a baby of your own.

Journalist and novelist Elizabeth Day talks about this in relation to her fertility journey on her podcast *How to fail with Elizabeth Day*. We only tell ourselves one story of who we should be, how our lives will make sense when we become mothers. We tie our life's purpose to that one wish and we don't invite ourselves to dream a different dream.

If you are reading this now, in the thick of your fertility fight or taking a pause, or if you know someone who is, I hope you know there is so much love for you right now. There is a whole community of women and men who know and understand exactly how you feel. Reach out to someone, share your heartbreak, allow yourself to be vulnerable with those who make you feel safe. There is a richness in sharing our stories. Really, it is our only purpose here.

I send love to you and those others who desperately want to be mamas. I send love to those who have had a similar battle to mine and those who had an easier time with fertility, but had other challenges in parenting.

Liesja x

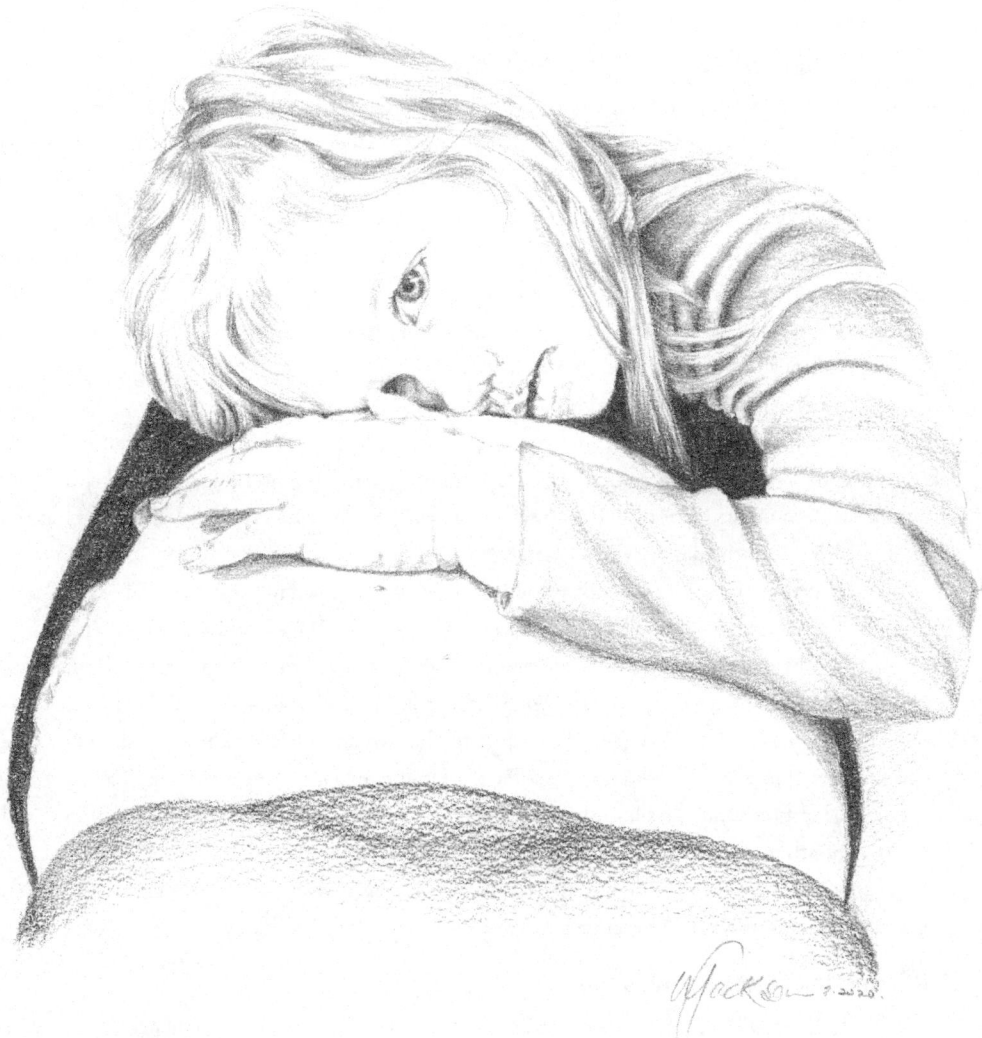

Liesja's pregnant belly is held tenderly and adored by Freyja, the child so longed for and birthed breech. Sadly, Liesja experienced more early pregnancy losses before her son, Lachy, was born. His big sister was beside herself with excitement to have an expected sibling, watching her mother's tummy grow and waiting for that new arrival ...

🌱 Dear Mother Becoming,

Dry your eyes and take some deep breaths after reading Liesja's extraordinary journey, offered with grace. As she wrote, "Reach out to someone, share your heartbreak, allow yourself to be vulnerable with those who make you feel safe. There is a richness in sharing our stories. Really, it is our only purpose here."

Take a moment now to sit with the feeling her words have provoked. Honour them. They are yours, very real, and to be acknowledged. If early pregnancy loss has been part of your experience, there are offerings of support in the spiritual section later in this chapter. We see you, Mama.

The letter at the beginning of each chapter tells the real experiences of a mother; their words are held with reverence, compassion and awe as I write to you now. Love,

Wendy

What does it feel like in early pregnancy?

How does pregnancy affect the way we see ourselves? These are loaded questions. The answers are individual and unique to each woman. There is utter joy, excitement and fizzing jubilation with a welcome pregnancy. There is the desolation, hollowness and grief in pregnancy loss. If the pregnancy is unexpected, there is the shock and then the decision to keep the pregnancy or not. If unwanted, the emotions of guilt, anxiety and grief are combined with being confronted with the choice of method to end the pregnancy. The experience of ending an unwanted pregnancy or a fetus that has anomalies can be traumatic. There may be conflicting emotions, held in secrecy.

This is a journey of discovery and change in all aspects of your life.

Imagine an invisible umbilical cord between you and your child, which weaves its way through every aspect of your physical, hormonal, emotional, cultural, economic, spiritual and social life. When we become pregnant, we don't see a cluster of cells. We see a child. That invisible umbilical cord influences our awareness, thoughts, actions and feelings for that possibility of a real child. It impacts us in every part of our lives until the day we die. We change.

We are in a state of suspension, not yet a mother, not recognisably pregnant, and yet not the same woman before the second line of the pregnancy test appeared. We begin to think differently and are affected deeply by our hormones. We become more aware of our body as it changes and feels the effects of pregnancy. We perceive ourselves and the world around us with new eyes. We see changes in how the world now perceives us. We privately adjust to this secret, our bodies not yet showing the signs, yet feeling the effects to a marked degree. There's fatigue, nausea, vomiting, constipation, emotional wobbles, fear of pregnancy loss and so much more. It's a secret shared between a select few until that magical 3-month marker when we feel it's safe to share our news.

Until then, we keep quiet, hide our symptoms as much as possible and make excuses for ourselves. We don't complain or want to be a burden. We can't be seen to be 'making a fuss'.

Suffering in silence. Why is that?

Maybe we keep quiet because we're more concerned for the comfort and convenience of others. We are raised with the belief we should keep our pregnancy quiet in case we have an early pregnancy loss. We are concerned about the reactions of our colleagues at work; maybe they will view us as no longer fully competent or committed to our job, and we fear being passed over for any advancement in our career.

So we suffer in silence.

In her book, *Silencing the Self: Women and Depression*, Dr Dana Jack, a professor of psychology, found that self-silencing begins in the early teens. This is when women begin to suppress their feelings, emotions and own identity to develop and maintain relationships and appear agreeable. However, their inner feelings are growing angry and resentful. All this is linked to depression and disconnection in women.[1] This tendency to keep quiet has profound effects on how we negotiate pregnancy, birthing and parenting in a world of experts.

Be a good girl …
Do as you're told …
Don't draw attention to yourself …
Doctor knows best …
Don't make a fuss …
No more.

You matter. Your needs and expectations matter. The aim of this conversation is to inform ourselves so we can speak up with autonomy and confidence, and question why we are being steered towards a certain mode of care, investigation or intervention.

It is time that early pregnancy is recognised in our society as a time of needing support. In early pregnancy, the body is undergoing massive changes while the embryo implants and becomes a fetus. Women must no longer suffer in silence for fear of judgement. We must support them in practical and emotional ways, such as helping with the school run for the other children when they can't get their head out of the toilet bowl, and dropping off meals because the smell of cooking makes them retch. And making sure they know rest isn't a dirty word.

From the very beginning of pregnancy, there is opportunity to create a village, where women can reach out and accept help. This needs to become normal. We are worth being held during these first months of pregnancy because they can be challenging and filled with change. It may even be the time when support is most needed.

Let's look into what's happening during the early months through the Tree of Matrescence.

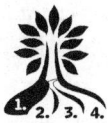

The Physical, Hormonal and Emotional Influences on Early Pregnancy

Hormones in early pregnancy

Hormones deeply affect the physical and emotional changes in your early pregnancy body. Understanding why and how you change is underpinned by the chemistry that affects your mind, body and soul. Hormones are given a bad rap, blamed for everything. In so doing, we sideline and diminish hormones as 'a female problem'. And yes, they are responsible for so much! Hormones are the major player during your pre-conception, pregnancy, birth and early mothering experiences. They will change you to your core.

A huge part of your matrescence is getting to grips with the effects of hormones. This will enable you to realise the normality of your feelings, emotions and actions, so you can navigate your way through pregnancy, labour and those early months with your baby.

Hormones need to be respected and reframed as incredibly powerful. There will be highs and lows in the extreme. By knowing what is happening to you, you will become so much more aware, and able to prepare yourself for a new type of surrender and acceptance of their role in your life. The intent is to navigate this life-changing rite of passage towards connection, intimacy, rest, peaceful transition, joy and tears. To become filled to the brim with recognition of your own worth, achievement and self-esteem.

In her Childbirth Physiology Course,[2] author, educator and former midwife Dr Rachel Reed uses the analogy of a symphony, where individual hormones are the musicians in an orchestra and the brain is the conductor. The body's organs are the musical instruments that the musicians (hormones) are playing. The rhythm and pattern – particularly in physiological labour – is the music we make when everything is in harmony. Drawing from this imagery, let's begin with our first musician.

Progesterone is produced by the corpus luteum after ovulation; it is the bit left over after your egg is released. The corpus luteum (often seen as a 'cyst' on early scans) maintains your pregnancy in the first 10 weeks while the fertilised embryo embeds in the lining of your womb and until the placenta develops enough to take over production of this hormone. It affects smooth muscle, relaxing it, preventing the womb from contracting – so maintaining your pregnancy. In doing this, progesterone causes dizziness as it relaxes the blood vessels throughout the body, lowering blood pressure. It also affects the smooth muscle in the gastrointestinal system, so hello heartburn, constipation, nausea and vomiting. Progesterone increases hair growth, so enjoy the luscious locks, but don't be surprised if some hair appears around your nipples and lower abdomen. Also, vivid dreaming can occur. While making you feel awful, this musician is also crucially helping your body's immune system tolerate the foreign DNA of your growing fetus.

Progesterone lights up the right side of the brain and is associated with intuitive knowing and creative thinking. In doing so, progesterone makes you more introspective and reflective; you might wish to withdraw from the external world, particularly in the second part of your menstrual cycle. As it floods the body in labour, progesterone also gives you an intensely powerful ability to withdraw into yourself, particularly during the separation phase of early labour (more with Ashleigh in Chapter 3 and Ally in Chapter 4).

Oestrogen is called the 'people-pleasing' and 'caregiving' hormone and here's why. Mostly produced in the ovaries and associated with the first half of our cycle and leading to ovulation, oestrogen is also maintained by the corpus luteum until the placenta takes over. Oestrogen promotes greater awareness of yourself and others, reducing risk-taking behaviours. It increases your ability to read your baby's and others' expressive cues to understand their needs. Part of maintaining placental function and preparing your breasts for milk production by enlarging the milk ducts, this hormone also enhances the role of **relaxin**, another hormone that softens ligaments.

Oestrogen plays its music in your developing fetus too, by triggering the growth of several organs and body systems, and stimulating hormone production in your developing baby's adrenal glands. It also adds notes of nausea, an increased appetite and is associated with what some women describe as 'glowing'. It helps the uterus respond to oxytocin in labour.

Introducing **human chorionic gonadotropin** (hCG) next. When your fertilised egg implants in your womb, the developing placenta produces hCG. This is the musician that tells your body you are pregnant, and informs your ovaries to stop producing a maturing egg each month. This is the hormone we look for to produce that double line on a pregnancy test. As a musician, hCG is loud and rises sharply in the first trimester, dipping and then levelling out at around 4 months. hCG keeps your embryo firmly implanted in your uterine lining.

Playing in harmony with the increased sound of the musicians progesterone and oestrogen, hCG helps sustain your pregnancy and builds nourishing blood vessels in the placenta. As hCG plays its merry way through your body, while maintaining the growth of your embryo, the accumulative effects of its side melodies are deep fatigue, nausea, vomiting, breast tenderness, light-headedness and emotional upheaval.

The hormone **human placental lactogen** (hPL) is the musician that plays your metabolic system to increase or maintain levels of energy flowing to your growing baby by reducing your sensitivity to the hormone **insulin**. Insulin transfers glucose into your cells for energy. If for any reason you are fasting or hungry, free fatty acids in your body are changed into glucose, ensuring your baby gets the required energy. This mechanism is particularly useful if you are so nauseated that consuming food is hard. hPL also has a growth effect on your baby, and plays in harmony with oestrogen and progesterone in later pregnancy to promote breast tissue growth. Produced by the placenta at 6 weeks, hPL levels continue to rise throughout pregnancy.

Further hormonal musicians will continue to be explored throughout the book.

After reading all this, if and when you feel fatigued, foggy, sick, emotionally wobbly and constipated, remember it's because your musicians are increasing the volume on the symphony that keeps your pregnancy in place. Your body is adapting to this new state of being and assisting your developing baby to grow. Hold your body with respect, nurturing yourself by whatever means you can. Understand that you feel this way for a damn good reason and take steps to do what feels right for you. Rest and support is calling. This is why I am suggesting we begin to speak up, ask for and accept help with grace, and begin to grow villages of support in the early months. Rest is not a dirty word.

Anxiety, fear and worry can be very real at this time. If they continue, please reach out to your care provider. Remember the tree leaves? Self-worth and compassion. Let them become a mantra. You matter.

Supporting you emotionally and physically early

As you are aware, the purpose of this book is to prepare you so that you emerge emotionally and physically well during and after pregnancy, birthing and the fourth trimester, (the 3 months after birth). The Centre of Perinatal Excellence (COPE) has produced the Ready to Cope app, which is on the **wishlist** 🌿. (Perinatal means the entire pregnancy, birth and postpartum period.) As a means of weekly support, COPE's app tells you what to expect each week, has an appointments calendar, and information that is trustworthy, insightful and comforting. The app is to help reduce the risk of anxiety in pregnancy, the chance of experiencing a traumatic birth, PND and postpartum depletion. COPE also has an antenatal email list for fathers that provides oodles of information and support for partners. It explains to them what is happening with you during pregnancy and what to expect. Please download the app. Your mental health is vitally important.

In her book *Liberating Motherhood: Birthing the Purple Stocking Movement*, lawyer Vanessa Olorenshaw states: "Women deserve to feel nurtured, seen, heard, and valued. There is not enough of this in everyday life, let alone during periods of greater, more intense need: pregnancy, birth, breastfeeding and mothering. Thing is 'needs' and 'mother' often equate to 'mothers meeting needs' rather than 'others meeting mothers' needs'. It is somehow shameful to be seen as 'needy'. As modern women, we have been schooled in disavowing our needs as women—our bodily needs and emotional needs—just as much as our foremothers were expected to be all self-sacrificing and subservient."[3]

We do deserve better, and a way to begin is with our first practice on loving yourself, reconnection and mindfulness.

How to be kind to yourself: Mindfulness

Being kind to yourself is a powerful place to start. Sarah Napthali, a practising Buddhist, mother and author writes in her book *The Complete Buddhism for Mothers*: "We need to look after our own health too by making time for quietness and rest. In practising compassion, we speak kindly to ourselves and notice whether our inner voices are supportive and friendly or judgemental and demanding. We are patient when we falter, for parenting makes amateurs of us all as we confront its never-ending new stages. It helps to cultivate self-awareness, not guilt."[4]

Why am I talking to you about being kind to yourself in early pregnancy? Typically, this is when we feel most challenged by the changes in our body. Often, we hold in all the physical effects, emotions and thoughts, as we have been conditioned to keep them quiet.

Like so many overwhelmed, exhausted and time-poor mothers and mothers-to-be, practising self-loving kindness may be entirely new. Or something you have tried with varying degrees of success, attempting to 'fit it in' to your hectic life. Starting now in this early phase sets you up for a deep inner knowing that being kind to yourself reduces your stress and anxiety levels.

A beautiful quote on loving yourself by Robert Van De Weyer from *Readings of Buddhism* goes: "If you investigate all external objects, you will find none is dearer to you than yourself. If you investigate all other living beings, you will find no one is dearer to you than yourself. When you understand this, you truly love yourself. And those who truly love themselves, never deliberately cause injury to others."[5]

A family benefits when a woman practices kindness to herself as a deeply held value. This is then witnessed and learned from the cradle by the child.

To begin practising self-loving kindness, you need to become present with yourself. This means catching the moment your inner critic talks nastily to you. The times you feel that big emotion, a knot of tension in your chest, the result of unkind words or judgement from others. I'm actually talking about mindfulness here, a buzzword right now and seemingly a bandaid to cope with life stresses. But what actually is mindfulness? Why is it suggested? How is it helpful in pregnancy, in life? And how do you actually do it?

Mindfulness means paying attention in a particular way, on purpose, within the present moment and without judgement.

Why do we need it?

When anxious, stressed or traumatised, we experience an *amygdala hijack*, and the stress hormones **cortisol** and **adrenaline** flood our body into survival mode, or fight or flight. The amygdala, part of our brain's limbic system, is a structure that affects our emotional and behavioural responses in stressful situations.[6]

In one study, mindfulness meditation training was found to alter stress-related amygdala activity. The practice of mindfulness is a potential neurobiological mechanism that promotes functional neuroplastic changes (neurological rewiring), resulting in stress reduction effects.[7] We know it works, which is why we do it. (It's important to mention that *eustress*, healthy stress, is also produced by these hormones, which we will discover with Samantha and Ashleigh in Chapters 2 and 3 respectively.)

How do we practise mindfulness?

Let's begin this practice by addressing your inner voice and biggest critic.

I must keep carrying on no matter what, or what will people think? That I'm making a fuss, being lazy, unable to cope and worthless?

This is where we change the inner conversation we have with ourselves to focus on things that are positive and nourishing without feelings of guilt. Understand that worth is not measured in what we do for others, how clean we keep our home, our performance at work, achievements, qualifications or how much money we make. Our worth is not in how we look, how busy we are seen to be, always doing, doing, doing. That is not our worth.

Begin to notice when that inner voice and critic talks to you. What is it saying? Something horrid? How does it make you feel? Catch it mid-sentence, acknowledge it, and breathe. You can tell it to take a running jump off a short pier into a deep lake and stay there, if you prefer. Notice the tension through your body, and soften. As you breathe in again, speak to yourself as you would a dear friend: gentle, kind, compassionate, loving and respectful. The 'inner vicious voice' needs to become your 'inner value-yourself voice' instead.

I offer you these words to begin with …

I am worth so much. Worth being loved, treated and spoken to with respect and dignity.

Stand in front of the mirror each morning, fully present with yourself, and say …

I love you. You are beautiful just as you are.

It's hard at the start and you might feel silly. However, find dignity and respect from deep within you to cultivate an attitude of self-worth, love and kindness. Only you can make this change and fully comprehend that your worth is immeasurable. You deserve kindness, respect, nourishment and love.

Mindfulness is a practice that takes time and effort to build. It's a simple concept, but not easy to do. Imagine learning to swim or a new language. The repeated practice over months and months? It's the same with mindfulness. We train our brain to rewire its responses to emotional stimuli. In truth, practising mindfulness is being present with whatever is happening to you in that moment. That might be anxiety, stress, frustration, overwhelm, sadness, anger, joy, embarrassment … We can't stop those experiences of feelings happening, but we can be present with them.

The idea that negative emotions will completely disappear during mindfulness practice isn't true. Yet we can be fully present with them, acknowledge them and name them.

I am feeling anxious at the moment. I won't bury it but be present with the feelings that arise, respect them and use the tools I have to help myself in this moment. It will pass in time, and with non-judgement I am going to treat myself kindly.

Also, our brains think about the past, present and future all the time. It is what our brains do. Mindfulness is not having a blank mind. Far from it. That belief only triggers self-judgement and failure. Noticing the constant stream of thoughts is part of the practice of mindfulness. With time, the power these thoughts have to pull you away from attending to your feelings and experiences in the present moment will lessen. If this resonates with you, check out the Headspace mindfulness app.

The practice of mindfulness is deeply, intricately connected to breath. One isn't separate from the other. Deep breathing directly affects the *vagus nerve*, de-escalating our nervous system. This action reduces our response to fight-or-flight surges of **adrenaline** and **cortisol** in our body, lowering our heart rate, blood pressure, anxiety and stress.

Yoga has also been proven to reduce anxiety in pregnancy with immediate stress reduction effects. Pre- and post-class saliva samples showed that **cortisol** levels (stress hormone by-products) were markedly reduced after each class. The women's mood also improved.[8]

- **Wishlist** 🌿 **Ready to Cope app.** https://www.youtube.com/watch?v=_XtjZL8CVcA
- **Ready to Cope website.** Antenatal email list for men
  https://www.cope.org.au/ready-to-cope-for-men-antenatal-emails/
- *Seasons of Matrescence* S1 #5. 'Postpartum Identity and Mum Guilt with Dr Nicole Highet' Apple 🎙 Spotify
- **Headspace mindfulness app.** https://www.headspace.com/headspace-meditation-app

Touch is important too. In his book, *Men, Love and Birth*, Mark Harris, a midwife of 20 years, writes from a man's and a midwife's perspective for men, helping them understand their partner's needs and experiences in pregnancy, birth and early parenting. He helps them realise how to be supportive and prepares them for fathering. Harris states: "Birth, for blokes, can be a rite of passage too."[9]

Harris has some practical tips for the man in your life. The first is to give you a massage twice a week! How nice would a neck, shoulder and upper back massage be? A foot massage maybe? Massage practice is a way to become more connected during pregnancy and birth, and a great way for your partner to be in the good books too!

Practice offering: *Yogic breath*

Pay attention to your body in the present moment, using one of our greatest friends: our own breath. Known as *pranayama* in the world of yoga, there are quite a few methods for breathing within yogic practice that are perfect for pregnancy and birthing. We will explore these throughout the chapters, but first we will relearn how to breathe.

Our breath is with us always. It is such a simple thing to do, but so powerful and effective. Relearning how to breathe is essential. We tend to take short breaths that fill the upper cavity of our chest, particularly when anxious and when the amygdala is hijacked. We want to harness the vagal nerve to de-escalate anxiety and stress. Deep breathing achieves this.

It is important not to hold your breath while pregnant, because a constant flow of oxygen to the baby is needed as you breathe for them.

The first breathwork practice is the 3-part breath, also known as *yogic breath*. It is the foundation for other methods of breathing practice that will help throughout pregnancy, birthing and mothering.

- Begin with breathing in and out of the nose, noticing your chest expand and fall.
- Inhale for a long count of 3, sending the breath down to expand the belly. The breath in is precious oxygen, lifeforce and the catalyst for producing energy. This lifeforce energy is known as *prana*.
- Notice the ribs move outwards and shoulders rise.
- Exhale for a long count of 3 out. Notice the belly soften, ribs draw inwards and shoulders release downwards. *Apana* is the release of breath. The release of carbon dioxide.
- Place your hands on your belly with middle fingers just touching.
- Breath in and notice how the fingers no longer touch. Imagine sending a thought of love to your growing child. Breathe out with softness. Repeat 5 times.

With this practice, we can break the habit of immediate reactions to strong emotions. Who cares if someone looks at you sideways while taking a few deep breaths? You do what works for you.

That's the physical side of the practice, but what about your busy mind? A way to start practising mindfulness is to harness your senses, meaning touch, taste, smell, hearing and sight. Focus on being present and mindful by saying to yourself:

- I am breathing in, noticing just that.

- Notice the cool air in your nostrils as you inhale.

- Feel the expansion of your chest and belly.

- I am breathing out, feeling just that.

- Notice the warmth of the air as you exhale.

- Feel the softening of your chest and belly as you release.

- Notice the environment around you. Notice the people, sounds, smells. Feel where your body is connected to the ground, any tension in your muscles.

- With each exhalation, allow your body to soften ... facial muscles released, shoulders down, rapidly scanning your body from head to toe for tension and softening.

- Notice your pelvic floor too and release, soften, because this action is just as important as contracted strengthening tone.

- **Pregnancy yoga YouTube.** Suitable for beginners and throughout pregnancy
  https://www.youtube.com/watch?v=bmsVXHUn0g0

- **Active Pregnancy Foundation website.** https://www.activepregnancyfoundation.org/

- **Pregnancy, Birth and Baby website.** Your growing baby week by week. https://www.pregnancybirthbaby.org.au/pregnancy-week-by-week

---

From early pregnancy, I don't advise any deep backbends for advanced yoga practitioners. Abdominal muscles separate in pregnancy to provide room for your growing uterus. This is called *diastasis recti*, and if they are overworked, the muscles may not come back together after birth. We will talk about this more with Samantha in Chapter 2 and with Clémentine in Chapter 7.

Yoga flow instructions

A sequence of 25 postures (Asanas) is offered. As you practise your yoga, try to be fully present, paying attention to your breath and how it feels to intentionally move with the breath. If your mind wanders off to your shopping list and other to-do things, just notice that it has wandered, with no judgement, and return your attention to your next inhalation. What is your intention for your practice? An intention, or *bhāva*, is a guide or theme that can make your practice more meaningful. It could be to find quiet or calm, to release discomfort, or connect to your body and growing baby.

If you are fatigued, feel free to skip the standing sequence 15–20. Move slowly through the sequence with your breath as a guide. Inhale with upward movement. Exhale with downward, sideways or gentle twisting. When holding a posture for a while, sink into it with each breath out, allowing ligaments and muscle to stretch.

Please don't force yourself into anything. It doesn't matter how it looks. It's all about how it feels.

Always be kind to yourself.

A yoga mat is useful because it is less slippery than a bare floor or a carpet. Use folded blankets and pillows, or a firm cushion or bolster, as props to maintain the upper body in a slightly upright position when reclined. When moving out of a reclined position, please roll to the left.

While in each posture, allow for at least 2 full breaths for extension into the stretch and time to soften into it. If you are enjoying a particular posture or feel you need more time to ease into it, take a few more breaths. There is no hard and fast rule. Do what feels right for your body at the time.

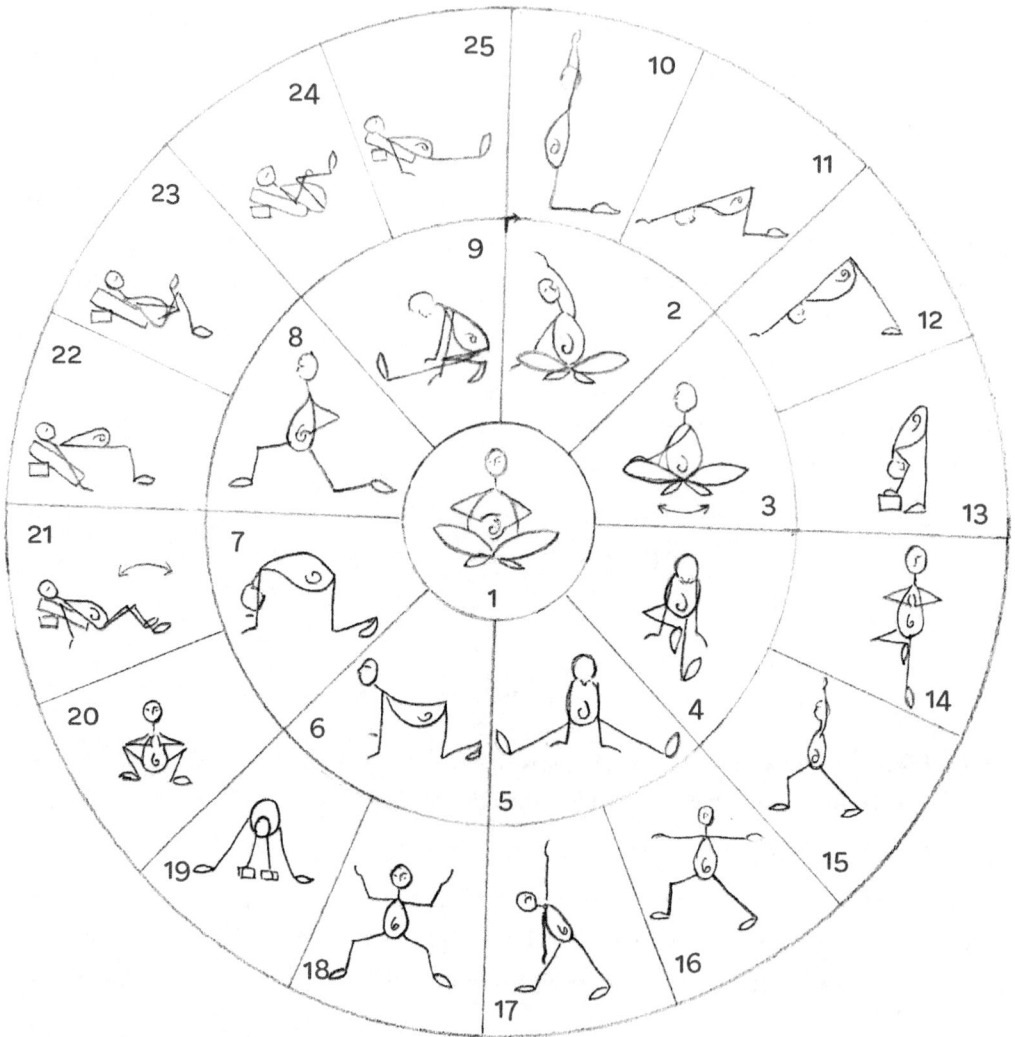

Early pregnancy yoga flow: Connection to mind and body

1. Sit cross legged in Easy pose. Scan through your body and find a comfortable position, supported by pillows if needed. If you wish, chant "Ohm" silently or aloud 3 times. Place your hands on your belly, middle fingers just touching and begin practising the 3-part breath. Repeat 5 times.

2. Inhale and raise the right arm over the head, leaning to the left. Turn your face to look upwards. Breath into the right side of the body. Expand the ribs to feel the stretch more fully. Press through the left hand as you exhale and release the right arm to the floor. Repeat on the left side.

3. Place the right hand on the left knee and left hand on the floor behind you to provide a gentle upper body twist. Inhale and expand the chest. Exhale and look over the left shoulder allowing a gentle press through the right hand to encourage a deeper twist. Exhale and release slightly. Inhale, fill the upper chest. Exhale, chin over right shoulder. Release the posture with a long exhalation. Repeat on the right side.

4. Lengthen the right leg in front of you, toes up to the ceiling. Bend the left knee and bring the sole of the foot to the inner right thigh. Inhale and lift from the pelvis to crown of the head to lengthen the spine, arms overhead. Exhale, keeping the spine straight, bend forwards and place your hands on the floor in front of you. With each exhalation, sink a little more. Look at the toes of the right leg, then allow the head to hang. Breathe. Press into the hands on an inhalation to rise. Repeat on the left side.

5. Place the legs in a wide arc either side of you with hands on the floor in front. Inhale, look up, lifting your body upwards from the pelvis to lengthen the spine. Exhale, allow the body to sink forwards, supporting the weight on your hands. With each breath move the hands away from the body and sink into the posture. Wide-legged forward fold. Allow your head to fall forwards for more spinal stretch. Press into the hands with an inhalation and move into an all-fours position.

6. Place a blanket under your knees for comfort. Tuck the toes under and press gently through the toes, knees and hands with spine neutral (a tabletop). Inhale to expand the belly and, as you exhale, sway your belly down towards the floor and look up to the ceiling. Open your chest outwards. Untuck your pelvis, so the tailbone is towards the ceiling. Cow pose. Exhale to all fours.

7. Inhale to expand the belly. Exhale, press through the hands and toes, tuck chin to the chest, tuck pelvis under, tailbone towards chin. Allow the shoulder blades to part, your upper spine upwards to the ceiling. Curl around your belly. Cat pose. Repeat Cow and Cat pose 3 times. Inhale into Cow, exhale into Cat.

8. Move to upright kneeling. Extend the right leg in front of you, with the foot further in front of the knee. Place hands on the right thigh, inhale deeply. Exhale and allow the body to sink. The right knee is at a 90-degree angle, left leg extends behind to stretch the hip flexor. Three breath cycles. Sink a little deeper on each exhalation. Inhale to slowly move out of the posture to transition to 9.

9. Inhale and tuck the toes of the left foot under. Exhale and sink the pelvis back over the left heel. Hands are placed on the floor either side of the extended right leg, toes to the ceiling. Three breath cycles. Sink a little more into a hamstring stretch. Repeat postures 8 and 9 on the left side.

10. Move to upright kneeling position. Knees hip width apart, toes untucked. Inhale, tuck the pelvis slightly under. Lift body upwards to extend the spine to the crown of the head. Shoulders back, arms hanging and hands soft. Exhale. Inhale, raise the arms wide to side, open the chest outwards, palms together in prayer above the head. Exhale, arms in a circle downwards as your pelvis sinks slowly to your heels. Inhale to upright kneeling. Repeat twice.

11. Inhale to upright kneeling. Exhale, bend forward at the hips, move through all fours, forehead to the floor and extend the arms in front of you. Puppy pose. Use a pillow for your head or under your chest for support. Knees are at 90 degrees. Breathe into the posture, shoulders stretch. If uncomfortable, cross the arms. With an exhalation, sink the pelvis down to the heels. Knees may need to move wider to make room for your growing belly. Rest your head on the floor or a pillow, arms either side of your body with palms uppermost. Melt into Child's pose. Rest as long as you wish.

12. From Child's pose, place your palms on the floor either side of the head and inhale to all fours. Hands firm, fingers wide. Tuck the toes under, knees hip width apart. Exhale, press equally through the hands

and feet as you lift your knees off the floor. Pelvis to the ceiling, lengthen through the spine, arms and legs. Allow the head to hang weightless. Downward Facing Dog pose.

Gently allow your heels to move towards the floor. Knees slightly bent with heels off the floor is fine. Untuck the pelvis a little. Three cycles of breath. If this is too strong, Puppy pose is an alternative. Exhale, bend the knees to all fours and sink into Child's pose. Rest a while.

If you feel like it, move to posture 20. Sometimes nausea and fatigue are just too much to move through a more energetic standing sequence. Be kind to yourself.

13. From Child's pose, inhale to move to all fours. Exhale, gradually move to a standing forward fold. Head hanging, knees slightly bent, feet hip width apart. Hands on a block or arms crossed. Each vertebra given space. Inhale and expand the rib cage. Exhale and just loll a while. Move the hips in little circles if you wish.

14. Transition to balance in Tree pose, inhale and shift your weight to your right foot. Find a point in front of you to gaze at to help your balance – your Drishti. Bend the left knee with toes lightly touching the floor. Exhale and note your shifted centre of gravity. Inhale and rotate the left leg outwards. Move to a wall for support if needed. Lift the left foot and place the sole on the inner calf of your right leg. If it is in your practice, place the left sole on the inner right thigh.

When comfortable in your balance and gaze, place the hands in Anjali mudra (prayer hands) at your heart. Inhale and raise the arms above the head, palms together. Exhale as you steady yourself into the posture and enjoy another 2 or 3 cycles of breath. Exhale, lower the arms, left leg rotates inwards, then place the left foot to the floor. Make small circular movements to settle the pelvis back to neutral. Repeat on the left side.

15. Transition to Warrior 1 pose. Step the right foot forwards and the left back to a wide-legged stance, pelvis facing forwards. Right knee slightly bent and left foot at a 45-degree angle. Inhale and reach the arms upwards, palms together, shoulders down. Exhale, sink the body down so the right knee bends towards a 90-degree angle. Widen your stance as you need to, and move to where your body feels good. Three breath cycles. Keep the muscles of your body taut, engaged and working, rather than passive.

16. From Warrior 1, with an exhalation rotate the pelvis to the left 90 degrees. The legs and feet remain as they are. Your body aligns with the long edge of the mat. Inhale. Exhale, lower the arms so they are parallel to the floor in line with your legs. The shoulders sink and imagine your middle fingers are pulled outwards away from your body. Turn your face to look along your right arm. Breathe into Warrior 2 pose. Feet firmly planted, left foot outer edge grounded.

17. Transition from Warrior 2 to Triangle pose. Inhale and straighten the right leg. Exhale, shorten your stance to your own leg length wide. Inhale, expand the rib cage and upper chest. Exhale, allow your body to reach slightly to your right foot and then bend at the waist. The right arm lowers to the right thigh. Left arm and fingers reach up to the ceiling. If it is within your practice, right hand on a block or the floor.

If your balance is stable, turn your face to look at your left thumb. With a slow inhalation, press into the feet to lift your body to an upright position. Exhale, arms down. Walk the feet inwards to a standing posture. Do small figure of 8 circles to release through the hips. Repeat the sequence 15–17 on the other side by stepping the left foot forward at the beginning of Warrior 1.

18. Move into Mountain pose, with feet grounded, spine long and crown of head to the sky, and face the long edge of the mat. Inhale deeply. Exhale and step wide to one side. Turn the feet outwards. Tuck the pelvis under, lengthen the spine, crown to the ceiling, hands on the hips. Inhale and lift the arms out to a star shape. Exhale, bend the knees and sink the body down. Bend the elbows with the upper arm parallel to the floor. Spread the fingers wide. Breathe into Goddess pose.

19. From Goddess pose, exhale as you bend forwards, hands to the floor, or on a block, firm cushion or bolster, then straighten the legs. Inhale and look forwards with spine and arms straight. Exhale, bend the elbows and allow the upper body to hang. Inhale as you lean into your hands, move your feet closer together. Exhale and put the props between your legs ready to squat.

20. Inhale, bend at the knees, feet turned outwards, pelvis towards the ground as you exhale. If you feel you can sink deeper, remove some props. Place the elbows to the inside of the knees and hands together in Anjali mudra. Breathe into the position, sinking a little more on each exhalation. Press the palms of the hands firmly together and downwards. Consciously soften the pelvic floor. Rock side to side.

21. Place props behind you ready to recline. Your back and head are supported in a semi-recumbent position with your sacrum on the floor. Bend your knees, feet on the mat. Take a few long, deep breath cycles and melt into a short rest. Place the feet to the edge of the mat. Inhale and, as you exhale, the knees fall to the right. Inhale and bring the knees up to centre, exhale and move the knees to the left in a windscreen wiper motion. Move with the breath.

22. Inhale, place your feet on the floor hip width apart, heels towards the buttocks. Arms beside you, palms down beside the hips. Exhale, tuck the pelvis under, lift your pelvic floor. Press into the feet, hands and upper back, lift your pelvis from the floor in Bridge pose. For a 3-breath cycle press into the hands and feet, clench the buttocks together and lift a little more. With the next exhalation slowly uncurl the spine from the shoulders one vertebra at a time, until the sacrum touches the mat. Untuck the pelvis, release the pelvic floor, soften. Repeat twice.

23. Return to the beginning of Bridge pose. Place the arms out on the floor like a cross. Put the right ankle on the left knee. Inhale and with the exhalation the legs move to the floor on the right. Keep the right ankle on the left knee. Turn the face to the left. If too intense over the left hip, place a pillow under the right knee. Breath into this posture to allow a gentle spinal twist and to lengthen the piriformis muscle over the left hip. With an inhalation, lift knees upright. Repeat with left ankle on the right knee.

24. While still reclined, place a hand on each knee. As you inhale, fill the belly and allow the knees to move away from the body as the arms lengthen. Exhale and draw the knees close to either side of the body towards the armpits. Repeat this twice. Rock side to side to massage your lower back if that feels good.

25. Sávāsana, the pose of meditative rest. Lengthen your legs and place a pillow under the knees for more comfort if you wish. Cover yourself with a blanket in cool weather. Arms to the sides, palms facing upwards. Slow, steady breaths. Scan through each area of the body and imagine a light gently flowing through you bringing comfort, softness, nourishment and rest. Release and soften. Allow the body to feel heavy. Gently close your eyes or maintain a soft gaze. Practise the *Metta Bhavana* meditation offered at the end of Liesja's chapter, page 47.

Cultural, Herstorical and Political Influences on Early Pregnancy

Much of what we believe to be true and acceptable in the culture of birthing is not, in fact, acceptable. Here we will explore the herstory, a word I first came across as an alternative to history in Dr Rachel Reed's book, *Reclaiming Childbirth as a Rite of Passage: Weaving ancient wisdom with modern knowledge*.[10] We will look at why and how the current early pregnancy norms in our culture evolved to have far-reaching effects on us today, and explore different topics in each chapter.

Discussing the estimated due date

Currently, in pregnancy, we live by due dates. We plan around them. We are asked, "When are you due?" and "Have you had it yet?" a thousand times. Due dates are ingrained in our cultural expectations. Our medical system works by them.

In 2000 obstetrician Dr Gerald W Lawson wrote about the current method (called *Naegele's rule*) used to calculate your estimated due date (EDD): "The idea that this rule can apply to every pregnant female – young or old, nulliparous (never given birth) or multiparous (has given birth), Caucasian, Asian, African or Indigenous – stretches credulity. In addition, many women regard the 40-week date as a deadline, which if crossed, may place the baby under stress. Forty weeks is a simple, round convenient figure that it has proved difficult to challenge, despite criticism. Nonetheless, what might have been an appropriate formula in Germany in the 19th century deserves to be revisited in the 21st."[11]

Yet, here we are over 20 years later!

Currently, we consider *term* (where baby is mature enough to adapt to life outside the womb without assistance) to be 37–42 weeks. *Pre-term* is before 37 weeks. We are given an EDD of birth at 40 weeks. *Post-dates* is after 40 weeks. *Post-term* is after 42 weeks.

Evidence now shows that the method we use to calculate our due date is out of date. I stand on the shoulders of giants here, drawing from Dr Rachel Reed's book, *Why Induction Matters,*[12] and Dr Sara Wickham's book, *In Your Own Time: How Western Medicine Controls the Start of Labour and Why This Needs to Stop.*[13]

Way back in our herstory, women expected to birth their babies within 10 moon cycles after their last menstrual cycle. The first written record of this method of calculating birth expectancy was 2,400 years ago by the Greek philosopher Aristotle. Each moon cycle is 29.5 days, so 10 moon cycles is 295 days or 42 weeks.

Dutch physician Hermann Boerhaave first developed a calculation in 1709 to estimate the due date of a baby by adding one week and 9 months to a woman's last menstrual period. That means 280 days or 40 weeks. There is some suggestion that this was formulated for legal reasons to determine the paternity of the child.

This was revisited and first published by Franz Carl Naegele in 1830. His method is the one we still use today. Naegele's rule is also for 280 days.

A glaring omission is that neither Boerhaave nor Naegele specified whether the EDD was to be calculated from the first or last day of a woman's period. If their calculation was meant to begin from the last day of a woman's menstrual cycle, then an entire week was intended to be added for an estimated gestational length of around 41 weeks.

However, writers of obstetric medical texts took it upon themselves to use the first day. This has become ingrained. On what authority or evidence did they do this? Apparently none. Aside from this tool being almost 200 years old, the main word used in these rules is 'estimate'.

Evidence shows that most pregnancies last longer than 40 weeks; just 35% of women birth in the week around that date. In first-time pregnancies, 75% of women who labour and birth spontaneously do so by 41 weeks and 2 days. In second and further pregnancies, we birth at around 40 weeks and 2 days. Most births are post-dates.

Applying Naegele's 200-year-old rule to all women today as one-size-fits-all is about fitting every pregnant woman into a controllable system, no matter her ethnicity or individual history. This is deeply flawed. With all the data we have now, it's high time the EDD calculation was reviewed.

While the key part of this is estimation, dates for induction of labour and caesarean sections are based on this old rule. The idea of a baby arriving at 40 weeks is so deeply embedded in our culture that we expect to give birth at 40 weeks. However, our bodies and our babies expect something else: to birth when they are ready! Currently, women are being induced into labour at 40 weeks +1 day pregnant, simply because they are past their EDD. The resulting cascade of intervention when a woman and baby are not yet ready to labour or birth is significant. Induction was originally intended for post-term dates, which was after 42 weeks.

Having this knowledge is part of working together towards reducing the risk of over-intervention, traumatic birth and PND.

There is a need for perceptive balance here, because sometimes induction is needed for medical indications for the mother, baby or both. Thank goodness we have the ability to assist in this way. We will be discussing induction for post-dates and more with Ashleigh in Chapter 3 and Katie in Chapter 5.

With this understanding, how do we get around the pressure of informing others of a due date? My suggestion is offering a *birthing month*. If it's good enough for royalty and celebrities, why shouldn't we do this too? You don't have to tell anybody your EDD, but you could give them the month you expect your baby to arrive. This is up to you, but it may save you a lot of stress, irritation and pressure when you get questions like, "Have you had it yet?" and "When are you getting induced?" Oh, and renaming the EDD the 'estimated date of birth' (EDB) would be a good start. You, the mother, give birth. No matter how. Nobody 'delivers' you.

- **Wishlist** 🌿 Great Birthing Rebellion #3. 'Due Dates' Apple 🎙 Spotify
- **Dr Sara Wickham website.** 'Why your estimated due date might need a rethink' https://www.sarawickham.com/?s=estimated+due+dates

---

Themes emerged as I researched this book, and one of them is that research into maternal matters is often outdated and based on flawed data. When good evidence is published, it can take up to 20 years for it to be put into practice. This needs to change.

Speaking of up-to-date research, this leads us into our next thought-provoking discussion …

Use of ultrasound and Doppler in pregnancy

Ultrasound scanning (USS) was developed from radar and sonar use during WWII. In her book, *Hail Caesar*, Dr Caroline de Costa talks about the rise of USS in pregnancy. She describes how Dr Ian Donald, Professor of Midwifery in Glasgow, served in the Royal Air Force as a medic during the war and had a deep interest in radar and sonar. In 1955 he borrowed an industrial machine to look at beef steak and then at abdominal tumours of his patients. Donald noted that the echo sound waves of different tissues and fluid could be adapted to USS in pregnancy. Commercial machines became available in 1963. By 1970 USS was firmly established in obstetric care.[14] (I mentioned before that it takes about 20 years for research that benefits the mother to be put into clinical practice; however, if it makes money or saves time, it's a different story.) Initially, Donald concentrated on the position of the placenta to diagnose placenta praevia, where the placenta covers the opening of the cervix.

Dr Sarah Buckley's book, *Gentle Birth, Gentle Mothering: A Doctors Guide to Natural Childbirth and Gentle Early Parenting Choices*, explains the use of USS in pregnancy and how it has become an expected, ingrained cultural norm. However, there is evidence that up to 49% of women having a scan are not aware it is a screening tool for abnormalities of their baby. Many think it is a routine check and many women expect a 'perfect' baby.[15] USS is now offered routinely in pregnancy in Australia. You can expect 3 routine scans, 2 of which are in early pregnancy, which is why we are discussing this now.

For every scan, women are meant to be informed about why they are having it and what doctors are looking for. There must be full disclosure of the effects the USS can have on body tissues and the noise it produces, and women must give consent.

Firstly, expect to be offered a very early dating scan, which estimates the gestation of the pregnancy (weeks and days) to give an EDD. If a mother is certain of her last menstrual period date, there is no evidence to suggest a USS for the EDD is a better measure. A dating scan at 7–8 weeks is accurate to plus or minus 3–4 days either side of the scan. That is a 6–8-day range either side of the USS date.

Say you are given an EDD of 15 March; the range would be as much as 11–19 March. A machine doesn't know your body like you do. When you are sure of your last menstrual period, consider whether you need a dating scan. Trust your body. It will be less expensive too as it's one scan fewer to pay for.

Secondly, a fetal nuchal translucency scan (FNT) is offered at around 12 weeks. This measures the thickness of the fold of skin at the back of the neck of the fetus as a possible indicator of Down syndrome. When done with some screening blood tests, a calculation of a risk of Down syndrome is given. If the risk is a chance of 1 in 250–300 of Down syndrome in the baby, the mother is offered further investigations, such as an amniocentesis. This is an invasive procedure which takes a sample of the fluid from around your baby that carries fetal cells with their DNA.[16] Please look at the Your Choice website on the **wishlist** 🌿 for information on screening.

Approximately 19 out of 20 babies diagnosed as high risk through FNT are found not to be affected. In addition, an FNT does not detect all babies who do have Down syndrome.[17] Before any screening, talk to your partner about how you may feel if an abnormality is diagnosed and what you would wish to do about the outcome, such as discontinuing the pregnancy. It's easier to go in knowing what you both think about the choices you may make afterwards.

There is an alternative to the FNT scan – the non-invasive antenatal test (NIPT), which is offered at 10 weeks. A sample of mum's blood is taken. Fetal cells cross the placenta into mum's blood stream. These cells carry the growing baby's DNA and a diagnosis of genetic difference, such as Down syndrome, can be made. It is a highly accurate blood test but not diagnostic. If a NIPT result is positive, further diagnostic tests, like amniocentesis or chorionic villus sampling (CVS), may be needed for confirmation. CVS involves taking a small sample of tissue from the placenta between 10 and 13 weeks. It currently costs between $400 and $500.

- **Wishlist** 🌿 Dr Sarah Buckley website. 'Ultrasound scans a cause for concern' https://sarahbuckley.com/ultrasound-scans-cause-for-concern/
- **Wishlist** 🌿 Your Choice website. Provides information about pregnancy screening. The what, why and how of screening, your choices and costs, if any. This helps navigate screening, depending on what you would decide with the outcome. https://yourchoice.mcri.edu.au/dashboard

Lastly, a morphology scan at 20–22 weeks' gestation can see the brain, heart, abdomen, limbs and other structural anatomy. If dating from this scan, the variation is a week either side of the EDD. Again, with an estimated date of 15 March using Naegele's rule, the range of accuracy means you should expect your birthing between 8 and 22 March. This scan does not always detect a structural anomaly and does not detect neurodivergence, such as cerebral palsy or autism.[18]

Some women choose to have as few scans as possible but still have this morphology scan. There are some babies who would not live once born due to structural abnormality or would be severely physically impaired. Again, the Your Choice resource may be helpful to you here.

Recommendation 37 of the NSW inquiry into birth trauma that I mentioned in the introduction suggests reviewing "guidelines for informing parents of fetal anomalies and genetic conditions ensuring that clinicians present unbiased options, offer ample time and support for decision-making". It also recommends providing "trauma-informed assistance and psychological support to aid parents in coping with the emotional impact of such diagnoses."[19] This needs to be adopted nationwide.

USS is undeniably an amazing tool to have when a pregnancy is outside the parameters of what is considered healthy. In the hands of a skilled ultrasonographer, it can be vital for monitoring the wellbeing of your baby. Further scans may be suggested for a medical condition of your own or of your baby. Good communication and feeling free to ask questions will assist in understanding why tests are recommended. Ask your care provider: "What are we hoping to learn and why?"

This next information is not intended to scaremonger, but it is important if you are planning non-medical 3D or 4D scans. When scans are offered or sought, it is important that women know the effects of USS and Doppler. USS is pulsed waves that have been recorded at 84 decibels – as loud as a diesel truck. Doppler is a continuous wave but quieter. Apart from the sound they make, these waves affect bodily tissue too. USS waves increase temperatures by 1–1.5 °C, and is presumed safe due to bodily temperature ranges up to 2.5 °C. However, the heat experienced in the body tissues is different from these bodily temperature ranges. Bones warm more than soft tissue. Depending on the settings and output of the scanning machine, heat will increase the longer the USS is used, and when the transducer is held in one place. As such, consider asking for the intensity and duration of exposure and maximum thermal index of each USS to be documented.

If you are offered any scan not for a medically indicated reason, please feel confident to challenge it. The commercialisation of 3D and 4D scans offered by walk-in, shopping mall, peek-in-the-womb-style, non-medical organisations is concerning. It's important to know about the exposure of your growing baby to sound and heat from the USS. Some professional bodies criticise this 3D and 4D non-medical keepsake as potentially harmful and they suggest reporting non-medical organisations.[20]

There is a lot of money to be made from pregnant women, which is a theme I found in my research for *Mother Becoming*. If every pregnant woman in the USA had one routine scan, it would amount to US $1.2 billion in spending.[21] You have a choice about how many scans you have and should be fully informed about the ambiguity of dating your pregnancy via this method, the nature of the estimation, the reasons the scans are being conducted, the side effects and the out-of-pocket costs. Only by being fully aware of these facts can you give your consent for the procedure.

The evolution of maternity care in Australia

How has maternity care in westernised culture evolved to create the current attitudes, beliefs and choices we have available in Australia? Why is it that women, upon finding they are pregnant, first go to a doctor rather than booking in with a midwife? Research overwhelmingly shows that midwifery continuity of care (COC) has better outcomes and satisfaction for mother and baby.

Birthtime The Handbook highlights the better outcomes: "The recently published Australian Birthplace study looked at 1.25 million births over 13 years, and found that women birthing in birthing centres and at home had lower incidence of induced labour, epidurals, ventouse and forceps births and caesarean sections, with no difference in the stillbirth rate."[22]

Part of the reason for this comes down to the herstory. The development of modern midwifery and obstetric practice in Australia is partly defined by what happened between 1950 and 1985. During this time, there was a large increase in specialist obstetricians taking over from where general practitioners had formerly had the monopoly over childbirth. Specialists oversaw the care of women admitted to their institutions, but most of the work was done by junior doctors and midwives. Until the early 1980s, specialists worked in public hospitals in an 'honorary capacity' where they were paid nothing or a token amount. They had to make a living though, so made their money from private practice.[23] This is when private practice and public obstetric medical models of care flourished, with largely male specialist obstetricians. By the time Medicare arrived under the Hawke Labor Government, the roots of private practice were already firmly established.[24]

Currently, when you discover you are pregnant, you make an appointment with your GP. This exposes you to a pathological (looking for ill-health, disease, risk) based model of care. The model of care you receive when seeing a midwife is physiological (based in health and wellness) Why? Because there is no provision for seeing a midwife first, unless you employ a privately practising midwife or are lucky to be one of the 10–15% of women offered midwife COC. Throughout history, women have been attended to and supported by other women during birthing, but with the wholesale transfer of birthing to hospital, this continuous support reduced dramatically. The result is the fragmented care of the hospital system.

As Professor H. Dahlen states in *Birthtime*, "We are blindly walking into an increasingly medicalised system. We keep inventing new technologies. We keep not testing them and trialling them properly. We keep not asking the long-term research questions about what we're doing to women. And it's an escalating process."[25]

As doula Maddie McMahon states in *Why Mothering Matters*, "We have replaced kith and kin and clan with doctors and parenting 'experts'. Our first thought on finding out we are pregnant is to visit the doctor. Attempts to encourage women to book directly with a midwife seem to be continuously thwarted, by GP receptionists, by women who feel only a doctor can confirm their pregnancy, and by society at large, which perpetuates the idea that pregnancy is an illness."[26]

A midwifery COC model resolves this fragmented care issue. A reciprocal relationship of respect and trust builds over time, with the warmth, compassion and wisdom a midwife brings. A relationship forms that offers to fill the spiritual experience of 'mother becoming' with meaning, acknowledgment and wonder. Midwives are present for the whole experience, particularly the postpartum period. Known birth support is vital. It is important to have trust in, and know, a person who believes in you, will advocate for you and walks hand in hand with you. No matter how you give birth and mother, it is of infinite value when someone knows your story, wishes and fears.

This is what is needed, instead of a medical conveyor belt of measurements, paperwork, different faces, different advice and time constraints. The video animation by Birthsmart offered in the goody box illustrates the fragmented care that most women experience in current Australian maternity health care. It offers some insight into what you may expect from your care. Have a watch and see what you think. It will assist you in considering what kind of care you would like.

In the UK and many European countries, when a woman becomes pregnant, she is asked, "Who is you midwife?" In Australia we ask, "Who is your obstetrician?"

Having continuity in your midwifery care is particularly important for our culturally and linguistically diverse (CALD) community. Australia is a nation made up of migrants. Some families are refugees, fleeing conflict or oppression. Many do not have English as their first language. Knowing one or a few midwives with the use of interpreters, instead of having fragmented care, is incredibly important for mother and baby wellbeing.

Maternity Choices Australia (MCA) provides resources and support for your journey. The MCA illustrates some important truths about the positive effects of continuity of midwifery care in Australia as it currently stands. With COC:

- there are 16% fewer *episiotomies* (a cut to the *perineum*, which is between the vagina and anus)
- there are 24% fewer pre-term births
- there is 15% less chance of instrumental birth
- women in labour need and use fewer pain medications
- there are lower mortality rates
- care is culturally responsive
- there is a higher chance of breastfeeding at 6 weeks and 6 months.

However, less than 10–15% of our birthing population has access to midwifery COC and there is only 1% growth per year.

Another great resource is the blog from the Transforming Maternity Care Collaborative (TMCC). Its goal is to "drive reform of maternity services to provide a primary care model that is midwife-led in the community, is accessible to all and is centred around respecting women's choices".

In its article 'Place of Birth: What if all low-risk women planned to birth in a birth centre or at home?', it highlights that women want home birthing, known care midwifery, little to no intervention, and choices and autonomy over their body and birth. Despite this, fewer than 1% have access to this kind of care. Birth centre care provides a proven midwife-led care environment aimed at less intervention, and less instrumental and caesarean birth. Yet currently, fewer than 3% of women have this choice.

Aside from improving maternal experiences and satisfaction, and more positive outcomes of birthing, the financial cost of birthing centres is less to the taxpayer.[27] The International Confederation of Midwives (ICM), in its Bill of Rights for Women and Midwives, states: "Every woman has a right to choose the place where she gives birth."[28]

In her book, *Reclaiming Childbirth as a Rite of Passage*, Dr Rachel Reed writes: "The legacy of herstory is rooted in centuries of appropriation and medicalisation of women's bodies and birth."[29]

The Midwives' Cauldron podcast, hosted by Dr Rachel Reed and Katie James, who is a midwife and lactation consultant, humorously explains the 'Herstory of Modern Birth Practices'. The podcast is an excellent source of reliable information and great to have in your goody box. I'm biased because they are midwives, but whatever I suggest for you is geared towards you and your wellbeing.

Hospital-based care and private practice are firmly established in Australia. The Royal Australian and New Zealand College of Obstetricians and Gynaecologists (RANZCOG) has published 'Maternity Care in Australia'. This document is about the provision of ideal maternity care, and states: "Maternity care is fundamental to the health of society. It should be based on the best available evidence applied with the individual woman as its focus."[30]

The intention behind these words is good, yet the achievement of this has a very long way to go and isn't being done quickly enough.

In *Birthtime*, Professor of Midwifery Hannah Dahlen states: "We could transform our maternity system in Australia tomorrow if we looked at the evidence and we realised what top-level evidence in the world is saying now, which is women need to have a midwife they know provide their care during pregnancy, during birth and the postnatal period. Women who are well and who are healthy should not be birthing in our big, complex hospitals that are geared towards problems. So, get them out."[31]

- Birthsmart YouTube, animation. https://www.youtube.com/watch?v=p4t9lmTU_Ng&t=336s
- The Raising Children Network video. Describes pregnancy care options for the CALD community. https://raisingchildren.net.au/pregnancy/pregnancy-birth-videos/pregnancy-multicultural-services
- Pregnancy, Birth and Baby website. Support for migrants to Australia, including information to assist with navigating care and financial assistance. https://raisingchildren.net.au/pregnancy/pregnancy-birth-videos/pregnancy-multicultural-services
- Wishlist ✿ MCA website. http://www.maternitychoices.org/resources
- Wishlist ✿ TMCC website. https://www.transformingmaternity.org.au/
- *The Midwives' Cauldron* S1 #3. 'The Herstory of Modern Birth Practices' Apple 🎙Spotify

Take a few long, deep, 3-part breaths. That was a lot to take in. Allow this knowledge to settle with space for mixed feelings, then gently explore how this has made an impact on you.

Social, Economic and Media Influences on Early Pregnancy

A time of steep social and behavioural change

The invisible umbilical cord is now embedded in our consciousness and helps us become aware of the growth within. It makes us want to provide a nourishing, safe environment and rethink what we put in our bodies. We start staying hydrated, taking supplements, eating healthily. We cut out alcohol, unpasteurised dairy, raw eggs, undercooked meat and all deli foods to prevent listeriosis. We cut down on caffeine and stop smoking. We may think about what we put on our body too. Our skin is the largest organ and we absorb everything that goes on it.

We may begin thinking about how pregnancy affects hobbies, work, sporting activities and social engagements. We have heightened awareness of the world, suddenly seeing pregnant women and babies everywhere! Our behaviour changes in terms of what we read, follow, join, subscribe to and learn. We become hungry for knowledge and affirmation that we are doing all the right things.

When do you tell people your news and why? It's entirely up to you, of course. Some will guess because you keep ducking out to the loo, are too sick to work, or they will notice that you no longer drink alcohol and are avoiding certain foods etc. Maybe you just seem different. If they do notice, you can ask them to honour your privacy until you are ready to share your news.

Be aware that sharing the news can be quite a social minefield to negotiate. One thing to consider is whether those you tell would be supportive if you were to have an early pregnancy loss. Would your privacy be acknowledged? Are you ready for all the questions about due dates, stopping work, returning to work, staying home, going part-time, your childcare plans, your birthing arrangements?

Are you ready for: "What type of birth do you want?" and "Who is your obstetrician?" (This needs to become: "Who is your midwife?") Do you know how you will answer: "How much will your partner be involved?" and "Are you going to find out the sex?" Or do you need time?

The choice to share the news of your pregnancy and when you do so is entirely yours. Sometimes holding that secret within until you're ready to share it feels deeply spiritual and private, no matter how pregnancy is affecting you. Even when feeling wretched, that connection to the change you feel in every cell of your body, mind and identity is profound.

On top of that, when you haven't had time to catch your breath or even really consider those questions, suddenly everyone feels they have the right to tell you their personal pregnancy, birthing and mum horror stories. Privacy ... poof!

At the same time, if you are suffering significantly while your hormones are at work, then speaking up, reaching out, accepting support with grace and without a sense of failure is how we change the narrative. If this is you, could your days of suffering in silence (and those of future pregnant women) be rewritten?

Your social circle is going to widen with entirely new people, especially when you meet your care providers. The relationships formed are vital; there must be a reciprocal attitude of respect and trust between you and them. Doulas, midwives, obstetricians, or a combination of all of them, need to work for you, whatever your circumstances are. The relationship should respect your agency, intelligence and choices. Hopefully, there will be a genuine wish to guide, support and provide information in a non-biased manner to support your choices throughout your experiences in pregnancy, childbirth and beyond. These people will become part of your new village.

Talking about widening your social circle and creating connections for your village, you might start to find your people in other pregnant women. Connections made now can last a lifetime, as you become authentic support for each other. Joining a pregnancy yoga class, swimming or going to another exercise group to meet people extends your village while nourishing your body. It's too early to chat about antenatal education classes in the early pregnancy stage, but not too early to begin to connect with others. Which of your friends and family members say, "Just call and I'll help where I can"? Which ones actually follow through with no judgement or expectation of return? These are the people who you call with the truth of how you are feeling. You can ask them for help in these early weeks.

- **Mamatribe website.** A COPE initiative to support new mothers
  https://www.mamatribe.com.au/jointhetribe/

The cost of childbirth and maternity care access

The economics of pregnancy, birth and becoming a mother are important to consider. The Australian Broadcasting Corporation (ABC) article 'The cost of childbirth and hidden bills to prepare for', found that public care is free in Australia if you have a Medicare card. However, you can expect to pay approximately $0–$1,500 out-of-pocket costs depending on how many tests and scans you have. If you have private health insurance, you are generally directed to an obstetrician, where out-of-pocket costs are estimated to be $2,500–$20,000.[32] Once you earn above a certain income threshold, you are encouraged to have private health insurance, and there are tax penalties if you don't. However, private care more often means a medicalised, time-controlled birth, with a higher chance of induction, interventions, assisted vaginal and caesarean birth.

The TMCC found that private care increases the chance of caesarean section in low-risk women. Women in private care have fewer choices. They are not offered homebirth, COC with a midwife, independent midwifery, midwifery group practice or birth centre facilities. Lack of care options and birthing place sets women on a course of greater intervention. In private care, the schedule fee that obstetricians receive for attending a birth is the same no matter the type of birth. On the other hand, while birth and intervention costs are set, antenatal appointments can vary in cost. Many obstetricians charge more than the schedule fee and this is unregulated. Medicare is also claimed when a women has private care and is currently set up as fee-for-service for both private and public care. In public health, obstetricians earn a salary, so there is no incentive to do more interventions.[33]

The belief that paying for care is best for women and their babies has become culturally embedded. In the documentary *Birthtime*, the culture of birthing in the private sector is summed up by obstetrician Dr Andrew Bisits, when he says: "You end up with these highly resourced women having all this intervention that then becomes the standard culture, because they are paying for it. Once you pay for something, it's an economic reality that other people will perceive this as being necessarily good."[34]

If choosing an obstetrician, consider asking about their induction, caesarean section, instrumental birth and episiotomy rates. You can also question their philosophy around supporting spontaneous labour and physiological birthing (birth without intervention, or as little as possible) as a way of choosing your care provider. Ask them to be transparent about how many weeks and days they suggest for induction of a healthy term pregnancy. What is their stance on external fetal heart monitoring (EFM), mobility, using complementary therapies and doula support in the birthing room?

Consider more than just the obstetrician your GP refers you to. There are a few absolute gems in private practice who are matricentric in facilitating physiological birthing and vaginal breech birthing, have a midwife working with them for continuity and truly 'stand by'. Unfortunately, they are the minority, but they are there. You can also elect to be a private patient in a public hospital, which means the public hospital receives your private health funding to supplement the public health care. However, this does not allow you a private room.

If you wish to choose independent midwifery care, do check how many appointments you receive, the range of care they provide, their back-up midwife and access to hospital if needed.

Maternal Mental Health Matters has a video called *The right maternity care for you*, which explains different models of maternity care.

- **Pregnancy Birth Baby website.** An overview of 'public versus private' care and some guidance if you have private health insurance. https://www.pregnancybirthbaby.org.au/public-vs-private-care-during-pregnancy

- *Australian Birth Stories* #399. 'Public and Private Care and Costs with Dr Natalie Elphinstone' Apple 🎙 Spotify

- **The Birth Project audio.** https://www.abc.net.au/listen/programs/healthreport/the-birth-project-an-online-tool/101700160

- **Maternal Health Matters YouTube.** https://www.youtube.com/watch?v=c4nA1Vtxdi8&t=3s

Early pregnancy is when you begin to wonder what sort of care is available to you. I put forward this information now so that you know the full spectrum and are prepared; I set out below the available choices of care. It is a postcode lottery as to what is available in your area and provision may depend on some socio-economic factors. The ABC's *The Birth Project* audio describes the postcode lottery of provision and the outcomes of those models of care from the voices of mothers and health professionals. I have made it as brief as possible because I don't want to fry your brain!

Public care choices are offered within the current model of pregnancy assessment (low-, medium- and high-risk) as categorised by the RANZCOG 'Maternity Care in Australia' guidelines mentioned earlier.

Public Care Choices

- **Community Midwifery Program** (CMP) or **Midwifery Homebirth Care** (MHC) is for 'low-risk' mothers, is provided in your home and wherever the midwife holds their clinic. There are currently 20 national publicly funded homebirth midwifery group practices attached to hospitals as part of a consortium.

- **Caseload midwifery COC** is where all care is provided by a small team of midwives who have access to a birth centre or hospital for low-risk pregnancies; however, there isn't much availability of these care options. Only 0.6% of women birthed at home in 2022.[35]

- **Midwifery group practice** (MGP) is mostly available to low-risk pregnancies, although all-risk MGP is also available, including Birthing on Country Care in some areas for Indigenous women.

  A group of midwives looks after you throughout, regardless of any risk you may have in your pregnancy; for example, if you need a caesarean section, you are still cared for by a midwife you know in hospital.

- **Birth centre care** is usually close to a hospital, and is staffed by midwives who look after you throughout at the birth centre. They have access to the hospital and collaborate with doctors if the need arises. Birth centres accounted for 1.6% of births in 2022. This needs to change.

- **Clinic Care** is attending the hospital antenatal clinic, where you are seen by a midwife or doctor, usually someone different each visit. Birthing is in the hospital with rostered midwives and overseen by doctors. Postpartum care is with a hospital-based midwife who visits you at home.

- **General practitioner obstetrician care** is antenatal care provided by a GP obstetrician. Birthing care is provided in a private or public hospital by the GP obstetrician and rostered hospital midwives. Postnatal care is provided in the hospital by the GP obstetrician and hospital midwives and may continue in the home or community.

- **Public hospital high-risk maternity care** involves antenatal care in hospital outpatient clinics (onsite or outreach) by midwives and/or doctors. Birthing and postnatal care are provided in the hospital and postnatal care continues in the home or community, and is provided by hospital midwives.

- **Regional and remote area maternity care** is the provision of antenatal and postnatal care in remote communities by a remote area midwife (or remote area nurse) or group of midwives, sometimes in collaboration with a remote area nurse and/or doctor, with telehealth or fly-in fly-out clinicians and contracted GP obstetricians. Birthing and postnatal care is provided in a regional or metropolitan hospital by hospital midwives and doctors. It may involve relocation before labour and has a big impact on all families, particularly Birthing on Country for Indigenous women.

Private Care Choices

- **Privately practising midwives** are self-employed and offer pregnancy, home birthing and postnatal care, either as a team of 2 private midwives who support each other, or as a group of midwives. They primarily care for you in your home and/or their private consulting rooms. Birthing is at home, yet independent midwives have access to a public hospital and collaborate with doctors where needed. Some independent midwives offer continuity of antenatal and postnatal care only and therefore cost less. A Medicare rebate is available for appointments, birth in hospital and birth centres but not homebirth. Some private insurances provide up to $3,000 cover, so it is worthwhile shopping around for your insurance type. A BabyCenter article on homebirth provides comprehensive information about engaging a privately practising midwife and home birthing.

  According to BabyCenter, a private midwife is approximately $3,500–$6,000 before Medicare rebates or private insurance; however, prices vary across states. If you want to discover more, get in touch with your local independent midwives. When looking at costs of private obstetric care, if you are seeking continuity and as little intervention as possible, this may be the choice for you.

- **Freestanding birth centres** are where privately practising midwives work from; women go there to birth. They are a home away from home. In 2024, there is only one in Tasmania, the Birth House.

- **Doulas** specialise in all, or a combination of, pregnancy, birthing and postnatal care, and are an incredible source of support for COC, particularly if that option isn't available to you otherwise. They are not medically trained. Look up doulas in your area to ask what their care, support packages and costs are, as they range from a single day to throughout pregnancy, birth and postnatally. There is no Medicare rebate and they are not covered by private insurance. Choice.com.au has an article 'Do you need a doula?' that describes their role and effects on birthing outcomes.

- **Shared Maternity Care** is where women want COC before and after birth that is provided by a privately practising obstetrician and midwife, but wish to birth in hospital. Birthing care is provided in a public hospital by the privately practising obstetrician or midwife, and/or hospital midwives. Postnatal care is provided in hospital and may continue in the home, and is provided by the private midwife.

- **Private obstetrician and privately practising midwife joint care.** All care is provided by a privately practising obstetrician and midwife from the same private practice. Birthing care is provided in either a private or public hospital by the privately practising obstetrician, midwife and/or hospital midwives. Postnatal care is provided in hospital and may continue in the home, where it is provided by the private midwife.

- **Private obstetrician** is where all care is provided by a private specialist obstetrician. Birthing care is provided in a private or public hospital by the private specialist obstetrician and rostered hospital midwives. Postnatal care is provided in hospital and may continue in the home or a hotel.

Freebirth is a choice some women make for one of many reasons. Here the woman chooses not to have a professionally trained person in attendance at the birth. We will talk about freebirthing with Ally in Chapter 4.

- **Wishlist** 🌾 *Great Birth Rebellion* #125. 'The Medicalisation Spectrum' Apple 🎙 Spotify Explains the choices available to women – from no professional care to complete medical overview.
- 'What is a doula and do you need a one?' Choice.com.au. https://www.choice.com.au/babies-and-kids/getting-ready-for-baby/planning-for-baby/articles/do-you-need-a-doula
- *Great Birth Rebellion* #109. 'The Birth House' Apple 🎙 Spotify

Media influences on pregnancy

From early pregnancy, the media has a massive impact on our self-image, identity and body consciousness in pregnancy and postpartum. The fallout from its huge influence isn't pretty.

COPE states: "Despite the fact that we are often inundated with images of expectant mothers with perfect baby bumps but otherwise unchanged body proportions, for most women this simply is not the reality."[36]

This is compounded by celebrity motherhood profiles showing the ease with which they are juggling work, family and mothering. They have 'bounced back' physically to their pre-pregnancy bodies in no time and look fabulous. The promotion of 'celebrity mums' in the media as a representation of motherhood *seem* to celebrate pregnancy and mothering. The truth is, this practice promotes standards of perfection that are unattainable, not based in reality and do not represent real-life mothers. These unreachable norms and values create a sense of failure and guilt for not being a 'good enough' mother.[37]

We know media imagery isn't authentic, but still feel compelled by it. Let's be real here. Most of us don't have an army of personal trainers, personal assistants, food prep chefs, stylists, makeup artists, hairdressers and childcare to make this celebrity momdom possible. In this early stage of pregnancy, there is an opportunity for you to do some social media cleansing. Here, I'm asking you to be very circumspect about what you feed your brain and soul. Media influence is phenomenally powerful and much of it is set up to make women feel like they've failed. It promotes a sense of not measuring up to social ideals of what pregnancy and mothering 'should be'. It sells an unattainable illusion, ingrained from childhood and heightened by media.

Think deeply about what aligns with your values and find a social media family – authentic networks that make you feel good, are grounded in reality and nourish you. This social media family should champion your pregnancy and prepare you for mothering in positive, respectful and supportive ways. They should celebrate you just as you are, lend support, and include positive imagery and helpful attitudes where your own life experiences are celebrated as you become a mother. Self-worth and compassion – breathe those in deeply.

This could be a catalyst for change, where we choose not to believe unattainable ideals that set woman against woman. Instead of constant 'comparisonitis' and feelings of coming up short, let's choose to be kind, accepting and non-judgemental towards ourselves and others. It's tough enough out there, but we can champion each other and choose not to subscribe to false media bullshit anymore. It has caused devastating harm.

- *Seasons of Matrescence* S2 #12. 'Body Image for Mums with Dr Zali Yager' Apple 🎙 Spotify
- **Tell me a good birth story website.** Facebook page. http://tellmeagoodbirthstory.com/
- *Australian Birth Stories* podcast. Apple 🎙 Spotify
  A resource to tap into and learn from the experiences of other women.

Self-identity, Beliefs and Values, and Spiritual Influences on Early Pregnancy

You are in a liminal state of in-between, evolving, adapting, learning and transitioning across so many differing aspects of life. Who are you now? How do you fit being pregnant into that? You are not who you once were, but not yet a mother. Mother becoming …

Recreating your identity with core values

It's important to reflect on questions around your shifting identity. Now that you understand the effect hormones have on you emotionally, physically and psychologically, how do you express emotions? How do you process changes in diet, heightened bodily awareness, thought patterns and the drive to learn more about pregnancy? What economic implications are there for you? Who do you want involved in your care? What will you do with your awareness of how herstory, culture and media affect how we see ourselves, our expectations and knowledge? How are you feeling in relation to social activities and interaction changes?

How do you see *yourself* now?

How are you seen and treated by others?

And what is your philosophy around birth and mothering? What have you been exposed to so far? What do you know about birth and mothering at this point in your life?

There is a lot to take in right now. One way of navigating these questions is to begin with what you value in your life. Self-identity affects the way we think, act and interact with loved ones and the outer world. Let's go through a process of determining your values so you can answer all that for yourself, gradually building your self-knowledge with each chapter as your identity continues to change.

Start by naming 4 things that really matter to you, that are integral to the way you live or wish to live. How have these changed now that you are in early pregnancy? How will they help guide you?

Now we'll look at finding 4 core values to help you navigate your pregnancy, birthing and mothering journey. Your core values will form a foundation to guide your decision-making, thought processes and choices. They provide a way to ground yourself when feeling confused, frustrated or overwhelmed.

You choose how to see and value yourself within the social, economic and cultural world you live in. You choose what you value and how you interpret those values as you wish them to manifest in your life. Below, I offer a list of examples that you can choose as your core values, but this is by no means exhaustive. You might want to look further. There are plenty more online. If it's hard to choose, start with more than 8 and then reduce it down.

Adventure	Environment	Honesty	Partnership
Ambition	Equality	Intuition	Patience Recognition
Balance	Family	Integrity	Reliability
Belonging	Financial	Kindness	Respect
Communication	Freedom	Knowledge	Safety
Compassion	Friendship	Leadership	Spirituality
Competence	Fun	Loyalty	Stability
Confidence	Generosity	Love	Structure
Contribution	Grace	Making a difference	Understanding
Courage	Gratitude	Nurture	Uniqueness
Creativity	Growth	Optimism	Vulnerability
Curiosity	Health	Peace	

How can you apply these values to how you see yourself and how you wish to be treated by care providers?

Say you chose 'reliability'. Within yourself, reliability is an important value; you see yourself as steadfast, trustworthy and consistent, and are valued by family, friends and work for those qualities. Can you now reflect this value towards yourself? See the ways that you are steadfast and how you can show up for yourself with kindness, consistent self-love and compassion towards your emotions, your changing body and your physical symptoms in pregnancy. Perhaps you can become your own best friend.

Might you then reflect that value onto the type of care you want? Reliable, trustworthy, consistent, steadfast. Might you seek others who hold this same value to be part of your village?

Spirituality in pregnancy

Spirituality can be an integral part of our lives; it is celebrated in the rituals and ceremonies we gather together to witness at big events like weddings, birthdays, funerals, religious festivals and holidays. Private spirituality expressed in prayer, chanting, meditation and personal rituals is deeply important. Wouldn't it be great if we celebrated menarche,[1] pregnancy and the new mother in such ways too?

There is a spiritual and philosophical practice within yoga called *ahimsa*. Its literal translation is 'non-violence' or 'non-harming'. This is not just about physical and psychological harm as we understand violence today. It extends to the relationship we have with ourselves.

How do we treat ourselves? Do we talk to ourselves as we would a dear friend or a loved one? Do we measure ourselves against others and always fall short? How do we look after ourselves physically? Are we taking time to nourish our bodies with good food, go for walks in nature, chat with friends, do a slow exercise class or just read, play music, dance, listen to a podcast with a cup of tea or have a nap? Do we feel guilty for taking this time for ourselves? Are we busy doing rather than being? Looking after everything and everyone else, a busy, buzzing mind and body?

Take this concept and feeling of ahimsa as you read this book. You will need it at times.

Embodying the practice of ahimsa is realising that you are worthy of treating yourself gently, kindly and without guilt, particularly during your first trimester. Ahimsa is the opposite of harm in every

---

1   Menarche: The first menstrual period marking the onset of puberty.

aspect of life. Talk to yourself in a respectful, loving way. Tell yourself, "I am enough just as I am." Know you are worth nourishing and really believe it! Only you can change your mindset so that it restores you mentally, emotionally and physically. You deserve nourishment.

Throughout the rest of this book, I invite you to rediscover your natural ability to connect with your body, mind and spirit. To acknowledge and respect the power it has to create, grow, birth and nourish life as you journey through these pages. How beautiful and incredible you are in your capacity to do so and reattune to yourself, your inner knowing about your own body and thought processes. From that foundation, you may find a 'pull of purpose' rather than the 'pressure of push'. Begin to cultivate this promise of ahimsa deeply within yourself.

Spirituality in pregnancy loss

Here, I honour Liesja, the other mothers in this book and all women who have experienced early pregnancy loss. May they claim a space of respect and dignity in honouring the loss of dreams, perceived futures, and feelings of grief, rage, confusion, hollowness and soul-deep sadness.

Let's start by changing the term 'miscarriage' to that of 'early pregnancy loss', because the former implies you *missed* the carrying of your baby, or that it was your fault, or something is wrong with you. No more.

We need to honour pregnancy loss in its many guises, including medically induced pregnancy loss, for whatever reason, because the grief and suffering is real. Judgement has no place here. We must be honest that the physical sensations of cramping contractions in early pregnancy loss can hurt. Really, really hurt.

So many women suffer alone on their toilet, in unexpected pain and with no one to hold them through it. They may need to carry on at work, collect and care for other children, all while losing their pregnancy.

It's not just the physical sensation but the emotional sensations of grieving the loss. The place and time will always be remembered. Whether medically induced, naturally occurring, at home, in hospital for removal of retained products of pregnancy, or termination of pregnancy for any reason, those experiences are lived and remain. The silence around this suffering needs to be cracked open.

Let us hold them, being present, offering comfort through gentle words and touch. We'll provide the cups of tea and tissues, while holding the fort of home, children, life.

If this is you, ask for support from family or friends. Talk, cry, get help with children, shopping, meals. Have someone with you. Acknowledgment of your loss is vital. Draw on your faith and beliefs, whatever they may be. As an offering of ideas, you might form a personal ritual to honour your unique experience. Go to a place you love and usually feel at peace. Maybe that's a park, river or the sea. Find a poem that sings to your soul, write your own words or even make art. Perform a ritual symbol of release, like blowing bubbles, or scattering flowers, petals or native flower seeds. Place a letter to your unrealised child in the flames of a fire, sending the words upwards, outwards into the universe, to be forever held there. Plant something you love in your garden or on your balcony. Journal. Create a space in your home for candles, flowers, a simple statue, your written words. This may offer you some comfort.

There is a phenomenon called *micro-chimerism,* in which fetal cells pass through the placenta into the mother's body and remain. This means cells of the fetus you were carrying passed into you. You still hold them within. They are still with you.[38] This may be a confronting realisation and bring a myriad of emotions. Please reach out for support and nourish yourself if this is you.

Change and respect for pregnancy loss is happening, even if it is slow. Having birthed with no dignity in an emergency department in 2018, Karen Schlage gave evidence to a maternity inquiry about the loss of her 16-week son. She spoke of the devastation women experience in such loss when they are treated without kindness, respect or dignity. Canberra now has a 3-bed unit to care for women who experience pregnancy loss at any gestation.[39]

In 2021 the Australian Senate passed a bill to include 2 days' paid miscarriage leave in the Fair Work Act. "It comes after five years of campaigning by The Pink Elephants, a support network dedicated to miscarriage and pregnancy loss, to amplify the voices of those who have lost a child and ensure employers provide dedicated leave and assistance."[40]

The following podcasts are offered with a gentle notice, because listening in may trigger deep feelings; however, it may help you find some clarity and peace. The information provided as a means of support is authentic. You are not alone.

- *Seasons of Matrescence* S2#6. 'Misunderstandings of Miscarriage with Tahyna MacManus' discusses the topic with openhearted clarity, compassion, evidence and comfort. Apple 🎙 Spotify

- *The Shebirths Show* S2 #2. with Sam Payne from Pink Elephants, 'Making sense of losing the most important thing in the world' Apple 🎙 Spotify

- The Pink Elephants website.
  contact@pinkelephantssupport.com https://www.pinkelephants.org.au/

- Bears of Hope website. 1300 11 BEAR https://www.bearsofhope.org.au/

- Stillbirth and Neonatal Death Society (SANDS) 1300 308 307 https://www.sands.org.au/

- Red Nose 'Hospital to Home' and 'Guiding Light Peer Support' Phone: 1300 308 307 available 24 hours a day, 7 days a week, for early pregnancy loss for any reason.
  Online support is via intake@rednose.org.au and rednosegriefandloss.org.au/live-chat

- 'I need help' tick list PDF from PANDAS. If you are struggling with anxiety or depression during pregnancy or after pregnancy loss, use this to take to your GP or independent midwife.[41]
  https://pandasfoundation.org.uk/wp-content/uploads/2024/02/I-need-help-womenbirthing-people.pdf

---

Sending love to you, holding you in a long, enveloping hug, reminding you of self-compassion and tenderness in this **time of remembrance.**

Practice offering: *Metta Bhavana* meditation

Metta Bhavana is a Buddhist practice of compassion and universal loving kindness to yourself, to those in your world and towards all beings. It's a beautiful way to begin cultivating kindness and compassionate connection to yourself in body, spirit and mind. Here is a 4-part process of practising loving kindness for your pregnancy. The mindfulness we practised earlier will help here; in turn, this practice will increase your mindfulness.

- Beginning with you, practise your 3-part breath, becoming aware of all around you, harnessing your senses, softening and releasing your body. Say softly to yourself as you exhale, *May I be well and happy*, with a feeling of gentleness, kindness, patience and compassion towards yourself.

- Then with a hand to your heart and one on your lower belly, send loving kindness, nourishment and compassion to the growing life within you. See growing life in your mind. Say softly to yourself as you exhale, *May you be well and happy.*

- Mentally strengthening your sense of belonging, send love and compassion to your growing village. Picture this group of people. Say softly to yourself as you exhale, *May they be well and happy.*

- Extend your loving kindness and compassion outwards to all beings, picturing our revolving world, all continents and colours. (We might feel we are infinitely small in this practice of sending out to the world, but always remember, you matter infinitely.) Say softly to yourself as you exhale, *May we all be well and happy.*

- *May I be well and happy.*

- *May you be well and happy.*

- *May they be well and happy.*

- *May we all be well and happy.*

- Repeat this as many times as you wish. Picture what that looks like for you. Aloud, whispered, silent, there is no one way. Make this practice yours. Whatever works for nourishing you.

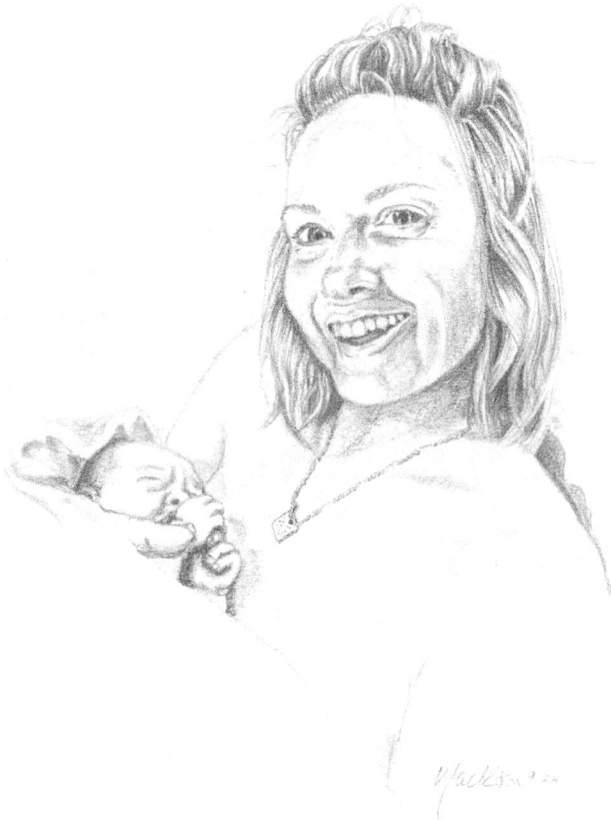

Look at Liesja. So triumphant after birthing Lachy. After all she went through to conceive, grow and bring him into the world, her joyous and powerful expression says it all. Now she is done.

Mother Becoming Insights and Actions in Early Pregnancy

The intention of this part in each chapter is to help you reflect on what you have read and learned, to explore what struck you deeply, how it made you feel and where you might wish to go with it. You may have felt confused, overwhelmed, enlightened, frustrated or angry. You are not alone.

Please sit with those reactions, feelings and emotions. Allow them to exist because they are yours to validate and feel. Please also try not to stay in them too long, because that isn't healthy. You can picture yourself on a long trek. We started with our boots and backpack. There are resting places along the way. Rest in sadness, anger or enlightenment, but don't stay there.

If you wish, you can journal, scribble notes on these pages or mull over your emotions for a while and see what lands as significant to you. Talk to your partner and friends. Meditate, go walk in the bush, whatever fills your cup. Reflect on the resources suggested throughout the chapter, then get your boots back on, shoulder your pack and move forward. There is no time limit to your journey.

How might it be for you ...

- If the process of mother becoming, matrescence, were known, understood, respected and supported in our westernised culture?

- If we relieved fear around pregnancy and birthing through this understanding?

- If feminism concentrated on conception, pregnancy, the birth room and early mothering too?

- If you were no longer self-silent and asked for support during your early months, particularly if you felt unwell or deeply fatigued?

- If you began your village in the early months?

- If you chose you first, realising you are enough just as you are, and worth nourishing?

- If rest were not seen as a weakness, but necessary, normal and embraced?

- If you took the time to practise the offerings to build resilience in mind and body throughout your pregnancy?

- If you knew your last menstrual period date and rethought the need for an early dating scan?

- If you remembered an EDD is just that, an estimate, with days either side, not a sudden cut-off?

- If we kept in mind that term is 37–42 weeks?

- If you offered a birthing month instead of a due date, taking the pressure off?

- If you felt confident to decline a quick look at your baby at each appointment where a scanner is available?

- If you didn't feel pressured by advertising to have a 3D or 4D USS, knowing the effects of sound and heat on your unborn child?

- If you could see a midwife instead of a GP when first finding out you were pregnant, normalising care from a physiological perspective rather than a medical pathological, risk-based approach?

- If you had midwifery COC throughout, referring to an obstetrician if needed?

- If COC with a midwife were the dominant model of care rather than obstetric?

- If you had more choices of places to birth and there were more facilitation of home birthing and many more birthing units?

- If there were more freestanding birth centres – a birth house "home away from home", where privately practising midwives offered their services.

- If Medicare provided rebates for homebirth with a privately practising midwife?

- If a midwife were also fully involved in private obstetric practice, filling your care with familiarity and closing that spiritual gap?

- If you chose to remove yourself from toxic media and surrounded yourself with those who champion you just as you are?

- If you were supported and respected with authenticity and integrity?

- If you chose to change your inner voice from vicious to deep value of yourself?

- If you saw yourself differently, worthy of being listened to, respected – enough just as you are?

- If there were a place of dignity and respect for women to go, other than the emergency department or labour ward, when losing their pregnancy at any gestation?

- If the term 'miscarriage' became 'early pregnancy loss' and we implemented the recommendation to ensure dedicated spaces were available for parents experiencing pregnancy loss or stillbirth in all healthcare settings?

Early Pregnancy References and Wishlist

1   D Crawley Jack, *Silencing the Self: Women and Depression*, Harvard University Press; 1991. ISBN 9780674808157

2   R Reed, Childbirth Physiology Course. https://www.rachelreed.website/childbirth-physiology-course

3   V Olorenshaw, *Liberating Motherhood: birthing the Purple Stocking Movement*, Womancraft Publishing; 2016, p62. ISBN 978-910559-192

4   S Napthali, *Buddhism for Mothers. A calm approach to caring for yourself and your children*, Allen and Unwin; 2003, p114. ISBN 9781742377018

5   R Van De Weyer, 366 *Readings from Buddhism*, The Global Spirit Library. Loving Yourself. 3/26 Udana 5.1 The Pilgrim Press, 2001. ISBN0829813853

6   Healthline. Amygdala Hijack. https://www.healthline.com/health/stress/amygdala-hijack#prevention

7   A A.Taren, PJ Gianonaros, CM Greco, E K Lindsay, A Fairgrieve, K Warren Brown, RK Rosen, L Ferris, E Julson, A L Marsland, JK Bursley, J Ramsburg, J D Cresswell, 'Mindfulness meditation training alters stress-related amygdala resting state functional connectivity: a randomised controlled trial'. Social Cognitive and Affective Neuroscience, 2015, 1758-1768 https://doi.org/10.1093/scan/nsv066

8   KM, Matsuzaki M, Shiraishi M, Haruna M, 'Immediate stress reduction effects of yoga during pregnancy: One group pre-post-test'. Women Birth. 2016 Oct;29(5):e82-e88. Epub 2016 Apr 17. PMID: 27094980. 10.1016/j.wombi.2016.04.003

9   M Harris, *Men, Love and Birth*, Pinter and Martin, 2015, p20. ISBN 9781870662251

10 R Reed, *Reclaiming Childbirth as a Rite of Passage: Weaving ancient wisdom with modern knowledge*, Word Witch, 2021, p24. ISBN 978-0-6450025-1-5

11 GW Lawson, 'Naegele's rule and the length of pregnancy - A review', Aust N Z J Obstet Gynaecol. 2021 Apr;61(2):177-182. doi: 10.1111/ajo.1325 Epub 2020 Oct 20. PMID: 33079400. p177. https://pubmed.ncbi.nlm.nih.gov/33079400/

12 R Reed, *Why Induction Matters*, Pinter and Martin, 2018. ISBN 9781780666006

13 S Wickham, *In Your Own Time: How western medicine controls the start of labour and why this needs to stop*, Birthmoon Creations, 2021. ISBN 9781914465024

14   C de Costa, *Hail Caesar. Why one in three Australian babies is born by caesarean section*, Boolarong Press, 2008. ISBN 97819210528012.

15   S Buckley, *Gentle Birth, Gentle Mothering: A Doctors Guide to Natural Childbirth and Gentle Early Parenting Choices*, Celestial Arts, 2009, p78-94. ISBN 9781587613227

16   Buckley, *Gentle Birth, Gentle Mothering*, p83.

17   Buckley, *Gentle Birth, Gentle Mothering*, p81.

18   Buckley, *Gentle Birth, Gentle Mothering*, p82.

19   New South Wales Parliament Legislative Council Select Committee on Birth Trauma, Report. 2024. p xix ISBN: 978-1-922960-38-2ii. https://www.parliament.nsw.gov.au/lcdocs/inquiries/2965/FINAL%20 Birth%20Trauma%20Report%20-%2029%20April%202024.PDF

20   Buckley, *Gentle Birth, Gentle Mothering*, p81.

21   Buckley, *Gentle Birth, Gentle Mothering*, p79.

22   *Birthtime The Documentary* and *Birthtime The Handbook*, 2021. Clark and Mackay; p101. https://www. birthtime.world/

23   C de Costa, *Hail Caesar. Why one in three Australian babies is born by caesarean section*, p23.

24   C de Costa, *Hail Caesar. Why one in three Australian babies is born by caesarean section*, p51.

25   *Birthtime The Handbook*, p39.

26   M McMahon. *Why Mothering Matters*. Pinter and Martin, 2018, p35. ISBN 9781780665900

27   Transforming Maternity Care Collaborative https://www.transformingmaternity.org.au/2021/09/what-if-all-low-risk-women-planned-to-birth-in-a-birth-centre-or-at-home/

28   ICM. Bill of Rights for Women and Midwives (ICM) 2024. https://internationalmidwives.org/resources/ bill-of-rights-for-women-and-midwives/

29   Reed, *Reclaiming Childbirth as a Rite of Passage*, p24.

30   The Royal College of Australia and New Zealand (RANZCOG). https://ranzcog.edu.au/wp-content/ uploads/2022/01/Maternity-Care-in-Australia-Web.PDF

31   *Birthtime The Handbook*, p39.

32   Article. 'ABC Cost of Childbirth'. https://www.abc.net.au/everyday/the-cost-of-childbirth-and-the-hid-den-bills-to-prepare-for/10350778

33   TMCC. 'Private Obstetric Care Increases Risk of Unplanned Caesarean for Low-Risk Women'. https:// www.transformingmaternity.org.au/2022/03/private-obstetric-care-increases-risk-of-unplanned-caesare-an-for-low-risk-women/

34   *Birthtime The Handbook*, p40.

35   Australian Institute of Health and Welfare. Australia's Mother and Babies 13.12.2024 https://www.aihw. gov.au/reports/mothers-babies/australias-mothers-babies/contents/labour-and-birth/place-of-birth

36   COPE. 'Body Image in Pregnancy'. https://www.cope.org.au/expecting-a-baby/staying-well/body-im-age-in-pregnancy/

37   L O'Brien Hallstein, AO'Reilly, M Vandenbeld Giles, Editors, *The Routledge Companion to Motherhood*. 'Mediated Celebrity Motherhood'. LO'Brien Hallstein, Routledge Press, 2020 Chapter 10, p133-146

38   R Martone. 'Cells living in mothers' brains: the connection between mother and child is even deeper than thought'. Scientific American website, 4 December 2012, https://www.scientificamerican.com/article/sci-entists-discover-childrens-cells-living-in-mothers-brain/

39   ABC Article. 'Mother's devastating experience of maternity care sees Canberra open dedicated early pregnancy loss unit'. https://www.abc.net.au/news/2023-03-24/canberra-early-pregnan-cy-loss-unit-opens/102134498

40   Australian Senate Bill. Miscarriage leave. https://www.austpayroll.com.au/senate-passes-bill-to-include-miscarriage-leave-in-australias-fair-work-act/

41   I Need Help. PANDA Perinatal Mental Health toolkit to Take to Your GP. https://pandasfoundation.org.uk/wp-content/uploads/2024/02/I-need-help-womenbirthing-people.PDF

�🌬 Wishlist

1. Ready to Cope app, You Tube video. https://www.youtube.com/watch?v=_XtjZL8CVcA
2. *Great Birth Rebellion* #3 'Due Dates' Apple 🎙 Spotify
3. Dr Sarah Buckley's website article 'Ultrasound scans a cause for concern'. https://sarahbuckley.com/ultrasound-scans-cause-for-concern/
4. Antenatal Screening for Chromosomal Conditions-It's Your choice. https://yourchoice.mcri.edu.au/dashboard
5. Maternity Choices Australia https://www.maternitychoices.org/
6. TMCC website https://www.transformingmaternity.org.au/2021/09/what-if-all-low-risk-women-planned-to-birth-in-a-birth-centre-or-at-home/
7. *Great Birth Rebellion* #125 'The Medicalisation Spectrum' Apple 🎙 Spotify

Chapter 2
The Middle Months with Samantha

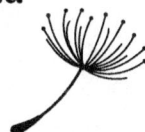

Meeting Samantha

Samantha and I met at pregnancy and postnatal yoga classes. Her absorption during class and willingness to take it all into birthing and mothering was lovely to witness. Her calm and gentle nature, with a deep need for soul-searching, came through.

Samantha is a registered nurse, but felt her energy would be better directed towards something else. She was not sure what at that time. Her journey of mothering her children and 3 stepsons, her struggle with motherhood, change in identity and feelings, all while experiencing life-altering health issues, is inspiring. Coming to understand matrescence had a profound effect on Samantha's life.

During the time of this book's evolution, Samantha has evolved too. While still nursing, she has found energy, passion and purpose for supporting other women and mothers. She is now a postnatal doula, aromatherapist, matrescence mentor and gentle, yet fierce, advocate for the wellbeing of mamas. Her role in that space is growing slowly, as the pull of responsibilities of a young family is very real. Yet she feels she is on her path.

Mama to Casey and Layla, here is Samantha's letter to you.

"Soon-to-be Mama"

Dear Mama or soon-to-be Mama,

I have put off writing this letter to you for a very long time. I wrote one version, but that was before the birth of my second child. It no longer captured my whole experience. In all honesty, no number of words or style of writing ever could sum up motherhood. In fact, my birth doula, Bonnie, once said to me, "We don't have the words in the English language to describe birth." I completely agree with this for birth and postpartum. The closest word I have come to know that fully encompasses this powerful transition is 'matrescence'.

Here, I share honestly and from the heart, but please remember this is but a small part of my journey to becoming a mama.

I believe there's a reason you are sitting here reading or hearing my story, so take what resonates and leave the rest. I also acknowledge that simply being in this space of reflecting on my journey so far, writing the words you see before you, has opened a floodgate of deep emotions. Take a moment or as many as you need to pause, breathe, stay hydrated and grounded while reading this and all the stories in this book. I will too.

I am also reaching out to my mentor, friend and yoga teacher Wendy, the phenomenal author of this book, to walk beside me as I share with you. I could write a whole book about the importance of my mama friends, those who don't judge or criticise, but love and acknowledge.

Let's start somewhat at the 'beginning' of my transition to becoming a mama. Between 5 and 9 months, carrying my son, Casey, then my daughter, Layla, was the absolute best experience. The constant nausea and bone-aching tiredness of the first trimester had passed. In its place, I experienced the heavenly pregnancy and placental hormones. I could feel and see bubba moving and just felt that glow that we often (but not always) see in pregnant women.

I felt this was a 'safe' stage for me, as I had experienced numerous early miscarriages before, between and after both of my full-term pregnancies. Through my experience as a theatre nurse, I had also seen traumatic births firsthand. It's not that I was afraid of birth. There were just heaps of unknowns, things out of my control, which unnerved me a little.

My second and third trimesters felt relaxed and exciting, especially with Casey, when I was involved in antenatal yoga with my beautiful Wendy and another mama who shares her story in this book. I was in anticipation, preparing the nursery, choosing things for him and connecting with my stepsons about our journey.

Shortly before I gave birth to Casey, we had the most connected, loving seaside holiday as a family. I planned to prepare some food when I began maternity leave, but both Casey and Layla arrived earthside 'early', giving me little to no time to prepare. However, I honestly felt so beautiful – and thought life itself was beautiful – during my pregnancies. So, I didn't give much thought to my postpartum phase. I placed no importance on building a framework to support me.

My second and third trimesters left me feeling the most connected to my body I think I have ever been in my whole life. Again, I know that is not the case for every mama. But for me, the feelings of beauty, strength, miracles and connection I had about my body at this point was something I'm truly glad I anchored in as best as I could at the time. I am still working on feeling this connection to my body again, now over 6 years after giving birth for the first time.

Although I enjoyed my second trimesters in both pregnancies, they were very different. The environment was also very different with each. With my son, we were in our own home; I had time to nap, do yoga and nap again between working shifts at the hospital. With my daughter, we were living with relatives, as we were building our farm about 200 km away. This alone was extremely stressful, as I didn't have my own space to nest. My profession was no longer aligned with me during this time, but it was necessary to keep the bills paid and my maternity leave covered. The work, especially being called in overnight, was debilitating.

At almost 3, Casey was (finally) sleeping through most nights, but with early pregnancy I was up and down during the night with nausea and my bladder. I was so exhausted I asked my GP to repeat my blood tests as I thought I was seriously iron deficient! These factors, along with what I'd learned since birthing Casey, led me to push (against my husband's wishes) for a birth doula with Layla.

I connected immediately with Bonnie and felt this reassurance as I entered the final weeks and days pre-birth. My intuition was spot on. Casey came earthside in 4 hours, while Layla took her mama to the extremes of exhaustion through 27 hours of posterior contractions and presentation! Bonnie was an essential part of my birth support, keeping me fed, hydrated, and helping me rest and move positions often. It is my firm belief that her support was fundamental in allowing me to give birth vaginally with only minimal medical intervention.

My body was different between Casey and Layla too. With Casey, I felt fit and slim, with a forward, round bump. With Layla, I felt huge, like I had widened at my hips, and my face and arms felt fuller. Perhaps that's why I 'knew' I was having a girl, while I didn't have an inkling with my son.

I felt more confident in my second and third trimesters with Layla as well. However, I am still dealing with the disappointment that I didn't know as much then as I know now. What I did know was that I wanted to co-sleep with Layla, wanted the support of a birth doula, wanted to include more natural remedies like essential oils, wanted to have a photoshoot as I knew the time was passing so quickly and wanted a mama blessing rather than a baby shower.

I knew how much I was rebirthed with Casey; this was not just about the little human coming earthside, but about recognising my journey as well. I was fortunate enough that all of those particular wants turned into reality in that second pregnancy.

There's honestly so much more I could share even within the experiences of my second trimesters, but I will instead highlight one of the biggest things that has impacted my journey. (There are a few big things!)

Motherhood has been innately woven in duality for me, in all of my experiences, from the moment I knew I was pregnant with my first angel baby and even before that in my step-mama journey. Duality for me means feeling and experiencing seemingly opposite things at the same time or in comparison. My first pregnancy with Casey was in our own home, with me following as much of my body's cues as I could. But with my daughter, I felt like I was walking on eggshells, with no privacy or space to relax. Both births were so different, but each was incredibly transformative – portals where I found the deepest depths of resilience, strength and, in many ways, going with the flow.

I had minor medical intervention – I believe unnecessarily – with both of my hospital births. I wish I had the opportunity to birth at home on our farm, but still feel I had empowered births. I was more confident in my second (completed) pregnancy, but also more fearful of how hard postpartum was for me the first time. I was torn between knowing what my baby, body, mind and soul wanted for nourishment (rest, nutrition, birth and postpartum doula etc.) and then needing to do what was required to pay the bills (work) and build our home. Recognising the fear, guilt and worry I had in all the unknowns, I found the deepest layers of myself that provided all the 'knowns' I needed. I still feel lost, lonely and like I am drowning some days, but I also connect to the richest love, compassion and confidence I have ever felt.

This is the duality I walk with every day.

I also want to briefly touch on my postpartum seasons, although I believe every mama is forever postpartum, hardly the '6 weeks' as it is so often called. In the days, weeks, months and years following the birth of Casey and later Layla, I felt like I'd been slammed into a brick wall. The hardest was following the birth of Casey. My bright, beautiful firstborn bore the brunt of a mama not coping in a system that was never designed to support her. From an otherwise smooth and glowing pregnancy and empowering birth, having been raised around little children with lots of aunties and cousins, having practised as a registered nurse for more than 8 years and being in touch with my strong maternal instinct, the thought that postpartum would be an onslaught never even crossed my mind. Let alone planning for support, nourishment, rest or recovery.

I fell into a space where I had no diagnosed mental health condition. I distinctly remember my GP saying, "You just need some sleep." Yet I didn't, on the other end of the spectrum, feel supported, nourished or understood.

So many mamas fall into this space, where there is little to no true understanding of what happens following birth. I fell deeper and deeper into a kind of survival trauma that I am still healing from. I had broken sleep of maybe 4 hours a night, screamed out in pain every time Casey latched onto my breast, and was trying to be the 'good' mama and wife, still holding on to most of the housework and home organisation duties. I had no supports close by. And did I mention little to no sleep? This all made me a shell of a human being.

What I now know as postpartum rage hit me in the wee hours one morning as I was trying my best to settle Casey. The hot, wet tears, the uncontrolled shaking, the horrific words of my inner voice labelling me and the silent screaming only lasted a few minutes, but the (unnecessary) guilt lasted so much longer. I was so worried that expressing what I was feeling to any health professional would mean Casey could be taken from me, or I would be forced to undergo treatments I didn't want. I had a myriad of fears.

These episodes of rage were not frequent, thank goodness, but they rocked me to my core.

My feelings of inadequacy and craziness have taken years to dismantle. I have mourned the connection, time and intimacy with my husband. I have grieved for the freedom to sleep, eat or do anything when I wanted. I resented those mamas in the mothers group who had babies that slept. Honestly, I even struggled to enjoy postpartum yoga. Wendy held such beautiful space for us mamas postpartum, but just not having any personal space, alone time or peace (while practising yoga or doing anything at this stage) led me to feelings of guilt.

I knew what a miracle it was to have a happy and healthy baby, so why couldn't I just be happy?

With loving hindsight, I can see now how stripped bare I was. I suffered major postpartum depletion, yet at the time I had no idea such a thing existed. For me, it looked like this ...

Physically: I was almost malnourished and dehydrated constantly. Mentally: I was a wreck; sleep deprivation alone can do that, never mind the massive hormonal and psychosocial shifts that occur as I transitioned to being a mama in our community. (I know now that the changes in a mama's brain are so significant that they can be seen in medical imaging; I just thought my brain power had evaporated.) Emotionally: I was on a rollercoaster, riding a seemingly never-ending train of high highs and deep lows, sometimes at the same time! Spiritually: I questioned everything I once held to be true; my priorities, beliefs and values all shifted at warp speed. It was an achingly heartbreaking time for me. As much as I loved (and love) babies, I found it difficult to absorb much happiness with my own. I am still working through how much guilt and regret I have from my early postpartum days, and how my little man has held me as much as I have held him.

When Casey was around 6 months old, divine timing would have it that I was introduced to a coach, mentor and mama whose work and community I am still part of today. I made the decision that I needed to find another way. Motherhood was not meant to feel this tortured every day.

Together with Wendy's gentle encouragement and mention of the word 'matrescence' more than once (which I famously dismissed the first time I heard her say it), I slowly began rising into the richest tapestry of a woman I have ever known myself to be.

I am still deep in this journey and more determined than ever to live a life where my peace and joy is the first priority, leading by example for Casey and Layla, now and into the future, showing them there is another way.

Matrescence for me has been the hardest thing I have ever experienced and keep experiencing. Yet it is the most profound catalyst for my personal growth, emotional transformation and finding the joy in the everyday moments with my children. I have lost and found more of myself than would ever have been possible for me without becoming a mama. I have found my passion and soul's purpose to nurture and support mamas in ways that I couldn't or didn't even realise I needed or deserved.

This is the single biggest journey I have ever undertaken, and coming to a place where I can now openly and with courage share my challenges, struggles, beauty, lessons and joy in mamahood is a wonderful place to be. Connecting to my maternal wisdom and strength, while linking arms with likeminded mamas, is truly a blessing and has helped me curate peace and joy within the seemingly never-ending turbulent chaos in mamahood.

I truly hope parts of my story have resonated, reassured and perhaps opened your eyes to the essence of matrescence and especially postpartum. I hope you find the safety, courage, love and support that every mama deserves.

Lots of love, Mama,

Samantha

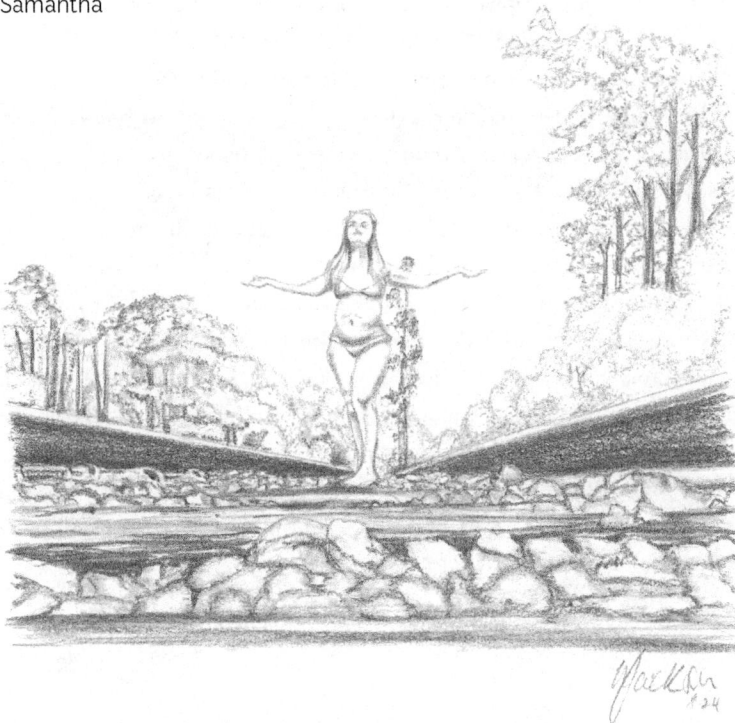

The joy in expansion held in the image of Samantha on a derelict railway line says it all. Glorying in her body and capturing the essence of that time forever.

Dear Mother Becoming,

Got your cup of tea? Warm your hands and feel the heat permeating through your palms. Take a pause and tune into your breath. Take a few long breaths. Inhale for a count of 5. Exhale for a count of 6.

That was raw and insightful reading, wasn't it? That's the reality of what mothering can be. Samantha's words need to be held close right now: "I have lost and found more of myself than would ever have been possible for me without becoming a mama." This transition to mothering, no matter how many times experienced, needs to be fully supported. In this chapter, the middle months, we will discover more deeply what 'mother becoming' means. The impact of early consideration of a well-prepared fourth trimester, (the first 3 months after birth) can't be emphasised enough. Fourth trimester planning needs to begin here.

Welcome to the middle months of your pregnancy, which Samantha enjoyed. Well, mostly! This time is not quite the limbo period of early pregnancy with its invisibility, because your body is physically expanding. You are now no longer one individual, but 2 lives, nourished and growing together. Your pregnancy gradually becomes visible, completely out of your control, and that's okay. You are becoming more every day.

We continue to learn about the intertwining influences that affect this stage of your pregnancy and life through the tree of matrescence. We shall hold this information with gentleness as we explore more of the tree roots of knowledge, and you will find your unique strengths to build resilience. Through meditation and yoga practice you will get in touch with your pelvic floor, build on breathwork, physical strength, and become aware of the capacity of your body. The invisible umbilical cord becomes firmly established.

In continuing our herstory and cultural journey with Samantha, we go deep, but please don't throw the book at the wall just yet! It will explain why we have the choices we do and do not have in our maternity care and why it is top-heavy with medical obstetric practice.

We will discuss informed choice and consent to help you find your voice, because this impacts your experiences in pregnancy and birthing. Understanding the power you have over your body and not self-silencing enables you to make assured decisions for yourself and your unborn baby. Care providers need to acknowledge and respect your decisions and consent. The resources and tools provided will assist you with decision-making; your empowered choice is matricentric feminism in action.

When your voice is heard and respected, it builds your confidence to question where research comes from, when statistics and risks are presented to you. You will be able to decide if routine screening tests are right for you. For example, we will look into the use of universal screening for gestational diabetes.

With Samantha, we will look into the nasty practice of mum-shaming, where the mythical, cultural ideal of 'the good mother' strips women of confidence and makes them judgemental of each other. We will discuss how to avoid this. We also dive into the financial effects of becoming a mother, with informative and supportive resources for you to explore. You will continue to build your village, preparing you for your fourth trimester. Here, in the middle months, we look at building your village through preparing for a beautiful ceremony called a *mother blessing*.

The Physical, Hormonal and Emotional Influences on the Middle Months

More hormonal musicians and their middle months melodies[1,2]

Relaxin plays notes to soften smooth muscle throughout your body, making your ligaments much looser, more pliable and easier to lengthen. This makes joints more mobile, particularly in the pelvis. It also lengthens your cervix and helps to prevent contractions in early pregnancy. Relaxin is produced by the corpus luteum in the luteal phase (after ovulation), then the decidua (part of the lining of the uterus), then the placenta.

Relaxin is 10 times louder than your non-pregnant levels in the middle months, which explains why you feel aches and pains in pregnancy. Relaxin is involved in how and why the 4 bones of your pelvis move to help your baby negotiate their way in birthing. This musician works in harmony with **progesterone**, playing your arteries to soften them. The effect of reducing blood pressure to cope with your increased blood volume in pregnancy is responsible for that lightheaded feeling and the occasional varicose vein.

Prolactin, the hormone in breast development and lactation, harmonises with **oxytocin** and **oestrogen,** stimulating a chorus of breast tissue development – particularly *alveoli*, where milk is produced. Prolactin is produced in the anterior pituitary gland in the brain. It promotes maternal behaviour, which is why it is so often called the 'mothering hormone'. This musician is introduced into the orchestra here, because you start to make breastmilk at around your fourth month. (It's okay if you don't see any; there is nothing wrong.) Fascinatingly, if you have a partner, they are in harmony with you because they also produce prolactin during your pregnancy and after birth.

Cortisol is a by-product of the hormone **adrenaline**, which is released after a fight-or-flight response. Cortisol is probably one of the least understood melodies being played around the body, because we often only hear about it as a negative by-product from stress. However, eustress (a moderate, positive form of healthy stress) is vital for our wellbeing. It controls blood sugar levels and regulates metabolism, helps reduce inflammation and assists with memory development. Produced in the adrenal glands, its effect on salt and water balance helps regulate blood pressure. Cortisol is at its noisiest in the morning to get us going, then quietens in the evening to promote sleep. (We will discuss **adrenaline** with Ashleigh in Chapter 3 in relation to slowing labour).

Talking about cortisol leads us nicely into emotional and stress-related effects that are transferred from mother to baby. The hormonal melodies of calmness, love, fear and stress filter through the placenta. As you begin to feel your baby moving, they become aware of you in these months. They can hear you and close family members, even taste the chemical notes of food through the amniotic fluid, all preparing them for what they will experience when born into your world.

If you are stressed or experience an adrenaline rush from sudden fright, please don't feel you are harming your baby. That's the opposite of what this chapter is about. All these hormonal responses happen in our lives. So, just breathe. Talk to your baby, if you like, and explain the fright, sadness or worry to them.

Remember, your experiences and environment are also preparing your unborn child for life, which isn't all sweetness and light. Your emotional and mental health during pregnancy is so important. Your emotional and physical health are intricately linked.

Exercise in pregnancy

Exercise in pregnancy is great, safe and releases yummy natural **endorphins** that make you feel good. (More on endorphins with Ally in Chapter 4.) You don't need wrapping up in cotton wool – that is a myth that persists today. Yes, rest is vital, but your physical health and preparing your body for birthing and recovery are important too.

A quick-reference guide for much of what you need to know about exercise in pregnancy can be found at the Active Pregnancy Foundation website, which is on the **wishlist** 🌾 .

In these resources, they promote pregnancy and postnatal exercise in swimming, dancing, belly dancing, Pilates, yoga, home exercise, running, walking, resistance training and cycling. Finding your own thing is excellent – whatever that is.

Quite often, it's pregnancy that propels women to seek information about exercise, and it can be their first time experiencing exercise. It's perfectly safe to try something new when pregnant, if you start gently. An exercise class is a fabulous way to connect with women experiencing much the same as you. The possibility of lifelong friendships and support can be made through this connection.

Remember, relaxin is playing through your body, so when it comes to stretching, move towards the limit you feel in your body and pull back a bit. If stretches are held for a period of time, such as a yoga posture on the floor, please support your body with blankets, cushions, pillows or whatever you have at hand.

For now and for the rest of pregnancy, it becomes important to not lie flat on your back while exercising. This is because the weight of your womb presses downwards onto a main artery supplying your baby with oxygen-rich blood. It's also common sense in the middle months to start reducing sports that can lead to a fall, such as off-road cycling, horse riding, skiing etc. You know your body. Ideally, avoid contact sports like rugby, football, kick-boxing, as well as sports in extreme heat and hot yoga. I also discourage weighted sit-ups and gym machinery that encourages deep abdominal twists. In yoga, avoid any deep back-bending postures that overstretch the abdominus recti muscles that run straight up and down from the bottom of your chest to your symphysis pubis. In pregnancy, these muscles naturally separate to allow the growing expansion of your uterus. Overstretching and overworking them can lead to diastasis recti, which we cover with Clémentine in Chapter 7.

Why do I keep coming back to yoga? As a yoga teacher, I'm biased of course, but there is a wealth of evidence to support the positive effects of yoga practice in this time of a woman's life. In a review of research on yoga in pregnancy, "The evidence highlights positive effects of pregnancy yoga on anxiety, depression, perceived stress, normal vaginal birth and shorter duration of labour."[3] In addition, a study on gentle yoga for women with high-risk pregnancies in hospital found all the women involved had reduced stress levels; this was confirmed by the nursing staff, who also said the yoga didn't disrupt medical care.[4] So, gentle yoga is positive in high-risk pregnancies too.

- **Wishlist** 🌾 Active Pregnancy Foundation website.
  https://www.activepregnancyfoundation.org/findyouractive

- *Birth-Ed* S1 #6. 'Yoga for Pregnancy and Birth with Obstetrician Dr Leah Deutsch' Apple 🎙 Spotify

- **Belly dancing in pregnancy YouTube.** If you fancy a go.
  https://www.youtube.com/watch?v=q1Tl-gHitF0

Our important pelvic floor

At this stage of your pregnancy, let's talk about getting in touch with your pelvic floor. What exactly do I mean by that? The soft tissues, ligaments and muscles within and around the outside of your pelvis connect to the structure of your pelvis, but also to your spine, hips, gluteal (butt) and leg muscles. These all play a part in assisting your baby as they negotiate the journey through the birth canal. It's so much more than your vagina and perineum stretching when giving birth, which is generally all women know.

Understanding the pelvic floor and pelvis dynamics, with awareness of how the tissues in and around your pelvis work together, prepares you for birthing and healthy recovery afterwards. A defining purpose of the sacrum and coccyx (refer to illustration A) is to move outwards during labour and birth; this is called nutation. This movement makes more space as your baby's head fills your pelvis. Outwardly, this becomes visible as a diamond shape in the mother's lower back (refer to illustration B). The sacroiliac joint is the strongest ligament system in the body. The ligaments and fascia that surround the joint provide structural reinforcement. The hormone relaxin assists them to soften and allow movement.

Practise releasing your pelvic floor – it is as important as learning to contract the muscles. Here's how to do it. When you go to the toilet to pass urine, allow as much release and softening as you can. You may notice that urine flow becomes faster. This is exactly the feeling I am talking about. Release, release a bit more, release and soften again.

I am asking you to do this now because, as I mentioned earlier, practice becomes embodied. It will be easier when birthing your baby to release and soften with the natural urge to bear down; this will help make more space. Combined with your inner knowing of the dynamic dance your body and baby do together in labour is powerful. Yoga allows for awareness of the interconnectedness of tendons, ligaments and muscles throughout the pelvis. Practising now also gives you a deeper awareness of this amazing part of your body for post-birth recovery.

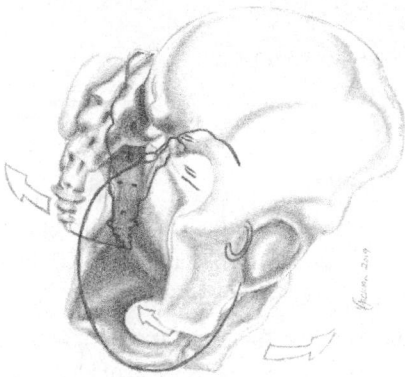

Illustration A. An internal view from the baby's perspective, this clearly shows the outward movement of the sacrum to make space for the baby's head. This is what nutation of the sacrum looks like and why a mother should be free to move to allow this natural process to occur.

Illustration B. An external view of nutation of the sacrum is illustrated as the shaded upside-down triangle at the base of the mother's spine. The sacrum can be seen moving outwards when the head of the baby is deep in the pelvis.

There is a practice offering at the end of this root of knowledge. You can release these structures through certain yoga postures, opening and making space for your baby for the emergence phase of birth.

- 'Anatomy and physiology of the pelvis' YouTube. https://www.youtube.com/watch?v=eK9-jWdUmVk

- 'A simple way to find your pelvic floor muscles' YouTube. https://www.youtube.com/watch?v=q0_JAoaM6pU&t=4s

- Wishlist 🔖 'Pelvic floor health for expectant and new mums', PDF by the Pregnancy Centre and Continence Foundation of Australia. https://continence.my.salesforce.com/sfc/p/#A0000000KUc9/a/5K0000003lek/nEDoZ3oU8.RlEab2f0E7RQ_RYNAeSA1rtAjEgDcSf0g

- Wishlist 🔖 *Beyond the Bump* S1 #35. 'All things pelvic floor (and why we shouldn't put up with pissing ourselves)' Apple 🎙 Spotify

---

Sex in pregnancy

Talking about the pelvic area, intercourse is absolutely fine during a healthy pregnancy. The release of the feel-good hormone oxytocin (which we talk about with Ashleigh in Chapter 3) with clitoral stimulation and orgasm, connection and physical touch produces calm and contentedness, which reduces cortisol. Your growing baby can't feel a penis or sex toy tapping on their head (or bottom)! They are cushioned by amniotic fluid. The hormones released are good for all of you!

Of course, if you have unexpected bleeding or fluid loss, please speak to your care provider before resuming sex. If your care provider suggests intercourse or orgasm isn't advised for medical reasons, do ask for a full explanation as to why. In other words, keep enjoying your sexual life. If you want more reassurance, pop onto this resource …

- **Pregnancy, Birth and Baby website.** Provides information on sex in pregnancy. https://www.pregnancybirthbaby.org.au/sex-during-pregnancy

---

Gestational diabetes screening. To have or not to have?

In Australia, there is universal screening for gestational diabetes (GD). In the UK and many other countries, it is not routine because research doesn't support the practice. The latest 2023 Cochrane Review about GD finds that sugar level targets from different professional organisations worldwide differ from each other and rely on consensus (agreed opinion) rather than high-certainty evidence. Diagnosis of GD varies between 2% and 26% worldwide, depending on the parameters of blood sugar levels used for diagnosis.[5] (The Cochrane database compiles best evidence.)

In Australia, diagnosing GD is done by general consensus rather than high-level evidence and has a low threshold for diagnosis. By screening everyone, rather than if there are risk factors, more women are diagnosed with GD. The blog post 'Gestational diabetes: beyond the label' provides information on the low threshold for diagnosis of GD in Australia.

GD diagnosis has become one of the major reasons for induction. The main cause for concern by obstetricians is when GD isn't picked up and the baby becomes *macrosomic*. This is a big baby who has more fat because they have received a higher amount of sugar in the blood from mum. A big baby is discussed in detail in the *Great Birth Rebellion* episode, 'Gestational Diabetes'.

GD screening is offered in such a way that it feels like you have to have it. It is generally done at 24–28 weeks. This is sensible if you have indicators, like diabetes in the family and/or sugar in your urine.

For reliable evidence-based information on GD to help you decide if you wish to have the screening test, the following resources are excellent. If you have been diagnosed with GD, the *Great Birth Rebellion* podcast provides lots of information about exercise with GD and emphasises the need for an individualised approach to your care. Please have a listen if this is your experience.

- Dr Rachel Reed Blog. 'Gestational diabetes: beyond the label' https://www.rachelreed.website/blog/gestational-diabetes-beyond-the-label
- Dr Sara Wickham website. 'Gestational Diabetes' https://www.sarawickham.com/articles-2/gestational-diabetes/
- *Great Birth Rebellion* #18. 'Gestational Diabetes' Apple 🎙️ Spotify
- *Great Birth Rebellion* #100. 'Movement for Management of Blood Sugar' Apple 🎙️ Spotify

Back to the benefits of yoga, research has shown: "Yoga and pranayama significantly decrease blood glucose levels, which in turn can prevent adverse maternal and fetal outcomes of GD. Safety during pregnancy is paramount and exercises such as low exerting forces such as yoga can be safe for both mother and fetus."[6]

To begin massaging your perineum or not?

The Cochrane database indicates that antenatal perineal massage reduces the incidence of trauma to the perineum, stating: "Women should be informed about the benefits of digital antenatal perineal massage." You can do this from around 35 weeks until you give birth, once or twice a week, but it is not advised if there is active genital herpes or placenta praevia.[7]

It is important to note that this technique reduces the incidence of episiotomy, but not of perineal tearing. There are devices out there being marketed that claim to stretch your perineum for you but there is no evidence to support their effectiveness. Consider if you really need to spend extra money on such a device.

Using your thumb is easier on your wrist, as your hand will not be as twisted as when using the first 2 fingers.

- **Pregnancy, Birth and Baby website.** The how, why and when to practise stretching your perineum if you wish. https://www.pregnancybirthbaby.org.au/perineal-massage

Mind–body reconnection and meditation

Mind and body interconnectedness are fundamental to our wellbeing, but we haven't been raised to believe that. For hundreds of years, medicine has separated mind from body. Much of this is due to René Descartes, the father of modern philosophy. In 1637 his theory of mind–body dualism (2 separate things) established their separate nature. He believed them to be 2 different substances: the body, unthinking, subject to the mechanical laws of nature; and the mind, free of these laws, a separate immaterial thinking substance. Although he wasn't the first to theorise the mind and body as separate, his work embedded that belief and heavily influenced medical practice.[8]

We need to reclaim our holistic mind–body connection, especially in pregnancy, birthing and mothering. The connectedness of the mind and body affects our perceptions of self; physical, mental, emotional and spiritual health are particularly needed for the wellbeing of pregnant women. The loss of this connection is partly responsible for our anxieties and fears around birthing. Returning to Sarah Napthali's 'Buddhism for Mothers', she clearly and beautifully explains this mind–body connection. She quotes the Buddha: "To keep your body in good health is a duty, otherwise we shall not be able to keep the mind strong and clear."[9]

· The *Birth-Ed* podcast S2 #8. 'Holistic Birth Preparation' Apple 🎙 Spotify

You could create a space in your home that is yours in which to rest, read, breathe, practise mindfulness, meditation and yoga postures, and otherwise do your thing. Be kind to yourself. Fill this special space with personal things, candles, flowers and plants, images and inspirational quotes that give you courage, inspire you, calm you. This space has your books, a note pad for ideas and questions that pop into your head to look up and ask of care providers, a journal to write in or a sketch pad. Add whatever floats your boat, lifts you up, nourishes and inspires you.

Extending meditation understanding

To begin this next practice, we take what we experienced with Liesja to another level, building on the 3-part mindful breath and becoming 'meditative'. Please don't fret. This isn't about your mind going blank or reaching total inner peace within half an hour. It is about being in the moment, with a gentle awareness of your breath, all your senses and any thoughts that pop into your mind. It is learning to notice thoughts with non-judgement, being kind, and returning to the awareness of your breath again.

Setting an intention may be useful. Intentions are simple, achievable things that are not meant to feel as though you are adding to your mental load. They are a way of reducing the stress of your worries or bringing a drop of brightness to low mood, fatigue or uncertainty. An intention before a meditation can be a single word: calm, gentle, rest, present, insight, strength, wisdom, resilience, compassion. It's whatever you need, or nothing at all.

Life is not happiness all the time. The pressure to 'be happy' and 'put on a good front' so you don't drain others or bring down the vibe is real. This leads to withdrawal from others, isolation and depletion – not so healthy and certainly not realistic.

For the purposes of meditation and mindfulness throughout this book, the practices aim to help you become embodied. What do I mean by *embodied*? Embodiment harnesses your innate ability to form an automatic connection between your mind, thoughts and intentions, and body awareness of discomfort, pleasure and comfort. Embodiment happens when you notice your senses, use body scanning, breath, visualisation and learned techniques of release and softening to help you be in the moment. They can become second nature when placed into practices that soothe, calm and strengthen.

This means we can experience physical and emotional sensations that are pleasurable, painful, emotional or fear inducing, and not bury anxious responses or run away from them. Sometimes, sitting with and embracing sadness, grief, frustration or anger, rather than pushing them away, can help. Here, you are learning the opposite of ingrained automatic responses like tensing up and breathing rapidly. Amygdala hijack increases the experience of unpleasant physical sensations. You intuitively know that the mind and body are connected, and that they are deeply affecting and responding to each other.

Breathing techniques are used as a method to bridge the gap between your mind and body when discomfort of mind, body or both occur. This active process of encouraging the quieting of the mind helps you temporarily withdraw into yourself to bring awareness of what that discomfort is. Maybe that means attending to racing thoughts, anxiety or physical discomfort by body scanning. This allows you to begin to discover a method unique to you that brings you calm, courage, peace, confidence and nourishment. With practice of your technique, it gradually becomes easier to drop in. This reduces cortisol and increases lovely oxytocin. You don't always need to be in a quiet place, still and undisturbed. Life just isn't like that. It's preferable of course to find time for yourself, but please don't beat yourself up if you are time poor and mentally overloaded! This only adds to your guilt.

These practices can be done anywhere, anytime. Even while you shop, cook, drive, have a cuppa or are at work, you can breathe and practise awareness. You can be present with your thoughts, body movements, sensations and sounds, and talk to your baby in any moment of the day or night.

Anxiety in pregnancy is very real. Many women suffer from thinking there is something wrong with them, that they will be making a fuss if they tell anyone, that other women are coping, so they should too. All of this is not true. Pregnancy can bring many anxieties, sometimes even depression, due to a multitude of factors. Some anxieties stem from social pressures, but there are others too, such as pre-existing anxiety, financial stress and physical and emotional abuse. Each is unique to the individual woman.

In Australia there is a digital screening tool called iCOPE, which is available to all public hospitals and maternal and child health services. This is a way to screen you for symptoms of anxiety and depression with your unique psychosocial risk factors. It provides an automated clinician and patient report, and offers resources. I hope your health provider is using it.

Please don't wait, suffer in silence or neglect your emotional wellbeing. You are the most important person. There is no failure or judgement here.

- *Beyond the Bump* S1 #159. 'What is Antenatal Depression and Anxiety with perinatal psychiatrist Dr Fran' Apple 🎙 Spotify

- **Digital screening iCOPE.** https://www.cope.org.au/health-professionals/icope-digital-screening/

- Please also check in with your **Ready to Cope app.**

Practice offering: Extending the breath

This pranayama practice notices the breath in more detail than we have before.

- Find that comfortable position again, practising the shoulder and neck roll, spinal stretch, hip wiggle, jaw unclenched. Soften through your body, using your senses to notice everything in your present moment. Soft gaze or closed eyes …

- In this practice, we begin by noticing and counting each breath out. As you breathe out, count one. On the next breath out, count 2. And so on up to 10. You can use a gentle press of your fingers and thumb in the count.

- The second part is to notice and count the in-breaths, a subtle change in concentration as awareness shifts. Again, one to 10.

- Then notice the entire breath, in and out, one to 10, with gentle awareness of the stillness in the pause between each breath.

- In the final stage, you choose where you wish to fix your attention in your breath cycle. It could be in the pause between, the cool air as you inhale or the softening of your body as you exhale. Count one to 10 ... Gradually build the count if and as you wish.

- Return to breathing without counting. Slowly reintegrate to the outer world, opening the eyes and maybe staying for a while ... maybe journaling some thoughts. See what you notice in your body, what comes up, or continue this practice and add the following part.

Practice offering: Bonding and connection to your baby with visualisation

- Place one hand on your heart and the other on your belly.

- Begin your 3-part breath, become heavy as you notice your body releasing, melting, secure.

- Extend each breath in to a count of 10. Visualise your love, nourishment and gentleness as a light, or your favourite colour, passing through the placenta, along the umbilical cord and infusing your baby.

- Each breath out, find a sense of softening, holding, and notice the connection of your palms over heart and firm growing belly.

- Picture your baby in your mind's eye, suspended in and nourished by your body.

- Breathe in, sending comfort and warmth, picturing them enveloped in the constant hug of your womb. Breathe out to a count of 10, softening further. Notice intrusive thoughts and return to your breath.

- Send an intention, a wish for them, if you like ... It could be a cherished childhood memory of your own to your child.

- Be in deep connection to the wonder and amazing capacity of your body and mind. Stay in this practice for as little or as long you like.

- Yoga for second and early third trimesters. YouTube.
  https://www.youtube.com/watch?v=dVFANV1oJeA

Practice offering: Yoga flow for connection to your pelvic floor

Directions for the poses in Liesja's early pregnancy yoga flow are not repeated. The poses are just named. Feel free to skip the standing sequence 15–20 if fatigued or your body says "no" today.

1. Begin this sequence kneeling on a bolster, or a block with a cushion on it. Hands together in Anjali mudra or resting on your belly. Use the pranayama practice to lengthen the exhalation count from one to 10. Repeat 5 to 10 times.

   Notice the pressure of where the bolster connects to the groin area. Sense where the urethra, vagina and anus are. Move from side to side and you may feel the sit bones of your pelvis. Notice if you hold

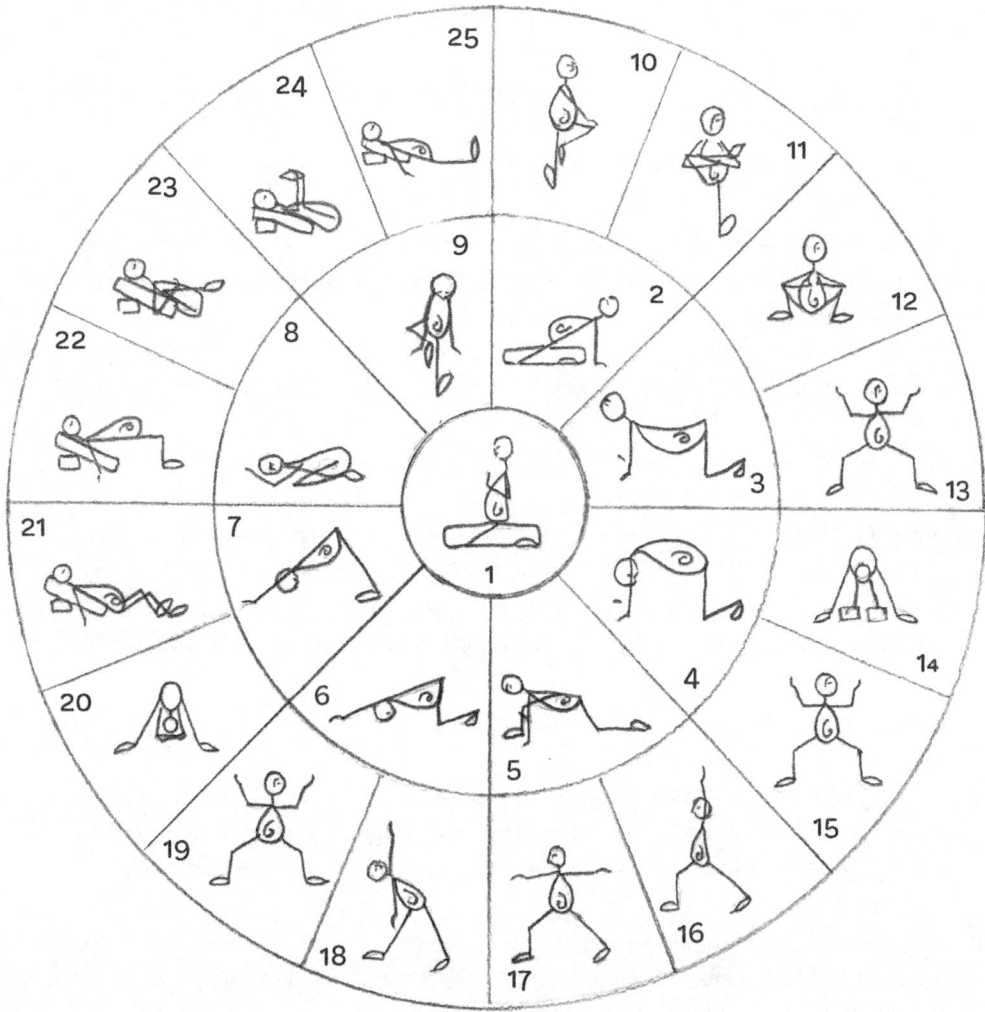

any tension in this area and soften. Pelvic floor exercise is offered in Alysia's chapter on page 231. Practise 3 rounds of these now.

2. Inhale. With the exhalation place your hands behind you on the floor, fingers towards or away from the body. Tuck your pelvis under. The stretch along the top of the thighs may feel enough. Inhale, press into the hands and lower legs, lift the buttocks slightly off the bolster. Lift the pelvic floor. Exhale, lower the body and soften the pelvic floor. Repeat twice.

3. Move to all fours for Cow pose.

4. Cat pose. Repeat Cow and Cat poses 3 times.

5. From all fours, step the right foot forward to the outside of the right hand. Foot turned outwards at 45 degrees. Inhale. As you exhale, sink your body forwards and allow the left leg to extend into a low lunge. Using the breath, explore this posture. Rock forwards, backwards and in small circular motions. With an inhalation, press into the hands, step the right foot back to all fours. Exhale and wiggle to realign the hips. Repeat on the left side.

6. Puppy pose.

7. Downward Facing Dog pose. Alternative is Puppy pose if Downward Facing Dog feels too strong. Transition to Child's pose.

8. To make room for your growing belly, move the knees apart, toes touching, and rest your pelvis on the heels into wide-legged Child's pose. Rest your head on the floor or a pillow, or place a pillow under your chest. Rest your arms and hands wherever feels most comfortable. Melt into the pose. Rest here for as long as you wish. Then move to a seated position.

9. Seated forward bend with bent right knee, sole of the foot to inner left thigh. Repeat on the left side.

10. Lengthen legs in front of you, toes to the ceiling. Bend the left knee and place the sole of your foot to the inner right thigh. Right hand on left knee and left hand on the floor behind you. Inhale and lift from the pelvis to crown of the head, lengthen the spine. Exhale with gentle pressure on the right hand, twist from the belly button and look behind you. Chin over left shoulder. Release upper body twist with next inhalation. Exhale, look a little further behind you. Repeat on the other side.

11. Lengthen legs in front of you, toes to ceiling. Bend the right knee and bring the foot to the top of left thigh. This might be a deep enough stretch. Scoop the right foot up to rest on your left forearm. Reach your right arm around the bent right leg and interlink the hands, or as near as possible. The leg is being held as though cradling a baby. Gentle rock side to side. Repeat for the left leg.

12. Move to squat and face the long edge of the mat. Feet straight. Two long breath cycles here. Exhale, place the hands in front of you, lift your pelvis up, widen your feet. Inhale and, with power through your legs, press into your feet and rise to Goddess.

13. Goddess. The Goddess posture is held 3 times in this sequence to strengthen the legs. Hold for 3 breath cycles.

14. Wide-legged hanging forward fold. Exhale as you bend forwards, hands on the floor, a block or firm cushion, then straighten the legs. Three breath cycles. Inhale and, with power through your legs, press into your feet and rise to make a star shape. Move to posture 21 if too fatigued to do the standing sequence.

15. Exhale, bend the knees and elbows and sink into Goddess again. Hold for 3 breath cycles. Move side to side while the knees are still bent. Inhale, stand upright to a star shape. Exhale and rotate the body through 90 degrees to face the short front edge of the mat.

16. Inhale, front foot to front of mat, back foot 45 degrees. Exhale, sink into Warrior 1. Two breath cycles.

17. Transition smoothly to Warrior 2. Two breath cycles.

18. Shorten stance and flow into Triangle. Two breath cycles. Repeat 16–18 on the other side.

19. Inhale, lift from Triangle, widen your stance and sink into the final Goddess. Hands on hips. Inhale, reach right arm up and lean over to the left. Exhale, right hand to hip. Repeat for the other side.

20. Hanging forward fold. Use props if the stretch is too strong.

21. Place props on the mat and recline. Windscreen wiper motion with bent legs, moving with the breath.

22. Bridge pose. Breath in and, as you exhale, tuck the pelvis under. Notice your pelvic floor and lift it as practised in posture 1. Lift to Bridge, hold for 2 breath cycles. Slow descent with exhalation. Repeat twice.

23. Place a hand on each knee. Inhale, knees move away from the body as arms lengthen. Exhale, draw the knees towards the armpits. Repeat this twice.

24. From previous posture, with knees bent towards the armpits, reach each hand to the sole of each foot. Unbend knees so soles of the feet are facing the ceiling. Happy Baby pose. Breathe here a while, explore the posture and soften the pelvic floor.

25. Sávāsana. Meditative rest. Scan through your body and make yourself comfortable. You may wish to lie on your side. Body supported, cosy. Place one hand on your heart and the other on your belly. Practise the ocean meditation offered at the end of Samatha's chapter, page 84.

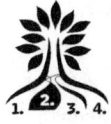

Cultural, Herstorical and Political Influences on the Middle Months

It is very difficult to say no to a doctor. This is why we return to self-silencing here. In these middle months, we are going to build confidence through understanding informed choice before consent.

Our herstory of losing our voice

Feminist historian and author Amanda Foreman, in her 'Ascent of Woman' series, uncovers the silencing of women. This herstory is as old as civilisation itself.[10]

4430 BCE	The Sumerians of Mesopotamia, in what is now modern Iraq, had an egalitarian, thriving society where Sumerian women owned their property and had control over their dowries. Silencing women really began 4430 years BCE, when Sargon of Akkad conquered this abundant place, imposing his masculine hierarchy that passed power, fortune and position to the sons. It is here, in the earliest known law codes, that we find one that says, "If a woman speaks out of turn, then her teeth will be smashed by a brick."
3375 BCE	Over time, women were barred from any commerce or sexual freedom and the 286 Law Codes of Hammarabi written in 3375 BCE clearly show the law legalising patriarchy.
3200 BCE	By 3200 years BCE, the 112 Laws of Assyria illustrate that men could now do what they liked with their wives, and over half the codes were to do with marriage and sex. Women and daughters became the property of husbands and fathers, and virginity became a pre-requisite for marriage. Law 40 is the first known written law about the veiling of women – long before Islam. Only slave girls and prostitutes were to be seen unveiled.
0000	There is no judgement here in mentioning religion and its profound effects on beliefs and culture. The rise of 3 monotheistic faiths – Judaism, Islam and Christianity under one Father God – suppressed and subsumed the worship of Pagan gods, goddesses and their ties with nature and nurture. Genesis 3:16 has become a touchstone of belief that women are deserving of pain and suffering in labour: "I will greatly multiply your pain childbearing; in pain you shall bring forth children, yet your desire shall be for your husband, and he shall rule over you."[11]
1200s	The Wise Woman, Midwife and Healer, knowledgeable in herb-lore, and called upon in illness, injury, birthing and death, was a respected figure in European history of the Middle Ages. Two radical changes occurred to alter her position in society and control her conduct in her role as a midwife. Firstly, in the early 13th century, women were barred from newly developed institutions of learning (early universities). This created the beginning of the male monopoly on health. Because women were not 'educated' in the field of medicine, they were punished for practising their knowledge of healing.[12]

| 1512 | To further control midwives in England, male physicians persuaded the English parliament and King Henry VIII in 1512 "that no woman is to use the practice of fysyk", and they legislated against women practising medicine or surgery.[13] |

| 1567 | In 1567 midwives were to be 'examined and admitted' by a bishop, and were required to take an oath to not use any kind of sorcery or incantation in the time of 'travail of any women' in order to practise. Licensing to practise was under the control of the church, giving it power over the activities of midwives, including scrutiny over their private lives. Midwives had to pay for that licence and were usually reviewed yearly. And so, church, state and male physicians controlled birthing.[14] Competition for births and income has become firmly established. |

| 1700 | The first 'lying-in hospitals' were established across Europe and North America in the 1700s; here, male medical students could practise their midwifery/obstetric skills as part of their training to become a qualified medical practitioner. A new disease named 'childbed fever' (puerperal sepsis, a severe infection that can cause death) arose due to frequent vaginal examinations with unwashed hands, and the use of contaminated instruments, such as forceps and scalpels, for assisted birth in unhygienic conditions.[15] |

| 1760 | The Industrial Revolution began in 1760 in Britain. It changed a largely agrarian cotton and wool economy into an era of iron and steam. Massive cultural upheaval occurred as people moved from villages and towns to areas of work in newly founded cities. New small units of mother, father and child/children lived in social isolation from extended family and friends, which led to the loss of lived knowledge and support. In addition to this, increasing pollution, overcrowding, poverty and disease from contaminated water led to higher mortality (death) rates.[16] |

| 1841–1843 | Maternal death rates due to infection was 16% for women in medical care, yet 2% with midwife and student midwife care in Vienna in 1841–1843. Maternal death hardly ever occurred in women birthing at home. The initial claims from concerned doctors were poo-pooed by their peers. In 1843 OW Holmes, a physician in the USA, advised '8 rules' for reducing infection for obstetricians, including hand-washing, changes of clothing and not attending autopsies while also caring for labouring women. His conclusions were ridiculed by many of his contemporaries. Charles Meigs, an influential obstetrician of the time, stated, "Doctors are gentlemen, and gentlemen's hands are clean."[17] |

| 1878 | In 1878 at the Dublin Rotunda Hospital, death rates from puerperal fever reached one in 4 women. "With reputations and income at stake, concealment of maternal deaths appears to have been tolerated."[18] |

| 1899–1902 | The government in the UK took an interest in maternity care only due to 'weak' recruits for the army.[19] The lack of fit men being available as troops for the Boer War led to a committee investigation, the Fitzroy Report. It found children were being breastfed less and less, largely due to the chronic ill-health and over-work of their working-class mothers, who were living in poverty in slum conditions. "Great harm is done and suffering occasioned to the women by their remaining at work too long before confinement as well as by their returning too soon after it." As many as one in 4 children died before their first birthday. |

1899–1902	"The heavy rate of infant mortality is said to be in large part due to the fact that infants are nowadays seldom fed from the breast."[20] By the 1900s, obstetric asepsis (extreme cleanliness as advised in 1843) was practised. Australia was quick to follow these changes and maternal mortality rates dropped to 5–6 per 1000 births between 1900 and the 1930s.[21]
1920s	In 1920s Australia, the removal of birthing to hospital under the guise of safety, less injury during birth and lower maternal death rates affected all women, no matter what race or class.[22]
1935	Enter sulpha drugs, the first antibiotic used in the early 1930s, and death from puerperal sepsis thankfully became very rare.[23]
1940s–1950s	As more women birthed in hospital, these institutions were in a prime position to educate nervous, isolated new mothers in scientific health care. Due to the fear of infection before antibiotics, babies were removed from their mothers, cared for in sterile nurseries and reunited for feeding every 3 to 4 hours. Mothers were told to wash their nipples to prevent infection, delivering a subtle message that they were a danger to their baby and only a sterile environment would do to raise them in. Mothers' time to care for, and bond with, their new baby in hospital and gain confidence in caring for them was restricted.[24]
	This practice of separating mothers and babies continued in westernised cultures for decades afterwards. Knowledge and wisdom in the art of supporting mothers in breastfeeding was lost due to the disruption to instinctive cues of baby-led demand feeding, which interfered with bonding. Doctors actively encouraged women to bottle-feed – the scientific method.[25] (Note: science is not the enemy, as it teaches us so much about ourselves, how incredible we are and how much we don't know yet. However, mothering isn't a science.)
1992	In *Birth as an American Rite of Passage*, Robbie Davis-Floyd describes the 'technocratic' model of obstetric care, likening it to an assembly line production of saleable goods. A woman's body (the factory) is treated like the machine that makes the 'goods' (the baby), to be tinkered with and modified by technicians (male obstetricians) in a timely, cost-effective manner to ensure an optimal final product. This separates the mother and baby by treating the factory (woman) and product (baby) as separate entities. In addition, Davis-Floyd discusses how women were blamed when something went wrong during pregnancy or birth, due to her refusal to follow doctors' orders, the defectiveness of her body, or her own inadequacy as a person.[26]
2019	Dr Clare Davison, independent midwife, writes in her thesis that "… the rise of obstetrics and its eventual dominance over midwifery in the western world was achieved by the argument that those who cared for the female body could only do so by viewing it as a machine to be supervised, controlled and interfered with by technical means."[27]

To date, women anticipate childbirth with a fear of the unknown. A shroud of silence about birth has persisted through the generations. The truth of the rawness, lack of dignity, vulnerability and intense physical and emotional experiences of women in hospitals during childbirth has remained largely hidden. This is beginning to change with awareness of birth trauma and postnatal depression.

We live in a technological world. We accept that technology will be part of monitoring our pregnancy and birthing. We expect it to intervene if necessary. This has become an integral part of our lives. And when needed, it's fabulous! But when overused, it has deep consequences. We must find a balance.

Hospitals need to run efficiently. With the influences of industrialisation, mass production and viewing women's bodies as machine-like, birth has become more of a production line, with time constraints and interference to speed the process along. The fact that labour is unique to each woman is rarely considered. In this environment we don't practise using knowledge of, or experience or faith in, physiological birth with mindful support.

I write about all this to provide a deeper understanding of our evolving herstory. In our modern culture, women are achieving more and have better health, living conditions, social power and education; yet there is the paradox of disempowerment and fear of birth. With this herstory of the rise of medicalisation of childbirth under a male domain, is it any wonder?

Women have been trained to adhere to societal expectations of the self-silencing 'good girl'. We hear, "Do as the doctor tells you." We're told not to question or make a fuss. We have even been blamed for taking too much time to birth our babies. We have felt an unnerving sense of beholding and submissiveness and we hand our bodies over to professionals who 'know better'. Women have had to allow their bodies to be intimately dealt with by health professional strangers, as if that is the only safe way to be pregnant, labour and give birth. Sometimes the health professional doesn't fully explain why a procedure is being done or ask for permission or consent to do it.

This section gives you the evidence you need for autonomy over your own body and the choices you can make. Because you have a voice that needs to be listened to and respected. Nobody has the right to make a choice for you without your being fully informed of all the options of care, and the risks and benefits of investigations and procedures. You need to know why tests are done and why certain care pathways are being suggested.

Writing this is a way to help you find the confidence to question and take up space, because you are the powerful person here, consenting, having your own free will, not being coerced or forced.

Phew! Take a full and deep breath in, with a long exhalation. Keep breathing this way as feelings arise from witnessing our herstory so far. Allow those emotions to be felt. Take a break for a while. Nourish yourself. Journal or chat with a loved one for support. As we continue now, we begin to find ways to make change.

Talking about informed consent and informed refusal

When a doctor or other healthcare provider recommends an intervention or treatment, they have a legal obligation to inform you of the risks and benefits of the full range of options of care without bias or coercive language. You are entitled to evidence-based, individualised recommendations, and to be supported in your autonomy to give genuine consent. Ask the provider to give you the evidence for their recommendations. Remember, the choice to accept or decline the recommendation is yours, based on your personal understanding, needs and values.

Human rights lawyer Bashi Hazard states in *Birthtime*: "Childbirth is absolutely a human rights issue. When you are making decisions about somebody's body, their personal autonomy, their right to decide, the circumstances in which they live, breathe, function, you have to abide by those fundamental human rights. What we're seeing in pregnancy and childbirth is women all around the world are reporting that as soon as they become pregnant, there is a presumption that those rights don't apply to them."[28] Part of the

Universal Declaration of Human Rights includes the right to decline any medical procedure that violates a woman's bodily integrity, even if that refusal increases her or her fetus' risk of death.[29]

In a submission to the Australian Human Rights Commission, Human Rights in Childbirth revealed a disturbing finding about the use of 'bait and switch'. This is when some maternity service providers 'bait' women into care, promising what the woman wants by " … misrepresentation or concealment of the healthcare provider's or the facility's intentions, practices, and preferences, in order to gain women's trust and custom during the course of the pregnancy."[30] They then 'switch' the care they said they would provide at the end of the pregnancy, when it is too late to change care provider.

Sadly, this was Samantha's experience. Women find it difficult to change their care provider or birth facility when a highly interventionist model is proposed in the last weeks of their pregnancy. So, women are experiencing "hospital policies or protocols that were not disclosed prior to booking to mandate routine interventions and invasive procedures during labour at a facility". Governments are currently refusing to mandate disclosure of intervention and complication rates of hospitals, including private hospitals and individual care providers.[31] This makes it hard for women to choose where they wish to birth and who with.

This is well described by Catherine Deveny, an author and comedian who imitates an obstetrician when interviewed in *Birthtime*: "'I'm really pro vaginal birth. I won't induce you or give you a caesarean section unless it's really necessary.' Then a couple of weeks out there's a bit of sucking air between the teeth, a bit of [inhales] as the blood tests come in, or the measuring is being done, or the heart rate is being listened to … 'Baby looks a bit big …' Just these tiny things being said to start to rattle these women."[32]

Coercion within the health profession and patient relationship can be done in several ways, such as withholding risks or exaggerating the benefits associated with a recommended treatment. Magnifying risk estimates to dissuade a patient from an option, or demeaning a woman's choice as putting her fetus at risk, or even threatening to involve child protection services make her feel like a bad parent. Threatening to withdraw care if a woman refuses medical advice is also unacceptable.[33]

The article 'Yes You Can Say No!', written by Rhea Dempsey, doula and Australia's own matriarch of all things birthing, is on the **wishlist** ✹. It discusses health literacy to help women navigate the practices, policies and procedures currently available in our maternity system. It gives you the confidence to say "no thank you".

Dempsey explains that women can enter what she calls a 'trance of acquiescence', because we wish to be sweet to everybody instead of speaking up for our wishes. Why is that? Well, flooded with oxytocin, our 'tend and befriend hormone' (particularly in labour), women are conflict-avoidant. We want to maintain good vibes and avoid conflict. So we put our wishes and needs last in tough negotiations about procedures and interventions.[34] Conflict causes anxiety, which creates an adrenaline response.

Dempsey suggests women need to get savvy about all that will be routinely offered – to be prepared and ready to give 'informed consent' or 'informed refusal' to protect themselves from any unnecessary interventions. Many women are unaware they even have a choice. Dempsey states: "What health literacy and medical decision-making should look like in practice is patient autonomy on the part of the patient – in our case the birthing woman – who will make her choices in light of the evidence provided and based on her values and research, her baby's and her own health, her sense of responsibility and her capacity. Now her choice might either be giving 'informed consent' – that is, saying 'yes' to what's suggested; or it may be 'informed refusal' – saying 'no' to what's suggested. In either case, there will be an expectation that her autonomous choice will be accepted without coercion or refusal of support and goodwill."[35]

The flow of information goes both ways too. For a medical professional to provide care, they need information from the mother. Building a relationship with mutual respect for each other's knowledge should happen without a power dynamic in the health professional's favour. We need to rethink the historical adage of 'doctor knows best'. Doctors know a lot. When complications arise in pregnancy, they are the experts. Ideally, as Dempsey states: "On the part of the medical caregiver, in theory they should practice in a way that honours patient autonomy and, in our case, provide the birthing woman with woman-centred care by sharing evidence-based information. They will quantify risk specific to the particular woman and her baby, and practice within the code of ethics of their profession."[36]

How do you negotiate this potentially negative environment and culture in maternity care? Please use the resources in the goody box. This all seems to have been doom and gloom. It's not meant to be. However, health literacy is very important. It is part of the change we are making to ensure better care, prevention of trauma and PND in you and other women.

- **Wishlist** 'Yes You Can Say No!' article by Rhea Dempsey
  https://www.birthingwisdom.com.au/yes-you-can-say-no-rhea-dempsey/

- **Wishlist** 'Right Birth Your Choice' PDF tool by Maternal Health Matters (MHM)
  https://maternalhealthmatters.org.au/wp-content/uploads/2023/02/Right-Birth-Your-Choice-Workbook-Jan-2023.pdf

- **MHM. Choice and Consent. YouTube.** https://www.youtube.com/watch?v=w1MvCFOrthc

- **Maternity Consumer Network (MCN) 'Respectful Maternity Care Charter' visual chart**
  https://www.maternityconsumernetwork.org.au/_files/ugd/76e9eb_1f0071e1a7044858a4c79ef5249e7415.pdf

- **Pregnancy, Birth and Baby website. 'Choice and Consent'**
  https://www.pregnancybirthbaby.org.au/understanding-informed-consent-and-your-rights-when-having-a-baby

- **MCN 'IDECIDE'.** Quick-reference tool that helps you make choices and decisions around consent. Save this link to your device to remind you, as it's especially useful in labour. https://www.maternityconsumernetwork.org.au/_files/ugd/76e9eb_898a2138549b4b478da372f8033a479f.pdf

- *Birth: The Forgotten Feminism* Issue #2. with Ellen O'Keefe on 'Maternal Health Matters'. This podcast discusses a survey which looked at dignity, consent information, procedures and lack of accountability on costs of maternity care. It's direct and honest. Apple Spotify

Recommendations 15, 16 and 17 of the NSW inquiry into birth trauma deal with consent. They recommend "urgently supporting maternity staff with appropriate local protocols and training to ensure that the Consent to Medical and Healthcare Treatment Manual is implemented". They also recommend: "review laws and consider any necessary legislative changes regarding informed consent" and "provide support through adequate funding to ensure all practising maternity health practitioners in NSW undertake informed consent training".[37] Bring it on nationwide.

Matricentric feminism on informed choice

Informed choice is a political conversation, because it means advocating to make change for women and mothers in the pregnancy, birthing and early mothering space. It begins with awareness, knowledge and understanding of what is currently offered to pregnant and birthing women, and how they are being made to fit into a healthcare system that is time-poor, staff-poor and costly. Indeed, the current model is more costly to government in its current unwieldy form than a midwifery continuity of care model would be.

More important is the emotional, physical and psychological cost to women that current maternity care inflicts. This conversation is about illustrating how the current patriarchal, neoliberal culture and institutional birthing systems need to change to make healthier mothers and families the focus.

Talking to Google about how her book *Give Birth Like a Feminist* came into being, Milli Hill discusses bringing back comfort and nurturing, with the woman as the central focus and medicine in the background. Her book is about empowering you in your journey for all types of birth. If you would rather listen to a podcast, Hill talks with Skye Waters, host of Positive Birth Australia.

- **Wishlist** 'Milli Hill: Give Birth Like a Feminist' YouTube. https://www.youtube.com/watch?v=sJ7xX3ZKkU4
- *Positive Birth Australia* S2 #57. 'Milli Hill, Author and Founder of the Positive Birth Movement' Apple Spotify

Social, Economic and Media Influences on the Middle Months

Everybody has an opinion. We are offered plenty of well-intentioned advice about what is good and bad for us in pregnancy, and best for birth and the early days. This comes via family, friends and media. As this advice comes, the pressure of being a good mother builds while gestating your baby. You may be judged for your choices, with well-meaning interference, but interference nonetheless. We are talking about this here in the middle months to help you avoid the pressure to be perfect and to reduce any associated influence and stress.

The toxic narrative of perfection

Despite decades of feminist critique, the prevailing attitude of 'the good mother' still exists in public policy, media, culture and the workplace. It starts as children, when society exposes us to the ideals of what a good mother is. This shapes the lives of Australian mothers and keeps them stifled. Women are called 'a bad mother' for not keeping to societal norms.

What does the ideal of a good mother look like then? The good mother is heterosexual, married, monogamous, white and native-born to Australia. She acts responsibly, is an intuitive nurturer always available for childcare, and never puts herself or her convenience before her children. She identifies as the child raiser. Ever patient, creative, kind, loving, filled with gratitude, satisfied, fulfilled and enjoying her role. In other words, " ... the good mother is known as that formidable social construct placing pressure on women to conform to particular standards and ideals, against which they are judged and judge themselves".[38]

Woe betide the mother who does not possess one or more of these amazing attributes. If she feels anger, isolation, frustration, apathy, regret, boredom or maternal rage, then she is a failed mother. Regulation of women through 'good mother' versus 'bad mother' ideology in our society continuously rates mothers through endless media and content. There are quizzes that ask: Are you a bad mum? There are 'bad mum' chat rooms and websites where women 'confess' their bad mothering behaviour and feelings. Thankfully, this provides alternative narratives of what mothers do, and how they behave and feel. The reality of modern mothering. Phew!

Matrescence is all about normalising the myriad of feelings a mother has. Mums are not broken and do not need fixing. They need recognition and support. This is all about understanding and identifying where to make the changes, both on an individual and cultural level. There are a few challenges to break through on the way though.

One of these challenges is the nasty phenomenon of mum-shaming. Society criticises women's decisions about childbirth, feeding, parenting styles, working or staying at home, childcare and education, body recovery post-birth and more. Shame is an intensely painful feeling. Believing we have failed or are flawed in some way makes us feel unworthy. With unrealistic external and internal expectations placed on mothers, judgement feeds mum-shaming. Some mothers feel they are being genuinely helpful with their comments, while others get a boost to their own battered ego by putting others down. This all leads to insecurity about pregnancy and birth choices, and parenting abilities, loneliness, emotional and physical burnout, anxiety and depression.

Social media outlets vomit up garbage pictures of the perfect, hallowed mother, who has 'bounced back' and got all her shit together, making real mothers extremely vulnerable to 'comparisonitis'. This takes mum-shaming to another level.[39] Coming back to words from Sarah Napthali: "Whether or not we're aware of it, we often treat others in a similar way to how we treat ourselves. If we avoid exploring our own pain, we don't tend to look deeply at the pain of others. If we are harsh and judgemental with ourselves, this can extend to others as well."[40] Treat yourself gently and allow all the external nonsense to dissolve around you.

It's already challenging enough becoming a mother and being a woman in a patriarchal society. How about we change the narrative? Women support women, holding each other up, championing each other and cheering each other along. We provide for each other in emotional and practical ways. Let us no longer judge each other or ourselves constantly with the vicious inner voice. Media bombardments suck. 'Perfect mother', 'mother shame', imagery about our bodies and how we should behave. Telling us what we need in the way of 'stuff' in order to be a perfect mother. All this isn't even real, but an illusion of impossible attainment. It has been deeply embedded in women's psyche, making us feel worthless. It's utterly toxic.

As Vanessa Olorenshaw writes, "If women felt empowered and interested in pursuing a sisterhood which actually valued, nurtured, supported and loved each other with compassion and kindness, that would be a start wouldn't it? Wouldn't that at least challenge the patriarchal system in which we operate to 'man down' a bit? Can we lead by example? We really do have the right. We have a lot to be proud of. By ignoring, with each woman, the needs of that mother even during pregnancy, we are setting the scene for the role of the mother to be sidelined in society, economics, politics and media."[41]

- **Wishlist** 🌿 *Beyond the Bump* S1#146. 'Why being a 'Good Enough' Mother is more than good enough – debunking the perfect parent myth with Dr Sophie Brock' Apple 🎙 Spotify

Building boundaries to bring kindness and protection for yourself

Changing this narrative starts with kindness and compassion to yourself. Not judging yourself. Not comparing yourself to others. Acceptance of who you are, your genetic makeup, beautiful in your individuality. Seeing your strengths and the strengths in others. Offering support even if all the energy you have is for a few kind words.

Life is going to change as you become a mother. Matrescence is change to the core of your being. What we cover next will assist you in navigating these changes. It is vital to set boundaries as part of resilience-building, protecting yourself, being kind to yourself and putting your needs first so you have the energy to care for yourself and family. Setting boundaries, putting them in place and sticking to them can be hard, but doing so reflects your values towards yourself and for others to witness.

So, how might this look?

- **Emotional boundary:** How emotionally available you are to others at any given time. Expressed as, "As much as I want to be there for you, I don't have the emotional capacity right now," or "Everything I have is invested in my own emotional health/mother becoming".

- **Internal boundary:** Your self-regulation of energy spent on yourself and baby versus others. Expressed as, "I'm recovering from birth, bonding with my baby and don't wish to have visitors, but I'll gladly see you briefly and accept your offer of a meal, or to do some washing, tidy my home, or hold my baby while I shower," or "I'm having a nap with no feelings of guilt".

- **Mental boundary:** The freedom to your own thoughts, beliefs, values and opinions. Expressed as, "I respect your perspective on how you wish to feed and parent your child. Shall we agree to disagree?"

- **Physical boundary:** Privacy of body and personal space, including touching your pregnant belly or your baby. Expressed as, "Please don't touch my belly," or "Please don't touch my baby," or "I decline consent to that particular physical examination or procedure or test," or "I am uncomfortable being hugged by strangers".

- **Time boundary:** How much time you spend with others and on doing things. Expressed as, "I have had a full week; I'm having a quiet weekend," or "My time is precious and consumed with my newborn. I'm fatigued right now, so can we keep this concise or arrange another time?" or "I'm having a nap".

- **Conversational boundary:** Topics and media threads in which you are uncomfortable being part of the discussion. Expressed as, deleting the media minefield of demoralising, disrespectful, judgemental meanness and "I don't want to hear your uninvited horrible pregnancy, birth and mothering stories," or "I would rather not be involved in this conversation," or "I don't have the mental space for this".

- **Economic boundary:** Your financial capacity, monetary choices. Expressed as, "I'm not in a position to afford [...]. I will join you for dinner/buy your birthday present/lend you some money another time".

Parental leave, super and the economic implications of becoming a mother

Women are placed at financial disadvantage when taking time away from work to be a mother. This is particularly true with superannuation, where women's security is affected on becoming a mother, because they are handicapped from achieving an equal superannuation balance with men. This is because they are more likely to take on unpaid care work (mothering), work in a reduced capacity (fewer hours), or leave the workforce altogether. In Australia, the shift towards a greater emphasis on self-provision in retirement is limiting to women because current structures of superannuation policy in Australia privilege a full-time and uninterrupted career.

Returning to Vanessa Olorenshaw: "The focus on workplace economic participation and equality loses something rather important: our humanity, how we want to live our lives, and the inconvenient truth: that many mothers want to spend time with their children, many of them exclusively for at least the first few years of life. The traitors that we are. We are punished financially as a result because of the stark truth that what we do is not recognised as worthy, worthwhile, or as work."[42]

The 2016 Census reported that the number of women over 55 experiencing homelessness increased by 31% from 2011 to 2016 and is still increasing. Why? Because of the greater risk of financial and housing insecurity due to a combination of low superannuation from having taken time out of the workforce to care for family, working part-time or casually throughout their lives and being at the mercy of the gender pay gap.[43]

This is called the 'motherhood penalty'. When women become mothers, they are penalised financially due to maternity leave, reduced working hours and diminished career trajectory. Women retire with 40% less superannuation than men. The economic value of unpaid childcare work is estimated at around $345 billion and the burden of providing this care falls disproportionately on women. The Workplace Gender Equality Agency (WGEA) highlights and champions strategies to reduce the financial inequality of women, stating: "We need to place much greater value on the contributions mothers make in our workplaces and to our nation's economic wellbeing through both their paid and unpaid work."[44]

It isn't all doom and gloom! An ABC article, 'Superannuation isn't fair for new mums. Here's what couples can do to even it up', highlights the very underused superannuation 'contributions splitting'. The working partner applies to the Australian Taxation Office (ATO) and contributes from their own superannuation to the mother's. The mother is still working after all, harder than ever before. By doing this, her superannuation and financial security doesn't suffer.[45]

Have the conversation with your partner about contributions splitting now. You should not be penalised for having a baby. Taking a career break to stay at home or returning after parental leave should not be to your detriment. Protecting your future and heightening your own sense of security is important. You are worth it. Mothering is valuable.

- **WGEA website.** For the gender pay gap, flexible work, support for parents and carers and more. https://www.wgea.gov.au/

- **Australian Tax Office website.** Contributions splitting. https://www.ato.gov.au/forms-and-instructions/superannuation-contributions-splitting

- **The Pregnancy, Birth and Baby website.** Pregnancy in the workplace, parental leave, Medicare claims and returning to work. https://www.pregnancybirthbaby.org.au/paid-parental-leave

- **Fair Work Ombudsman Parents and Families website.** For those experiencing difficulties with their employer. https://www.fairwork.gov.au/find-help-for/parents-and-families

- *Australian Birth Stories* #401. Georgie Dent, executive director of the Parenthood, discusses a step-by-step guide through the financial support systems available to parents and recent changes to paid parental leave (PPL) (especially the use-it-or-lose-it model). Apple 🎙 Spotify

- 'Paid parental leave is changing' ABC article. From July 2025, the total weeks of paid parental leave will increase to 24, but at least 3 of those weeks must be used by the second parent. https://www.abc.net.au/news/2023-10-19/how-does-expanded-paid-parental-leave-scheme-work/102996982?utm_source=abc_news_web&utm_medium=content_shared&utm_campaign=abc_news_web

Drama sells: media and mum marketing

Childbirth and mothering have been internationally marketed as a commodity. Media and advertising exploit parental insecurities, fears and the social construct of 'good enough' parents. What capitalist institution wouldn't take the opportunity to make money out of something?

It started early in our herstory. From 1893, *Babyhood* magazine stated in its editorial: "There is a science in bringing up children and this magazine is the voice of that science."[46] This created a perfect platform to advertise goods by undermining a mother's confidence in herself. For example, Lysol, a disinfectant, was aggressively targeted at women and mothers. One particular advert for Lysol sees a worried mother looking over her unwell child, while the doctor states: "Madam, you are to blame!" The male doctor is telling the mother that she is the cause of her child's illness by not being sanitary enough and using scientifically inspired Lysol to keep her home clean and germ-free.[47]

Childbirth has become packaged and sold to women as scary and unsafe, and only the medical establishment can save women from it. Women grow up with imagery of birthing in hospitals: red-faced, pushing hard, people coaxing her with raised voices. Lots of fear and screaming and panic in the partner. All while she is on her back, legs apart under bright lights exposing her entirely. She is in a hospital gown, depersonalised, strapped to monitors that beep and ding, a drip in her arm and doctors with gowns on all around her. Draping the woman with sterile linens with just her vulva and anus on show, a barrier between herself and the 'deliverer'. Instruments applied, and babies pulled out and resuscitated.

Drama sells.

The narrative of childbearing as seen in films, TV, books, blogs and so on needs to change. This imagery fuels negative, ignorant, fearful perceptions. It should be replaced with knowledge, dignity, respect for the strength of women's bodies and birthing. It ought to reflect the reality of undisturbed physiological and supported birthing.

In addition, women are inundated with advertising for all the 'stuff' needed during pregnancy, birthing and postpartum – from fashion to furniture, nipple shields and pumps, prams, baby bottles, formula milks etc. Most of it is not needed or can be sourced second-hand. Yet women are pressured to buy it for fear of being judged as a not-good-enough parent, placing an unnecessary financial burden on the family and feeding into the one-upmanship, competition and comparisonitis.

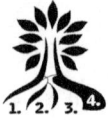

Self-identity, Beliefs and Values, and Spiritual Influences on the Middle Months

Finding your strengths for greater confidence

Women naturally have a lot of strengths, but we don't always identify them in ourselves. These strengths are not always recognised, celebrated or valued, yet they keep our world revolving and make us incredibly efficient at home and in the workplace. As I mentioned before, we become more risk-averse when pregnant and mothering, but that does not mean we are not brave. We listen with empathy and are good communicators, making others feel heard and understood. Even if we raise our voices when tired, or have already asked children to do something, to hurry up, to get in the car, for the gazillionth time. Mothers are superb problem solvers, able to get to the nitty gritty of an issue and rapidly form a plan. We are seriously resilient, hard-working, persevering through challenges of pregnancy, birthing and mothering. We take resilience to an entirely new level.

Mothers are multi-taskers extraordinaire, juggling so much with physical, emotional and organisational brilliance. We are compassionate, natural-born nurturers able to give so much love, with empathy for family, friends and those around us. We are creative, we often excel at arts, brainstorming and collaboration. We join creativity with problem-solving and apply that to getting a toddler to engage, making a meal last 3 days or negotiating all manner of things day and night. Such skills make us phenomenal in the workplace as well. Mothers are totally awesome!

Here's the cautionary note. Our strengths, when not fully recognised and valued, are also our downfall. In a world of comparisonitis, frantic mothering busyness, and a huge mental load where we are taken for granted, our bucket will leak until it is empty. Burnout. Depletion. We need to be aware of this to avoid it. We should guard against being taken for granted, not just by ourselves, our families and communities, but by society.

Here I propose doing a strengths exercise to boost self-worth, respect and identity. This is a mental tool to use alongside values to help in decision-making and to prevent burnout. As we did with values, see what resonates with you from the list on the following page and whittle it down to 4. See how you can apply them alongside your values for greater confidence and autonomy.

Next, journal how you would use your strengths alongside your values for your pregnancy, birthing and mothering. This is all about building you up and assisting you to navigate this new world. Believe in yourself.

Jessie Johnson Cash, midwife, academic and shamanic craftswoman, when interviewed in *Birthtime* said, "We need love. We need women that love themselves, that know their bodies, that are okay in their own skin, that grow up feeling that it's alright to say the word 'vagina', and to gain pleasure, and to live in a body that is not always the ideal of what it should be. We need care providers, and we need women to actually just be real and to love women."[48] Totally true.

Adaptable	Diligent	Kind	Persevering
Ambitious	Efficient	Leading	Persuasive
Articulate	Empathetic	Listening	Polite
Artistic	Energetic	Loving	Practical
Aspiring	Enthusiastic	Mature	Punctual
Brave	Ethical	Methodical	Realistic
Calm	Experienced	Meticulous	Reliable
Capable	Friendly	Modest	Resilient
Caring	Generous	Non-judgemental	Resourceful
Cheerful	Grateful	Objective	Responsible
Clear-headed	Hard-working	Openhearted	Respectful
Communicative	Helpful	Flexible	Self-confident
Competitive	Honest	Forgiving	Self-disciplined
Considerate	Humble	Focused	Self-reliant
Cooperative	Imaginative	Optimistic	Selfless
Courageous	Independent	Organised	Sensible
Creative	Innovative	Outspoken	Serious
Curious	Insightful	Open-minded	Sincere
Decisive	Intuitive	Passionate	Sociable
Determined	Inventive	Patient	Sympathetic
Devoted	Involved	Perceptive	

Celebrating you in your 'mother blessing' rite of passage

When mum thrives, so does the baby. Remember I mentioned reclaiming lost knowledge and wisdom? Navaho women hold a sacred spiritual ceremony for pregnant women that celebrates this immense rite of passage; they call it a 'Blessingway'. It's wonderful that we can relearn from other cultures to reclaim lost knowledge and wisdom. With respect for the Navaho and not wishing to appropriate their culture we call this ceremony a 'mother blessing'.

Instead of a 'baby shower', a mother blessing is a beautiful way to honour the woman before she becomes a mother. It is usually held in the later months of pregnancy with a gathering of friends and family, birth and future postnatal support. Others, like your midwife and/or doula, may attend if their professional commitments allow. This is matricentric rather than baby-centric. It is a very feminine ceremony, but of course male partners, friends and family are welcome too. After all, you are building your village. It's your celebration, so do what you want.

A mother blessing is all about providing for you, the mother becoming, in practical, emotional, sensible, supportive and more sustainable matricentric ways. This is village-building that meets your needs. It is not about receiving more baby outfits, hats, booties and stuff that you will never use. You are the centre of attention, as you should be in a matricentric approach. You are made visible again in society.

As Vanessa Olorenshaw so potently writes: "Where is the ceremonial marking of this momentous transition – social and biological – which happens in the journey from woman to mother? We celebrate marriage. We celebrate the birth of a baby. But nowhere is there an adequate celebration of the transformation of a woman in waiting for her baby. Why not? Can we dare to suggest that it is because pregnancy is seen at once unremarkable and a nuisance to business interests? Because motherhood is not respected or valued? Because women themselves have forgotten that we are allowed to celebrate and support our sisters? Because to want, as a woman and mother, is to want too much ... something involving a woman's body and her power; a woman which is growing and sustaining life inside her body? The nurturing of that woman? Nah, skip on. Get back to work!"[49]

We deserve better. We matter. Let's embrace our worth to celebrate ourselves and our sisters to make way for a better future for our daughters.

A few ideas that may tickle your fancy for your mother blessing

So, how would you go about arranging a mother blessing? How would you hold one? Firstly, there is always the option of finding someone who provides this service and a place to gather, or even hold the ceremony outside. They send invitations to all the people you wish to be there, telling them what to expect and bring. They act as the space holder, fulfilling the role of facilitator of your mother blessing. Alternatively, you can ask a friend or relative to arrange it for you or do it yourself. It doesn't have to be elaborate and expensive, with 'stuff' that goes into landfill. That's not the point. The mother blessing should not become another thing added to your mental load. It's supposed to be joyful.

For a start, everyone brings food. Generally, the gathering is a circle with a centrepiece of flowers, greenery, candles or whatever you want, with cushions and blankets around the outside for comfort. You may want some aromatherapy. Ask someone to act as mistress or master of ceremony. Begin with a grounding meditation to focus the energy and intention towards this serious yet utterly joyful celebration of you. You could add a few gentle yoga stretches to get everyone comfortable.

Activities can be things like a belly cast where your bump is covered in plaster of Paris. This sets quickly and can be decorated at a later date (even with your child!) as a keepsake. You might choose belly decoration in the form of a mandala with non-toxic henna that lasts for weeks. If you want, you could wear a crown of flowers! You could have a foot bath with flower petals scattered through, feet rubbed with sea salt and coconut, or olive oil massaged into your feet. Yummy.

Have your favourite soothing music playing in the background and even sing along with a happy song! Have guests write affirmations on cards or a piece of cloth (maybe calico) to be hung up when you are in labour to remind you that your loved ones are with you in spirit.

A soulful thing to do is a 'string ceremony' with your favourite colour in thick embroidery thread. Here, as you gather in a circle, the string is passed around, wrapped around each person's wrist (or ankle) 3 times, connecting all of you. Then, scissors are passed around to cut, then tie the threads. The string remains on everyone's wrists. Each time they see the string around their wrists, it is a reminder of you, the pregnant mum, continuing the connection between you all. It's a thread of love and good wishes.

Another beautiful activity is selecting a bead, charm or something that can be threaded onto the embroidery thread to make a bracelet for you when you are in labour. As the string is passed around and each individual adds their bead, they express an intention for you and your baby (aloud or whispered in your ear). As each bead is added, the person may express why they chose that particular item for you.

At the mother blessing, guests can offer something practical for the future, something really needed in your postpartum. They could promise to make a meal or deliver a snack, be a shoulder to cry on, tidy up your home, get a load of washing done, give a massage or hold baby while you shower or nap.

Alternatively, everyone can give a little money towards a postnatal doula for a day if you would really like that. Friends can set up a meal train on a roster for the first few weeks after you give birth. Look up the Meal Train platform to organise meals delivered to your door. Better yet, ask someone else to arrange it! Friends may be overloaded with their own families, so the offer of a phone call check-in to say, 'I see you', is a powerful form of support too.

However you create it, a mother blessing can be a truly powerful experience for all involved – it is all about the wellbeing of the mother and raising awareness of what is really needed to support her after birth. Planning for your postpartum experience starts here. Go for it!

- 'Village for Mama' website. Mother blessing ideas.
  https://villageformama.com/mothers-blessing-ceremony/
- *Shebirths* S5 #3. 'Planning a great postpartum' with doula Naomi Chrisoulakis Apple 🎙 Spotify
- *Newborn Mothers* #10. '21st Century Village-Building' Part 1, with postpartum doula and author Julia Jones Apple 🎙 Spotify
- *Newborn Mothers* #12. 'Expectations vs Reality of Motherhood', which talks about a survey where 85% of women said they expected help and support in their postpartum and 100% said they didn't receive the support they expected. Apple 🎙 Spotify
- Organising a mealtrain.com. https://www.mealtrain.com/

Practice offering: *Nādī Śodhana* breath

Nādī Śodhana breath, also known as the wave breath, is where we connect to the feeling of a wave, a rhythmic flow of noticing what is happening in our body and mind. The practice eases a busy mind. It requires alternate nostril breathing, meaning you are physically connected by the action needed for the breath in a deeply mindful way.

- Raise your dominant hand and use your thumb and ring finger to rest lightly on the outside of your nostrils.
- Curl the other fingers in on themselves so they are out of the way. Close the right nostril, inhale deeply through the left, filling your chest as you have learned to do. Then close the left nostril and exhale fully through the right nostril.
- Repeat the action on the other side, closing the left, inhaling through the right and exhaling through the left.
- Do this 5 times, a full round being as just described, and see how you feel. You can build on this with time and practice.
- Rest your hand. Continue alternate nostril breathing, mentally picturing the breath flowing in the nostrils as if your thumb and finger were still there. Alternatively, return to the 3-part breath, lengthening the inhalation and exhalation as feels comfortable for you.
- Imagine the rise and fall of waves in the ocean. Rise with the wave as you inhale and fall with the exhalation.

Practice offering: Ocean meditation

- Go through all the mindful actions as described in the previous offerings, either seated or in a supported semi-reclined position.

- Visualise standing before the ocean, seeing the differing colours of the water and the quality of the light. Ground your feet into the sand as it spills up, between and over your toes. Feel the air flow over your skin and the temperature around you. Listen to the shushing of the waves, the bird cries and the wind. Smell the salty tang and freshness of the air.

- Step into the water slowly and feel the coolness as it rises up your legs, over your belly and under your arms. Lie back and float. Supported, light, timeless, maybe close your eyes.

- With each deep inhalation, feel the rise of a wave beneath you. Lifting you, holding you, strong and sturdy beneath you. As you exhale, sink, surrender, soften and release while knowing you are still held.

- Notice the colours behind closed eyes and the silky feel of the water holding you. The breeze dries the salty water droplets on your sky-exposed skin. Feel the prickle and pop. Hear the rhythmic sounds of the waves. Taste salt lightly on your lips.

- Stay here for as long as you wish. Harnessing all your senses, rising and falling with the wave in each breath.

- When you are ready, allow your feet to sink onto the firm ocean bed. Slowly, noticing the water fall away from your body, walk towards the land. Allow the breath of wind and touch of sun to dry your skin and hair, as the sounds and smells of land, sea and sky keep you bound to the earth beneath you.

Mother Becoming Insights and Actions in the Middle Months

As we did in Chapter 1, this section pulls together all the threads of what you have just read. How much of it is new to you? Has it made you angry, sad, emotional or inquisitive? What impact has this knowledge and the feelings it evokes had on you? How have the practice offerings made you feel?

Remember the hike with Liesja? Take a pause in your trek. Boots off, have a drink and snack. Again, you can journal, make notes, scribble on these pages or dot point discussion topics you want to explore further. Sit with the thoughts, emotions and possible actions you want to take, remembering to be aware of that inner voice, knowing you are worth recognition and support.

How might it be for you ...

- If you lost any embarrassment or inhibition about your pelvic floor?

- If you asked for help when anxiety overwhelms you in pregnancy, and you realised you are not a failure or less for experiencing it?

- If you didn't silence yourself in your own thoughts or with others?

- If you acknowledged what women in our past suffered?

- If you journaled or talked with others when you feel angry, sad and frustrated at our maternal history?

- If you honoured the women before us by not allowing such treatment and suffering in yourself?

- If you felt fully empowered in your knowledge of informed choice and consent?

- If you were not pressured or coerced into choices, tests or treatments you do not want?

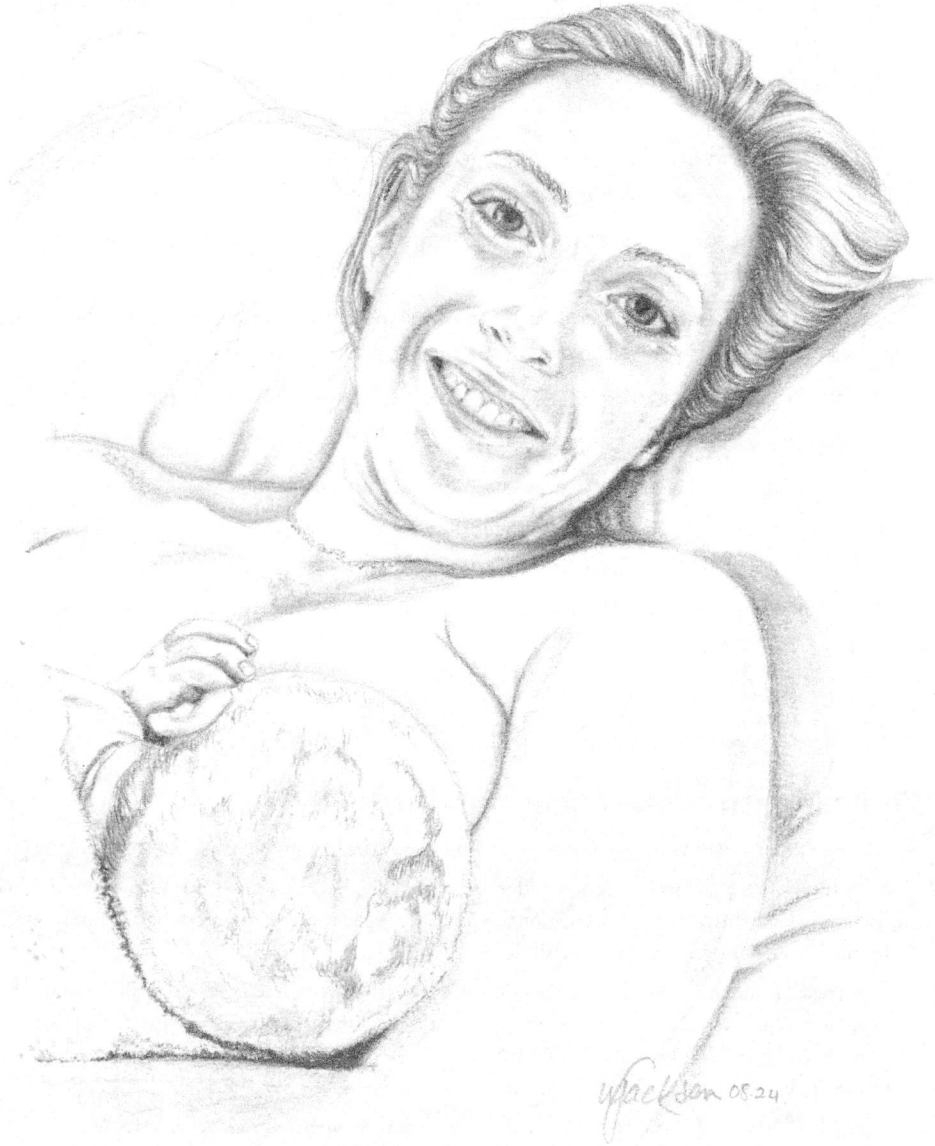

Samantha feeding Casey soon after birth. Such a sense of achievement and joy is expressed through her eyes. Her smile, an acknowledgment of wonder and love.

- If you realised the strength and capacity of your own body and, in so doing, reduced or removed fear around pregnancy, birthing and mothering?

- If the culture of self-judgement and comparisonitis did not give your inner voice permission to run amok, but embraced 'I am enough' and 'agree to disagree'?

- If you worked out the boundaries you need to survive for your mental, physical, and family wellbeing, and stuck by them?

- If you took up forward-thinking matricentric feminism and arranged superannuation contributions splitting so you feel secure in your financial future?

- If the NSW inquiry into birth trauma recommendations 15, 16 and 17 on informed consent were implemented countrywide?

- If you realised that 'scientific motherhood' and outsourcing to 'childcare experts' isn't your only option; that your intuition about yourself and your baby's wellbeing is powerful too?

- If you knew that your unique strengths mattered and you are a powerful woman in your own unique way?

- If you grew your village by choosing yourself first?

- If you celebrated a mother blessing and encouraged another mother becoming to do the same?

- If you planned for your postpartum with practical reality, setting yourself up to be supported, rather than with the impractical 'bliss bomb' the media throws at you?

- If you continued to take the time to practise the offerings here to build resilience in mind, body and spirit throughout your pregnancy?

Middle Months References and Wishlist

1   R Reed, Childbirth Physiology Course. https://www.rachelreed.website/childbirth-physiology-course

2   S Buckley, 'Hormonal Physiology of Childbearing: Evidence and Implications for Women, Babies, and Maternity Care' 2015 https://www.nationalpartnership.org/our-work/resources/health-care/maternity/hormonal-physiology-of-childbearing.PDF

3   L Corrigan, P Moran, N McGrath, J Eustace-Cook, D Daly, 'The characteristics and effectiveness of pregnancy yoga interventions: a systematic review and meta-analysis'. BMC Pregnancy Childbirth. 2022 Mar 25;22(1):250. doi: 10.1186/s12884-022-04474-9. PMID: 35337282; PMCID: PMC8957136. https://pubmed.ncbi.nlm.nih.gov/35337282/

4   AR Dangel, VO Demtchouk, CM Prigo, JC Kelly, 'Inpatient antenatal yoga sessions for women with high-risk pregnancies: A feasibility study'. Complement Ther Med. 2020 Jan;48:102235. doi: 10.1016/j.ctim.2019.102235. Epub 2019 Nov 4. PMID: 31987258; PMCID: PMC6989637.https://www.ncbi.nlm.nih.gov/pmc/articles/PMC6989637/

5   OJ Hofer, R Martis, J Alsweiler, C A Crowther, 'Different intensities of glycemic control for women with gestational diabetes mellitus'. Cochrane Review. 2023. https://www.cochranelibrary.com/cdsr/doi/10.1002/14651858.CD011624.pub3/abstract

6   PA. Balaji, SR Varne, 'Physiological effects of yoga asanas and pranayama on metabolic parameters, maternal, and fetal outcome in gestational diabetes'. National Journal of physiology and pharmacology. 2017; 7(7): 724-728 https://www.researchgate.net/publication/315470497_Physiological_effects_of_yoga_asanas_and_pranayama_on_metabolic_parameters_maternal_and_fetal_outcome_in_gestational_diabetes

7   Antenatal Perineal Massage for Reducing Trauma. Cochrane Review. https://www.cochrane.org/CD005123/PREG_antenatal-perineal-massage-for-reducing-perineal-trauma

8   R Descartes, Meditations on the first philosophy, In: Hitchins R. M, editor. Great Books of the Western World. New York: Encyclopaedia Britannica; 1952. https://scholar.google.com/scholar_lookup?title=Great+Books+of+the+Western+World.&author=R+Descartes&publication_year=1952&

9   S Napthali, Complete Buddhism for Mother, A calm approach to caring for yourself and your children, Allen and Unwin, 2003, p194. ISBN 9781742378018

10   A Foreman, H MacGreggor, L Hooper, 'The Ascent of Woman'. BB2 series. https://www.ascentofwomen.com/the-series

11   Holy Bible. Genesis 3.16. Revised Standard Edition of King James Bible. 1901. Collins

12   R Reed, *Reclaiming Childbirth as a Rite of Passage: Weaving ancient wisdom with modern knowledge*, Word Witch, 2021, p12. ISBN 978-0-6450025-1-5

13   Reed, *Reclaiming Childbirth as a Rite of Passage*, p13.

14   Reed, *Reclaiming Childbirth as a Rite of Passage*, p13.

15   C de Costa. "The contagiousness of childbed fever": a short history of puerperal sepsis and its treatment'. MJA 2002. Vol 177 P668-671. p669. DOI:10.5694/j.1326-5377.2002.tb05004.x

16   M Jowitt, *Dynamic Positions in Birth. A fresh look at how women's bodies work in labour*, Second edition. Pinter and Martin; 2020. p34 ISBN 978-1-78066-690-7

17   de Costa, "The contagiousness of childbed fever," p 669.

18   JA Bergin, (2012). Birth and death in nineteenth-century Dublin's lying-in hospitals. In E. Farrell (Ed.), *She said she was in the family way: Pregnancy and infancy in modern Ireland*, (pp. 91–112). University of London Press; p108. ISBN 9781905165650 http://www.jstor.org/stable/j.ctv51308f.14

19   Jowitt, *Dynamic Positions in Birth*, p34.

20   Fitzroy Report. 'Report on the Inter-Departmental Committee on the Physical Deterioration. Vol.I. Report and Appendix'. p48, 51, 137. Printed for his Majesty's Stationary Office, By Whyman & Son, limited, Fetter lane. E.C 1904 https://education-uk.org/documents/fitzroy1904/fitzroy1904.html

21   de Costa, "The contagiousness of childbed fever," p670.

22   O Best, B Fredericks, Editorss. *Yatdjuligin*, Aboriginal and Torres Strait Islander Nursing and Midwifery Care. Third ED. Cambridge University Press, 2021, p142-3. ISBN 9781108794695

23   de Costa, "The contagiousness of childbed fever," p670.

24   RD Apple, 'Medicalization of Motherhood: Modernization and Resistance in an International Context'. *Journal of the Motherhood Initiative for Research and Community Involvement*, (2014). 5(1). p155-126. Retrieved from https://jarm.journals.yorku.ca/index.php/jarm/article/view/39323/35652

25   RD Apple, 'Medicalization of Motherhood', p124.

26   RE Davis-Floyd, *Birth as and American Rite of Passage*, University of California Press, 1992. ISBN 9780520229327

27   C Davison, 'Looking Back and Moving Forward: A History and discussion of Privately Practising Midwives in Western Australia'. PhD 2019, p26. https://australianmidwiferyhistory.org.au/wp-content/uploads/2021/11/-2019-Looking-back-Moving-forward-THESIS.PDF

28   *Birthtime The Handbook*, Clark and Mackay, 2021, p81.

29   A Kowtoska, Informed consent and refusal in obstetrics: A practical ethical guide, Birth. 2017. 44(3). P195-199. https://doi.org/10.1111/birt.12281

30   Human Rights in Childbirth submission to the Australian Human Rights Commission to the Free & Equal: An Australian Conversation on Human Rights. 2019. p12. https://humanrights.gov.au/sites/default/files/2020-09/sub_149_-_human_rights_in_childbirth.PDF

31   Human Rights in Childbirth, p12.

32   *Birthtime The Handbook*, p72.

33   Human Rights in Childbirth, p12–16.

34   R Dempsey. 'YES, YOU CAN SAY NO!' Birthing Wisdom, 2018. https://www.birthingwisdom.com.au/yes-you-can-say-no-rhea-dempsey/

35   Dempsey. YES, YOU CAN SAY NO! p1.

36   Dempsey. YES, YOU CAN SAY NO! p1.

37   New South Wales Parliament Legislative Council Select Committee on Birth Trauma, Report. 2024. p xvi-xv ISBN: 978-1-922960-38-2ii. https://www.parliament.nsw.gov.au/lcdocs/inquiries/2965/FINAL%20Birth%20Trauma%20Report%20-%2029%20April%202024.PDF

38   S Goodwin, K Huppatz, 'The good mother in theory and research'. Sydney University Press, 2010, Chapter 1. p1. ISBN: 9781920899530 https://www.researchgate.net/publication/305851753_The_Good_Mother

39   M Risser, 'Mom Shaming: Definition, Examples, & How to Cope'. https://www.choosingtherapy.com/mom-shaming/

40   Napthali, *Complete Buddhism for Mothers*, p132.

41   V Olorenshaw, *Liberating Motherhood. Birthing the Purple Stockings Movement*, Womancraft Publishing. 2016, p 61. ISBN 978-1-910559-19

42   Olorenshaw, *Liberating Motherhood*, p185.

43   Mercy Foundation https://www.mercyfoundation.com.au/our-focus/ending-homelessness/older-women-and-homelessness/

44   Removing the Motherhood Penalty. WGEA https://www.wgea.gov.au/newsroom/removing-the-motherhood-penalty

45   ABC article 'Superannuation isn't fair for new mums. Here's what couples can do to even it up'. https://www.abc.net.au/news/2018-10-16/superannuation-system-isnt-fair-for-new-mums/10363694

46   Apple, 'Medicalization of Motherhood', p116.

47   Apple, 'Medicalization of Motherhood', p119.

48   *Birthtime The Handbook*, p143.

49   Olorenshaw. *Liberating Motherhood*, p60.

Wishlist

1. Active Pregnancy Foundation website. https://www.activepregnancyfoundation.org/

2. 'Pelvic floor health for expectant and new mums PDF by The Pregnancy Centre and Continence Foundation of Australia'. https://continence.my.salesforce.com/sfc/p/#A0000000KUc9/a/5K0000003Iek/nEDoZ3oU8.RlEab2f0E7RQ_RYNAeSA1rtAjEgDcSf0g

3. *Beyond the Bump* S1 #35 'All things pelvic floor (and why we shouldn't put up with pissing ourselves)' Apple 🎙 Spotify

4. R Dempsey. 'YES, YOU CAN SAY NO!' Birthing Wisdom, 2018. https://www.birthingwisdom.com.au/yes-you-can-say-no-rhea-dempsey/

5. MHM. 'Right Birth Your Choice'. https://maternalhealthmatters.org.au/wp-content/uploads/2023/02/Right-Birth-Your-Choice-Workbook-Jan-2023.PDF

6. Milli Hill talks to Google YouTube Video. https://www.youtube.com/watch?v=sJ7xX3ZKkU4

7. *Beyond the Bump* S1#146 'Why being a 'Good Enough' Mother is more than good enough – debunking the perfect parent myth with Dr Sophie Brock' Apple 🎙 Spotify

Chapter 3
Ashleigh With You in Late Pregnancy

Meeting Ashleigh

Ashleigh and I met during our yoga teacher training. She created the most divine desserts when it was our turn to supply a delicious lunch for everyone (alongside Ally, whom you will meet next). Ashleigh has a gentle presence, an indefatigable nature, a curious mind and a cheeky sense of humour. She was so open to learning, while often fatigued from caring for her feisty, non-sleeping toddler, Bonnie, and her surprise pregnancy with Octavius during our training.

Ashleigh was going to join Liesja, Ally and me for the postpartum part of our specialised pregnancy, birthing and postpartum training. The day she was going to join us, Octavius decided it was time to make an appearance, 6 weeks before expected. I was then incredibly honoured to be part of her birth support for her third baby, Rafael, also known as Rafrascal.

Ashleigh said no to an infusion of Syntocinon (oxytocin) on admission to private hospital after her waters broke naturally in the early hours. She harnessed her capacity and worked with yoga posture stretches, rebozo, nipple stimulation, acupressure and upright mobile postures to get into labour before the time limit she was given for intervention. While her husband provided external pressure on her pelvis to provide comfort and support her labour, we witnessed Ashleigh's raw power as she articulated what she felt: "I can feel my baby in my pelvis" and "I am going to push."

While standing, leaning on the bed, Ashleigh birthed her son into the world.

Mum to Bonnie, Octavius and Rafael, here is Ashleigh's letter to you.

"To all the mothers who were, who are and who will be"

Dear Me Nine Years Ago,

Here's what I wish I had known. Motherhood is tough. It's relentless. Physically. Mentally. Emotionally.

Pregnancy – even the journey to pregnancy – can be full of doubts and fear, as well as joy and excitement. Terrifying, aching, painful. Happiness, joy and sadness. All this, bundled into a bump! And if there's one thing you can do for any new-to-be mum, it's to give her unwavering love and support. No matter the circumstances. No matter the journey.

It isn't so much about doing birth the 'right' way or using yoga and breathing techniques to go through it. It's about feeling supported, loved and respected, and being held in a sacred place to birth safely in, whatever form that may take; to move through the birth process without fear or trauma; to be at peace with whatever arises and whatever the outcomes; to send our newborn mothers off into the first days of motherhood feeling supported, nourished and capable.

When you become a mum, you think you're going to break, and it is a kind of breaking. A breaking of all your hard edges and exterior walls, breaking into a vulnerability and dependence upon others, breaking down the rigid expectations of a life you set in one direction, only to discover the joy and heartbreak of unexpected detours, road bumps and deviations.

I look back at those years of early mothering with much regret and pain. I struggled so hard and felt so much weight and pain on a daily basis. My body felt crumpled by exhaustion and depression. Some days, I couldn't stand without feeling dizzy, nauseated and sick. I snapped and I cried and I dragged myself physically. I yelled and I broke cups and I cried every day. I stopped laughing and I stopped feeling joy. I only felt relief when the babies were asleep. I was told I chose this life. "Babies are hard. You'll be fine." And I hung and I clung on and I felt like everything was too hard, so I stopped doing anything.

But we weren't meant to do this alone.

With no level of consistent support, I stopped being active. I had no energy. I couldn't cook, because to cook was to meal plan, was to face the shops with a toddler and a baby and an alternating sleep schedule, was to clean the fridge regularly and rotate the veggies and mince, was to mash and boil and bake while toddlers tantrumed and babies cried, was to do dishes and put them away and take out the rubbish. Groceries weren't delivered then. We had no budget for takeaway. I feared burdening my family and friends. I look back now and don't even remember what we ate. Just very simple, hopefully healthy and quick, food. Everything became basic, just to survive on our own. And that was how I managed to get through the thick of early motherhood.

Running errands became one errand a day, so I could rest and recover between. One meal covered multiple days. I accepted day naps, and still do, just to keep up with life.

And as the babies grew bigger, I learned to trust myself and reject everyone else's expectations.

It has been hard to process all the anger at rejection, resentment, frustration and betrayal. Of feeling trapped with no escape.

From family and friends who won't visit if you're sick, because they'll get sick too. From family and friends who will only visit for tea and biscuits and a nice social chat. "Oh that baby is lovely, but it's dinner time, so I've got to go." From family who are busy working, live too far away, who want to come, but also can't.

But when you're not coping, and you're in the thick of it, and there's no one by your side, when the toddler is projectile-vomiting and there's diarrhoea on the bed from gastro picked up from daycare or a playground, when your baby has been waking every 2 hours to feed and breastfeeds take 45 minutes or longer, when your eyes are blurry and your back is breaking and your partner is working away for another week or 2 or 3 …

Tell me …

Where are you supposed to find the strength?

Tell me …

Where was the village?

Our society has so much to answer for in its failings of first-time mothers. Every story I read of mothers who break, of mothers who run away or hurt or, rarely, kill their babies even – how they are treated with such disgust and contempt … "Oh those poor babies." I am disgusted. Those poor mothers! My heart breaks for every single one of them.

Absolutely no mother would dream of hurting her babies. Only when you are so depleted, so broken, so unsupported …

I know the brink of those edges, where to admit you can't cope is to fear your children will be taken away, but to stay is a relentless, grinding suffering.

And this is probably why a lot of the older generations wash their hands of helping out. They did their time. They were just as burnt out as the rest of us. They don't want to go back there, as much as I struggled for months to put all of this into words.

And during this time – making friends with other new mothers, who are also burnt out, struggling, unable to support you and you unable to support them – it so easily turned to anger on both sides.

There, I have been most lucky. I have found the most beautiful range of women who have encouraged me, who saw me as a great mother, who also saw me as more than a mother. As a woman with needs and wants and a right to a happy life too.

If it wasn't for you, who encouraged me, who sat with me, who listened to me, who checked in on me, who cried with me, who supported me and reasoned with me … If it wasn't for each of you, I would have been lost on those slippery slopes of burnout and breakdown.

You have no idea of the profound impact your belief and encouragement had on me, how that pulled me out of days of suffering and depleted spirits.

I never wanted to join a mothers group, to sit around and talk about nappies and sleep schedules and mundane daily living tasks. Yet it's so essential to be among others going through it too. I found my mothers group in women who have passions outside of the household, who taught me that mothers can do and that they can be more than cooks and cleaners and butt-wipers. Mothers can hike with babies on their back, go camping with toddlers in the same camp bed, teach their kids to climb and play and sit in baby bike seats and swim together in their undies on summer days at a rocky pool while babies nap in prams.

I remember one of our first catch-ups, hiking into a national park in winter, with three-month-old babies snuggled into baby carriers and anoraks, and a backpack with snacks and a thermos of hot chocolate. It started bucketing with rain and I felt breathless with anxiety and stress. How irresponsible! We would need to call our partners to come rescue us. The shame. These same women, though, they sat about laughing and talking. In the breaks of weather, we chatted as we hiked back to our cars, popped the babies in, and all went home. Fresh air, companionship and smiles had me glowing inside for days, weeks, and even now, years later.

I ache when I hear that a friend or family member is pregnant, because I know how much help our first-time mothers need. I cannot give them that help myself, because I am still in the thick of mothering my 3 beautiful children. I try to drop off one meal, or go and listen while washing dishes, or watch a baby while they shower.

If this is a letter to pass on to the next generations of mothers, if there's one piece of advice I can give, it's to find your tribe, find those women who blow your mind, who amaze you, who inspire and encourage you to be the better version of yourself, while telling you that you are good enough already. And don't just cling to one. We can't drag each other down. We may not be able to save each other, but we do need each other. In sharing our stories, our struggles, our laughter, and our tears, we create the support and community that helps us all grow stronger. Let's lean on each other, not to be saved, but to be seen, heard and understood. That's how we build our village together.

Build your village with all of the women who do all of the things and do them all differently. Look at these women as your friends, for all their different abilities, and their different strengths, and champion them too.

May words be solace. May love stream through.

Ashleigh

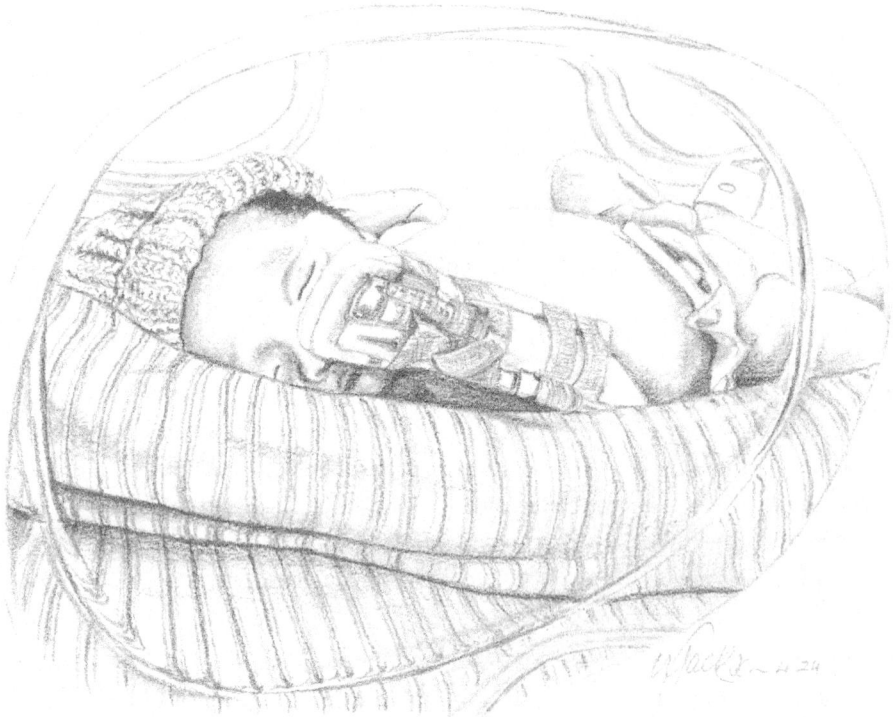

Little Octavius, being nurtured outside the womb in the neonatal intensive care unit (NICU), warm and comfortable, viewed through an access port, the shape of a womb in itself.

Dear Mother Becoming,

Reading Ashleigh's letter confirms that there are no rose-tinted glasses or bliss myths about mothering. Her honesty, given with such raw, emotion-filled vulnerability, makes the importance of preparing for the time after birth loud and clear.

Hear her words: " … if there's one piece of advice I can give, it's to find your tribe." That means finding your people early, feeling no shame in asking for help, seeking solace and love in doing these things, recognising that mum comes first. We are not meant to mother in isolation. Being connected to a community, a village, a network of support needs to be a normal part of the experience of early mothering. Mothering is the embodied journey for the rest of your life.

As we move into late pregnancy and preparing for birth here with Ashleigh, we need to invest as much time and energy into preparation for the fourth trimester too. An informed, prepared and supported fourth trimester will help reduce the risk of postpartum depression and depletion. We will be exploring this more in the social aspects of Tree Root 3, alongside finding deep trust in yourself.

All sorts of planning is happening, mostly for birth and a new baby. Much of that planning is going to be turned on its head in this chapter, because some things are out of our control. Sometimes, the dear little scamps come early, before the approximate of 37 weeks, and need some time in a neonatal unit. This was Ashleigh's experience with her second baby, Octavius. Sometimes there is a medical reason for induction or planned caesarean, making change necessary. It's still your unique journey, your birthing experience. Adapting to unforeseen, surprising or disappointing changes can still be made special.

We will discover a different way of planning for birth, which will make it easier to adjust to surprise changes, like planned inductions and caesarean birthing, and still make you feel safe, emotionally supported, listened to and respected. Whether you choose to birth by caesarean section or homebirth, for whatever reason, it's your choice. This is your mother becoming rite of passage. No matter how you birth, you have not failed.

Prepare for some fascinating information about the physical effects that hormones have on your brain and behaviour. I share some thought-provoking information about group B streptococcus (GBS), induction of labour, external fetal heart monitoring (EFM), and their associated risks.

Late pregnancy can be challenging and uncomfortable. Tears of fatigue will spill over, but they won't last. Surrendering to watchful, patient waiting is really important. Your body and baby are working together here to begin your unique birthing journey, when you are both ready.

The truth about how much money is made from women giving birth is going to be aired and shared. You will learn how it started, find out about the current exploitation of birth for financial gain and provider convenience, and we will begin to look at ways to change this situation. We'll also consider the disempowering and demeaning language that currently exists around birth and how it must change.

After that doom and gloom notification, bring on your mother blessing celebration! Yay! Mark this time of your life with honour and the mother-centredness it deserves. May it be fun, filled with emotion and commemoration. Build memories and strengthen the ties of your village.

Let's begin the next stage of our journey through the late phase of pregnancy with Ashleigh's words of solace and love enveloping us. Boots on, thermos of tea, snacks, pen for notes and doodling.

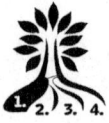

The Physical, Hormonal and Emotional Influences on Late Pregnancy

Pregnancy, labour and birth as a 'rite of passage'

Before we discover more hormonal effects of late pregnancy and early labour, Dr Rachel Reed's description of *phases of labour* is helpful here. This terminology replaces *stages of labour*. Her use of *rite of passage experiences* helps us understand labour and birthing in a different way. Currently, stages of labour are identified and used to measure for progress, which limits the time allowed for those stages and encourages intervention to speed things up.[1]

What are rite-of-passage experiences and why do we acknowledge their significance throughout matrescence? In anthropology (the study of humans, society and culture development), a rite of passage is a ceremony that acknowledges a person's change in status and identity, such as puberty and marriage, and marks the passage from one life stage to another. The ceremony usually involves *separation*, which is the leaving of the familiar, and *transition*, a time of testing, learning and growth. Part of the rite is *liminality*, the middle stage, like being suspended, evolving from *what was* to become *what will be*. When the rite is complete, *reintegration* into society occurs.

Pregnancy, labour, birth and becoming a mother are part of an ancient wisdom where we can use ceremony and celebration to mark an enormous physical, emotional and psychological change. A mother blessing as a rite-of-passage ceremony recognises theses phases of transition and change.

The first phase in labour and birthing is the *separation* phase, which is the terminology we will use to replace *latent and early labour stages*. This is where the woman begins leaving the familiar bustle of life with enough of the thinking part of the brain remaining active. Here, we are activating the village of support, arranging childcare and preparing the space for labour, and encouraging oxytocin to flow.

In this chapter, we will be recognising, valuing and supporting the importance of this phase, which may be weeks in preparation, with days of separation that you will forever remember. We acknowledge that this part of the labour experience is significant.

Then, we move on to the *liminal* phase, which replaces the *first stage of/established labour* terminology. This phase describes the importance of creating an environment of trust and safety to support transition, retreat and the ability for a woman to sink into the instinctive mammalian part of her brain. With Ashleigh, we will be exploring how to optimise and surrender into labour, as well as birthing in the environment and culture you choose or need.

Our orchestra of hormones in late pregnancy[2]

Introducing the musician **oxytocin,** the hormone most associated with birth. **Oxytocin** is produced in the more primitive part of the brain, the hypothalamus. It is secreted in pulses by the pituitary gland during labour, which is why contractions are at intervals. When first discovered, its association with labour and stimulation of the milk ejection reflex meant it became known as the 'mothering hormone' or 'the hormone of love'. Little further research was done on it until Dr Kerstin Uvnäs Moberg devoted her professional life to it. In her book *Why Oxytocin Matters,* Uvnäs Moberg suggests it should be renamed 'the hormone of health and life' as it is a powerful stimulant for social interaction and incredibly strong bonding with your newborn.[3]

There is a surge in energy towards the end of pregnancy and an instinct to prepare the home for a baby, which is driven by oxytocin. In labour, when working in harmony with the hormone **beta-endor-**

phin, oxytocin creates a mild euphoria. This hormone is powerful in the parent-partner too.

Oxytocin stimulates the release of **vasopressin**, which increases the potential for deeply meditative brainwave states. This action works to enhance your ability to withdraw into yourself during labour, to sink into liminality. **Vasopressin** cleverly heightens the responsiveness of the oxytocin receptors of your uterus ready for contractions in labour. It is oxytocin that causes the uterus to contract, starting at the top of the uterus (the *fundus*) and working its way down to the cervix. This action causes the cervix to thin and dilate while the fundus becomes thicker and pushes the baby downwards.

Oxytocin also reduces stress, fear, inflammation, the sensation of pain, and is necessary for digestion. It stimulates calm, growth and healing, and assists with reproduction by stimulating the release of eggs from the ovaries and helping sperm to swim. It is as much a male hormone as female and is present throughout our lives.

Oxytocin is stimulated by human interactions, such as touch, a social event, massage, hugs and laughter, and is heard loudly in labour, during sex and orgasm.

- **Wishlist** 🖋 Dr Sarah Buckley, *Ecstatic Birth. Nature's Hormonal Blueprint for Labour.* Free eBook https://sarahbuckley.com/newsletter/
- *The Midwives' Cauldron* S3 #7. 'Hormones from conception to pregnancy, birthing to feeding, bonding & attachment' Apple 🎙 Spotify
- **Wishlist** 🖋 Dr Sarah Buckley's Blog. 'Synthetic Oxytocin (Pitocin Syntocinin): Unpacking the Myths and Side Effects' https://sarahbuckley.com/pitocin-side-effects-part1/

Our next musician is **beta-endorphin**, the serious base note in this orchestra, that crescendos in this primal time of your life in labour and birth. This feel-good hormone provides physiological pain relief and, between contractions, a deeply withdrawing, resting phase. Produced in the pituitary gland, beta-endorphin acts on the central and peripheral nervous systems of your body as a reward and pleasure hormone. A naturally produced opioid, it is pain relief with an ability to respond to stress, supporting your immune function, psychological wellbeing and physical activity.

Beta-endorphin floods the body in response to pleasurable activities, such as sex and strong physical activity and exercise, especially when challenge brings an elated feeling. More on how this amazing hormone supports you in labour with Ally in Chapter 4.

Adrenaline is the musician that often gets a bad rap in this musical. However, it also has lighter and brighter notes that are purposeful and reassuring within the melody. Produced in the adrenal glands, adrenaline is released in response to stressful experiences, which can be positive or negative, triggering the body's fight-or-flight response. When we're excited but nervous, for example on a rollercoaster ride, a release of adrenaline occurs. Although frightening, we will find the rollercoaster exhilarating too, adapting in response to our situation.

Adrenaline provides a noticeable increase in strength and performance, and heightened awareness in stressful times, increasing mental concentration. In response to danger, it causes air passages to dilate, providing your muscles with oxygen, triggering blood vessels to contract and redirect blood to the heart, lungs and brain (our most-needed organs when in danger, because they facilitate fighting and fleeing). We discover more about adrenaline in Ally's chapter.

Melatonin, the sleep hormone, increases uterine sensitivity to oxytocin. Darkness and low lighting encourages the pineal gland in the brain to secrete melatonin. Working in harmony, melatonin and oxytocin make labour more likely to begin at night, when there is less busyness, other children are asleep, and retreating to a peaceful place is more possible.

Making their sound heard again here towards the end of pregnancy and in the separation phase are musical friends **progesterone** and **oestrogen**. **Prolactin** features here too, which we talk about more with Alysia in Chapter 6.

Oestrogen rises significantly towards the end of pregnancy. In the hours before labour, transference of certain hormones through the placenta from the baby stimulates increased oestrogen. It also stimulates the production of oxytocin receptors in the uterus and breast. This transference lets the mother's body know the baby is ready for the eustress of labour and transition to being born. The baby is able to adapt to the stresses of hypoxia during contractions, being born and transitioning to breathing and breastfeeding.

Oestrogen is needed to initiate the release of other chemicals, including relaxin, to begin ripening the cervix. 'Ripening' the cervix means softening it ready for the action of contractions, thinning it gradually, so it can open and pull over the baby's head.

Prostaglandins increase towards the end of pregnancy, playing on the cervix and softening it ready for labour. Prostaglandins are detectable in the amniotic fluid as labour draws closer.

Oestrogen then dominates, with progesterone fading into a background hum. Progesterone is no longer needed in its role to stop contractions. Oestrogen, working in harmony with uterine oxytocin receptors, begins creating the sound of strong, coordinated contractions needed in labour and to reduce bleeding after birth.

As labour begins, there is a huge surge in **prolactin**. It increases in the uterine lining (decidua) and is present in the amniotic fluid as it fills the fetal lungs and assists with respiratory preparations of the baby.

The fascinating neuroplasticity of our mother becoming brains

Understanding the physical neuroplastic changes that happen to a woman's brain during pregnancy and early mothering will help us understand this significant part of matrescence. These changes are caused by all the hormones we have been talking about.

Research shows that our brains change. On a magnetic resonance image (MRI), we can see if a woman is a new mother with 100% accuracy. The pituitary gland increases in size and grey matter shrinks by 5%. "Shrinks?!" I hear you say. Well, before allowing your inner voice to run riot with worry, let's begin at the beginning. By the end, you will be reassured and utterly amazed at our incredible brains.[4] We become so much more.

Dr Elseline Hoekzema, a leading neurologist in this field, says, "Brain changes may sound somewhat intimidating, but our findings suggest that there may be an evolutionary purpose to these changes that may serve you in some way when you become a mother … These findings provide some of the first evidence that these brain changes may in some way help a mother to care for her infant … It is not that mothers are losing brain cells, losing grey matter in these regions; it is that they actually have other cells come in to help reorganize and change up some of those connections to strengthen them, or at least make them more efficient."

Also, "It is important to stress that our findings do not suggest any link to changes in general cognitive abilities or intelligence."[5] So, our brain doesn't fall out with the placenta. Far from it!

> - **Wishlist** 🪶 *Great Birth Rebellion* podcast #140. 'Baby Brain' with Neuroscientist Dr Sarah McKay. Share this with your birthing partner and family so they understand the value of supporting you in your transition. Apple 🎙Spotify

Antenatal education

Who provides antenatal education for you? Hospital and midwifery group practice (MGP) midwives sometimes provide free antenatal classes. Your private midwife or doula may. Or do you want to do some private in-person or online classes? Antenatal classes are another source for village-building and for your partner to connect with others too. Find out what is available to you and what may be affordable.

> - **Pregnancy, Birth and Baby website.** Antenatal classes https://www.pregnancybirthbaby.org.au/antenatal-classes
> - **ABTA Preparatory resource called 'THINKNATAL',** which provides a series of educational PDF resources to fill the gap in topics such as recovery from perineal injury and caesarean birth, recovery from vaginal birth, which is not always fully explained antenatally. https://birthtrauma.org.au/thinknatal/

The NSW birth trauma inquiry made 2 recommendations for accessible, comprehensive, evidence-based antenatal education for all prospective parents and made available to CALD communities. The education should cover the different models of maternity care, aspects of birth, potential interventions that might occur and women's rights in birthing. The inquiry recommends reviewing consumer information about the options for pain relief, both medical and non-medical, during and following labour and birth.[6] Bring it on.

Group B Streptococcus (GBS) screening. To have or not?

In Australia, at around 36 weeks all women are routinely asked to do a test which involves placing a swab just inside the vagina and then around the anus. This test is for GBS, a type of bacteria. GBS naturally occurs in the vagina and rectum in approximately 20% of pregnant women without causing any harm. It doesn't reflect on personal hygiene and is not sexually transmitted. It just is. GBS comes and goes, so what may have been in the vagina at 36 weeks may not be present at birthing. If GBS is present at 36 weeks, antibiotics are given in labour via intravenous infusion.

In the UK, this screening stopped years ago because the evidence doesn't support routine testing.[7] It also ceased due to concerns about antimicrobial resistance with the overuse of antibiotics.

Babies develop symptoms of infection in the first 12–24 hours. When birthing in hospital and if you have GBS, your baby is monitored for 12–24 hours, whether antibiotics were used in labour or not.

One woman in 400 who is diagnosed as carrying GBS will have a baby who develops an infection. The baby will be treated with antibiotics. One in 3,400 babies will die due to the infection and 2 of those 3,400 will have some degree of disablement due to GBS infection.

At this point, listen to and read the resources provided. You can make up your own mind about having a swab done, and whether you want antibiotics in labour if the test comes back positive for GBS.

- *Great Birth Rebellion* podcast #6. 'GBS' Apple 🎙 Spotify
- Dr Sara Wickham website. 'GBS Screening: The Evidence' https://www.sarawickham.com/?s=gbs

Antenatal breast expressing and storing colostrum

Antenatal breast expressing (ABE) is a great way to have your own colostrum stored and ready to give your new baby if needed. Colostrum is the milk your body produces in late pregnancy and the first few days after birth. It is liquid gold and discussed in detail with Alysia in Chapter 6. Sometimes lactation can be delayed when having a caesarean, elective or emergency birth. If the mother has polycystic ovarian syndrome, has surgical implants or hypoplasia (little breast tissue), or multiple sclerosis, establishing breastfeeding may be delayed. Antenatal breast expressing is particularly useful if mothers have gestational or Type 1 diabetes mellitus; colostrum is used to maintain the baby's blood sugar until breastfeeding becomes established. It is also useful where a baby has a suspected cleft palate, or a cardiac or other congenital condition that may require separation for surgery, or lead to their needing assistance with feeding for a while.

Please have a listen to *The Midwives' Cauldron* about antenatal hand expression.

- *The Midwives' Cauldron* S3 #15. 'Antenatal hand expression with Anita Moorhead' Apple 🎙 Spotify
- Pregnancy, Birth and Baby website. 'Top 5 Tips for ABE' and more. https://www.pregnancybirthbaby.org.au/antenatal-expression-of-colostrum#how
- 'How to manually express colostrum' YouTube. https://www.youtube.com/watch?v=0fOZF9si_Us

Breastfeeding: informing yourself

Breastfeeding is undoubtedly the best for your baby and in many ways for you too, due to the feel-good hormonal influences of prolactin and oxytocin.

Breastfeeding requires support, not only while you learn and experience a new skill, but also because you need an environment that allows you time to feed, and nourishes you too. Your body uses a huge amount of energy lactating and as your body adjusts to a non-pregnant state of being. You need nourishment so that you can feed your child.

- Australian Breastfeeding Association (ABA) website. A great place to start. https://www.breastfeeding.asn.au/
- *Birth-Ed* S3 #6. 'Breastfeeding Preparation with Midwife Shaheda Khan' is rich in insights and wisdom. Apple 🎙 Spotify

Your circumstances are unique to you when it comes to support, time, family dynamics, work and financial demands. Breastmilk pumping time needs to be supported at home and in the workplace. Your choices on how you feed your baby are yours alone and shouldn't be judged.

I'll be talking a lot about breastfeeding with Alysia in Chapter 6 and Clémentine in Chapter 7.

While these are the postpartum chapters, late pregnancy is the time to begin thinking about it, to discover how you want to feed your baby, how you can support yourself in your choices, and what the physical, emotional and practical demands will be. If you passionately wish to breastfeed, look into breastfeeding support and a lactation consultant in your area now, as it will prepare you for any needs and complications, should they arise.

Empowering birthing experiences through birth support

Your birthing partner of choice walks the journey of this book with you. Trusted support is of infinite value to your emotional and physical wellbeing in labour and birthing. Research shows that teaching women and their partners holistic supportive techniques significantly improves outcomes and satisfaction. Holistic means using acupressure, visualisation, relaxation, breathing, massage, yoga techniques and practical partner support. The research shows the caesarean section rate declined by 44%, with 65% less use of epidural analgesia. There was a 50% reduction in medical intervention with augmentation.[8] Augmentation includes having an artificial rupture of membranes (making a hole in the bag of fluid around the baby) and starting synthetic oxytocin via an intravenous infusion. This is discussed in detail in Chapter 5 with Katie. Your birth partner and support is really significant.

> • *Great Birth Rebellion* #28. 'How to be a great birth supporter' is great to listen to together.
> Apple 🎙 Spotify

In addition to your dearest birth partner, one way to help negotiate continuity of care is working with a doula. What is a doula? A doula is a person who provides emotional and physical support and education to the woman and her partner during pregnancy, birth and postpartum in a non-medical capacity. As *Birthtime The Handbook* suggests: "Where the system prevents midwives from providing woman-centred care, women find a way to get support they deserve and desire. For some women, this means engaging the services of a doula."[9]

It is very important to define the difference between a doula and midwife. A midwife is a trained professional who has expertise in holistic personalised care that emphasises natural childbirth, while also being skilled in recognising and responding to complications. Midwives provide appropriate care while respecting the mother's autonomy, preferences and values.

It would be wonderful if doulas were embraced by hospitals. Continuing the unique relationship of trust and support for women who employ them. Yet many private hospitals are very resistant to doulas being in the birthing room. A labouring woman's experience shouldn't be affected by external egos or a 'them and us' mentality between care providers. Providers should work together to create the best environment, care, experience and feeling of safety.

Preparation for birthing

The results of the Australian Birth Experience Study (BESt) show that 77% of woman had made a birth plan. However, only 56% of those women felt supported in their birth-planning choices. Almost half where not supported in their hopes for labour and birth. This is so sad and has to change. Communicating your wants and needs to your health professional is really important. Some form of written guidance from you is essential to help them understand you. This opens up the conversation, sets the mood and is particularly helpful in our current system of fragmented care, where you may not have met the midwife or possibly doctor. Don't be fobbed off and feel you have to leave it in your bag. This is your body, your experience. Professionals need your consent to any care they give you.[10]

Here's an idea to get you started. Plans are quite structured and rigid. Any changes may lead to a sense of losing control or failure for not meeting the expectations of the plan. A map, on the other hand, can be seen from an aerial view, doodled on, paths changed according to the terrain, weather and circumstances. Prepare for different possibilities, and remain empowered during the journey. You might not end up on the path you originally plotted for your journey, but you navigated it your way to get to where you wanted to be. Birth-mapping for fluidity is a great alternative to a rigid plan.

So, yes, in a way you still write a plan, but you and your support person have navigated where you would like to go if different situations present themselves. You can inform yourself of choices you wish to make in different scenarios. Birth maps or plans or journeys, whatever you wish to call them, need to be supported by healthcare providers. This engages you in the process, and gives you realistic expectations about feeling emotionally and physically safe.

As part of your mapping, particularly if complications arise in your journey, RANZCOG's 'Women's Health Statement and Guidelines' is a source of information about changes to your mode of care. It gives insight into how your obstetric care provider may approach your care pathway. Ask for, or look up, the guidelines of the hospital you are birthing in too.

- Dr Catherine Bell, 'birthmaplife'. She has a mission "to provide all women with the means to make confident decisions regarding their pregnancy care, labour, birth and parenting." Explore 'birthmaplife', which has access to her book and online game in the member area. It "assumes nothing and prepares for everything". https://birthmap.life

- 'Women's Health Statement and Guidelines' website. Royal Australian and New Zealand College of Obstetrics and Gynaecology (RANZCOG) https://ranzcog.edu.au/resources/statements-and-guidelines-directory/

Movement in birthing

In birthing, movement is instinctual. There is a dynamic intuitive dance between the woman and her baby. The woman listens to her body and knows how, when and where to move to relieve the intensity of contractions. She is in control of her own body. She allows for the natural outward movement of the sacrum (nutation) to make space for the baby's head in the pelvis, as we saw in the illustration with Samantha.

This is a physiological achievement of evolution.

Our discussion with Samantha highlighted that the pelvis and soft tissues are deeply interconnected; it involves so much more than we currently consider in labour and birth. However, in hospitals, where 97% of births in Australia take place, the set-up of the room often restricts movement. This is due to the main feature of the room: the bed. Women are put on beds, on their backs, which provides convenient access to her by the care provider. This confining of movement constricts nutation, causing delay in labour and a snowball effect of interventions.

Sadly, many unassisted spontaneous vaginal births are in the *lithotomy* position, in which the woman is confined to the bed. Her legs are spread wide apart, her most intimate body is exposed, she is uncomfortable and unable to move when instinct takes her. As Professor Hannah Dahlen states in *Birthtime*,

" … look at our hospital systems. We have a big bed in the centre of the room, and we put women on it, and they never get off, so no wonder they're in pain. Once again, we fail women when we don't help them work with pain."[11] Birthing should not be about giving the care provider convenient 'access' to the woman.

Birth supporters can create an environment that encourages activity rather than passivity, by providing an environment where women freely choose movement that is right for them. Squatting, upright forward leaning, kneeling, on all fours, lying on their side – these positions make space for the sacrum to move outwards. Mobility and these positions also reduce perineal trauma, interventions, episiotomies, ventouse or kiwi cup (a suction cap applied to baby's head), forceps and caesarean births. Some suggestions:

- Move the bed to the side of the room, raising it up so the mother can lean against it.
- Use birthing balls, mats and cushions for the floor.
- Ensure low lighting and low noise.
- Create a private space: phones on silent, TV off, 'Please do not disturb' sign on the door.
- Provide water via a bath, birth pool or shower. In water, the labouring woman may move to a semi-reclined posture, floating, pelvis open, perineum supported by water.
- Provide a peanut ball to go between the legs, making space, if lying on her side.
- Use language that is suggesting and encouraging, to assist a woman's movements, while not being prescriptive.

These suggestions create a safe *mobile* space, where the labouring woman is actively supported and is able to move where her instinct directs her. Some women may choose to sit or lie down and that is their unique way of labouring and birthing.

Yoga is an accessible way of working with your body to move towards achieving an opening of the pelvic structures, creating space in the pelvic bowl for your baby's head as the sacrum moves outwards – releasing, and lengthening, and softening the ligaments and muscles.

None of this is meant to pressure you into feeling you must do lots of extra activity every day to prepare your body for birth. If it doesn't go the way you hoped, it's not that you didn't do it right or enough. I don't want you to feel as though you have failed! The intention of this chapter is to provide you with knowledge and practices that nourish you, make you feel connected to your body, and translate into labour, birthing and postpartum recovery.

- **The 'Dutch Pelvis' YouTube.** A fabulous demonstration to understand the movements your baby makes during labour and birth. https://www.youtube.com/watch?v=vZCvf5ggBxs
- **Midwife making a birthing room movement-friendly.** Facebook video. https://www.facebook.com/watch/?v=2188362614744534
- **Labour Hopscotch App with video.** https://labourhopscotch.netlify.app/

Also, know you can ask for the fetal monitoring machine to be placed outside of the room. It isn't needed in healthy labour and birthing, because a handheld Doppler can be used to listen to the baby instead. More about this a bit later.

Posterior baby and optimal fetal positioning. What is it all about?

There is some theory about how our sedentary lifestyles may have a link to what we term a *posterior baby*. This is when the baby's face is towards your pubic bone, as opposed to *anterior*, when baby faces the sacrum. While no clear evidence exists for the idea that sitting is a cause, there is negativity about this position, which is called *occipito posterior* (OP). Although a posterior baby may present into the pelvis in labour, it is important to know that this is a normal physiological position. Dr Rachel Reed notes in her blog 'In Celebration of the OP baby' that about 15–30% of babies start labour in this position, but fewer than 5% stay that way.

This posterior position may lead to longer, more intensely felt labour because the diameter of the head presented into the pelvis is wider. This is why midwives and doulas may use manoeuvres and other methods to relieve discomfort and assist the baby to rotate into an anterior position. This variation only really matters in deep labour if there is deemed to be 'delay in progress' in the hospital environment. In Chapter 4 with Ally, we will be talking about the physiological labour plateau, a natural rest or pause in labour that can occur at any time. We cover how these pauses can be mistaken for labour *dystocia*. Dystocia is a slowing of labour due to external and/or internal pathological influences. This is when medical assistance for labour and birth is needed.

During late pregnancy, if you experience lower back pain discomfort, you can help ease this with forward-leaning, hip-opening positions. For example, you might use a birthing ball at home and work, a kneeling stool, or even turn a chair and sit on a cushion with the corner positioned between your legs. It's a simple change to make you more comfortable.

- *Shebirths* S4 #4. 'Preventing Posterior & Breech Birth With Midwife and Spinning Babies founder Gail Tully' Apple Spotify

- **Dr Rachel Reed Blog**. 'In celebration of the OP baby' https://www.rachelreed.website/blog/in-celebration-of-the-occipito-posterior-baby

- **Wishlist** Dr Rachel Reed YouTube video series. https://www.youtube.com/@drrachelreed Including YouTube 'Occipito posterior position (back-to-back) in labour' https://www.youtube.com/watch?v=ZLUW85oiXeU&t=10s

- **Wishlist** 'Learning to facilitate birth with biomechanics – are we getting it right?' YouTube with midwife Molly O'Brien. Illuminating information about the dynamics of birthing. How to help yourself and those supporting you for your comfort and assisting the movement of the baby in the pelvis. https://www.youtube.com/watch?v=7cX58bXeEQ8&t=1046s

- *Birth-Ed* S2 #3. 'Your Baby, Your Pelvis and Labour Dystocia' Apple Spotify

---

When labour starts, how does the body know?

The physiological (spontaneous) beginning of labour is not yet fully understood and the timing is thought to be determined by the baby's maturity, via fetal cortisol production, and coordinated with the mother's readiness. It can't be predicted or controlled due to normal variations in the length of human gestation. There is a transition of the woman's conscious perceptive behaviour, and the physical irregular, low-frequency uterine activity in pregnancy, which transforms into the high-frequency, high-intensity uterine contractions of labour. This transference in emotional, perceptive and physical expression of behaviours usually begins during the night, when melatonin works with oxytocin to trigger contractions.

The separation phase of early labour

In this separation phase, the intricate dance, melody and interplay of notes of all the hormones discussed earlier are preparing the woman to begin separating herself from her external world. It can take weeks, days, hours, and is unique to each woman. It's her instinctive signalling to find a safe place with safe people, so she can labour and birth. Adrenaline has a purposeful surge in getting to this safe place and then isn't required. In the safe environment, she can finally sink deeply into her neocortex, the mammalian part of the brain, where beta-endorphins and oxytocin can flow. Prolactin also surges in early labour. As your body settles into this phase, rest, sleep, doze, snack ... rest, sleep, doze, snack ... rest, sleep, doze and snack again. You will need your energy for later.

An environment where oxytocin feels free to flow supports contractions to continue. The strength of the contraction is powered at the top of the uterus, compressing the placenta and amniotic sac, equalising the pressure around the baby and building gradually. This stimulates the body's release of beta-endorphins (natural pain relief) as labour happens. Contractions press the baby down onto the cervix, stimulating further oxytocin release, pulling the cervix open and descending the presenting part of the baby through the pelvis.

This incredible phase needs to be recognised as the whole of the woman's experience, because it is acknowledgment of her capacity. The work she has done to come fully into her labour and the implications of her separation phase experience are extremely important for the entire onward birthing journey.

The separation phase is often not considered worthy of note in obstetric practice. Only when labour is considered established is it deemed worthy of professional time and attention.[12]

Supporting oxytocin to flow at home

Please delete any apps for timing your contractions. You and those around you will know when the intensity of the contractions indicates it's time to call the midwife or transfer to the hospital. Timing is restrictive and keeps the thinking brain switched on.

You can prepare a safe and comfortable place to labour at home with your support for as long as possible. Oxytocin will be free to flood the body and adrenaline will lower. The following items and conditions can facilitate this:

- activating your village for supportive care of other children
- darkness, low light, blinds down
- quiet or gentle music, like a hypnobirthing soundtrack
- phones on silent
- meals, snacks, and plenty of fluids for everyone
- comfortable space, harnessing all your senses of sight, smell, hearing, taste and touch
- affirmations, pictures, music, aromatherapy lavender, yoga warm-up sequence and stretches, massage, gentle touch, stroking
- maybe a projection of stars and space
- mobilisation, position changes, TENS (transcutaneous electrical stimulation)
- shower, bath, pool, birthing ball, corner of chair, massage, pelvis pressure as illustrated in Chapter 4 with Ally
- dancing or moving your pelvis in a figure of 8

- Rebozo, a Mexican method that uses a long scarf for 'sifting' the pelvis and body for comfort
- the Hopscotch App on your phone, a great guide for moving. Have a look now, ready for labour.

There is no hard and fast rule for transferring to the hospital, if you're going there to birth. Waiting for '3 contractions in 10 minutes' is a poor guide, because it is impossible to know where a woman is in her phase. Go with how you feel. Intuit. Listen to your body. We will explore birthing more with Ally in the next chapter.

- *The Midwives' Cauldron* S4 #15. 'Early Labour' Apple 🎙 Spotify For confidence in listening to your body during this phase.
- **Rebozo techniques for an easier birth.** YouTube. https://www.youtube.com/watch?v=T_jSnrCXNtk

A change in the labouring woman's environment activates her neocortex into the 'thinking brain', which slows down contractions. Such changes might include the drive to hospital, arriving, and interacting with staff. This is a normal response. Once the woman's environment is restored, her hormonal song will harmonise again.

Prepare to minimise the effects of this by thinking about your move to hospital in advance and how you might keep the oxytocin flowing. You might wear sunglasses to keep that lowlighting feel and headphones with music to minimise distractions. You could consider your position in the car. For comfort, cushions can raise your sitting position to a more forward position instead of reclined. You can also place something in the footwell to raise your feet so you are in more of a squatting position. Try it out beforehand.

Empowered planned caesarean birthing

I am immeasurably grateful for the ability to plan the date of the birth of a baby by caesarean. This may be for women who have complications of pregnancy, such as placenta praevia (placenta covering the opening of the uterus), or women with pre-existing medical variations, such as a congenital heart condition where labouring may place too much strain on the heart. Then there are biological variations such as fibroids (growths in the uterus), or congenital variations of the pelvis where vaginal birthing isn't possible. There are also women who have *tocophobia*, a deep fear of giving birth and previous birth trauma.

I'm also grateful this exists for the unborn baby. A caesarean birth may be needed if there is a variation, in which experiencing labour would place undue stress on their condition, or if the baby will require surgery very soon after caesarean birthing, or in a twin pregnancy where the presenting twin (first twin who will be born) is in the breech position and the second twin is head down. Here, it prevents what is termed *head lock*, where the babies become stuck together and are difficult to birth vaginally.

I'm not writing any of this to frighten you, but to inform you that caesarean birthing, in an environment that is prepared for you and your baby, can be a beautiful experience. It is not a failing, but a blessing that we can birth in this way when it is needed, letting us optimise the health of mother and baby. We can empower your experience by birth-mapping for your own unique wishes, so that you experience a positive caesarean birth. You may choose, for example, music you love playing, quiet tones from the staff, watching the birth, having your baby on your chest skin to skin immediately, closely observed while on your chest, facilitating the first breastfeed, or having everyone sing 'Happy Birthday' to your child.

As I mentioned earlier, no matter how you birth, you haven't failed if it isn't a spontaneous vaginal birth. The following inspirational resources are information and support for a positive caesarean. Look into them now during the third trimester. Some mothers ask for a maternal assisted caesarean section, where they scrub up and lift their baby from their uterus. Your care provider may support this; it may not be your cup of tea, but it is worth asking if it does appeal to you!

- Dr Sarah Buckley Blog. 'How to Have the Best Cesarean' https://sarahbuckley.com/how-to-have-the-best-cesarean/
- *Great Birth Rebellion* #37. 'Positive Caesarean' Part 1 Apple 🎙 Spotify
- *Great Birth Rebellion* #38. 'Positive Caesarean' Part 2 Apple 🎙 Spotify
- *Great Birth Rebellion* #39. 'Maternal Assisted Caesarean Section' Apple 🎙 Spotify

Premature labour and birth

In honour of Ashleigh, whose second baby was born at 34 weeks and spent time in neonatal intensive care, let's talk a bit about premature labour and birth. Premature labour is when labour occurs before 37 weeks, where your body has prepared for labour earlier than expected and we don't always know why. The onset of regular contractions, abdominal tightening and pain, lower back pain, pelvic pressure and fluid leakage are all signs – separately or sometimes together. Calling your healthcare provider is an absolute must if this happens.

The chance of premature labour increases with twins, previous premature birth, infection, anomalies of the cervix, substance abuse and stress. Medication is administered to stop contractions. Steroid injections can be given to the mother to help the baby's lungs mature more quickly before birth. Care providers will investigate why premature labour has started.

In Australia, we are incredibly lucky to live in a country that has neonatal intensive care units (NICU). Being mum to a baby who needs extra care in the neonatal unit is an emotional and physical upheaval in so many ways. Not only is mum separated from her baby much of the time while in hospital, but the logistics of visiting from home, breast pumping and storing milk, arranging care of other children and the transition to breastfeeding need consideration and support. Add in anxiety and a myriad of other emotions with these physical demands, and mothering a baby in NICU makes this experience deeply challenging.

Here, as much skin-to-skin time with mum as possible allows for maximum oxytocin production for breastmilk. This should be supported, as research into skin-to-skin holding in NICU increases maternal milk volume and supports low birth weight babies.[13] We'll be chatting much more about skin-to-skin time with Ally and Alysia in Chapters 4 and 6.

- **Pregnancy, Birth and Baby website.** https://www.pregnancybirthbaby.org.au/supporting-parents-of-sick-or-premature-babies#resources
- **The Australian Parenting website.** https://raisingchildren.net.au/newborns/premature-babies-sick-babies/neonatal-intensive-care/coping-with-nicu
- *Birth-Ed* S2 #9. 'NICU, Neonatal Intensive Care with Dr Frankie Harrison' Apple 🎙 Spotify

Practice offering: *Svaha* and *Brahmari* – humming bee breath

The practice of svaha is to surrender. We like to know what is going to happen and when it will happen. Having some measure of control over our lives makes us comfortable. Yet so much of pregnancy, birthing and new mothering is unknowable and about adapting to sudden change. When there is an unexpected variation, complication or waiting … waiting … waiting... for labour to begin, it is difficult. This is why we cultivate the practice of svaha. So be it.

Svaha is to sit with what is uncomfortable – disappointments, changes and adaptations – with awareness, grace and patience. It is to sit with, and be in the joy of, the unknown of patient waiting. It is the discovery of your body's capabilities, and the love and confidence in you that is held in your support village. Svaha is surrendering into trusting your body's capacity and innate instincts, taking all that you have learned with you into any complications or variations that may occur.

Often, the sound mothers make in birthing is "oooooo", "aaaahhhh" and "uummmmm". These happen to be the 3 sounds of Om (Aum) fully pronounced. Birthing is primal. Sound expressed by a birthing woman is utterly normal and to be embraced, not suppressed.

Brahmari, the humming bee breath, is just that: humming. To become familiar with the normality of the sounds made during labour and birthing, try this practice.

- Sit in a comfortable supported pose, keeping your spine upright and top of your head reaching upwards. (Or just lie down comfortably somewhere … whatever you feel like.)

- Breathe normally, roll your shoulders and head, releasing through the neck, spine curved, almost tucking into a ball, then the opposite way, arching your back, chest out, chin to the sky, then settle to a neutral position.

- Wiggle about through your hips and pelvis until you feel your entire body soften and release in the posture.

- Close your mouth with teeth slightly apart to release any tightness in your jaw.

- Close your eyes or take a soft gaze if you prefer, and then block your ears with your fingers or some ear plugs.

- Take a slow, deep, breath drawing into the belly, letting it expand outwards, the side ribs expanding and the upper chest filling (an internal hug of your baby too).

- As you breathe out, make a humming sound for the entire release of breath, slowly squeezing the air from your lungs. Take particular notice of the vibration you feel through your head and body. The first time, be a bee and hum to your heart's content for 5 long, full breaths. Then, gradually increase the number to whatever feels comfortable for you.

- You may like to chant Om, or Aym (sounds like "I'm"), which is the feminine of Om, lengthening the "mmmmmmmmmmm".

- Or find a word that feels personal and strengthening to you. End with a long "ooooo", "aaahhhh" or "mmmm".

Another incredibly positive part of practising your humming, chanting, singing – whatever calms you and your baby – is listening to yourself. Remember the feel-good hormones passing through to your baby and how your baby can hear you? This association with sounds and your calming practice can be hummed or sung when soothing your baby after they are born. They remember. And, they associate the sound with the feeling.

Do a bit of a stretch and warm-up when labour is in full flow. You can prepare with an *asana* (yoga posture) warm-up and release through the pelvis using all you have learned to optimise your experience during labour and birth. In doing this, practise svaha, surrendering into the posture. Allow the body to soften, releasing, heavy yet supported.

One research study found that "the practice of yoga provided physical and psychosocial benefits for the women of this study, including strengthening of the pelvic floor, pain relief, improvement of breathing, reduction of stress and anxiety, and strengthening of self-confidence, self-esteem and autonomy in the management of the pregnancy and in caring for themselves".[14]

Practice offering: Yoga flow for late pregnancy and early labour

These postures can be used when in early labour to soften and lengthen the muscles and ligaments of the pelvis, spine and legs. Some provide deeply restful postures in late pregnancy and labour. They will also help you find relief from sciatic pain.

1. Sit cross legged in Easy pose. Scan through your body and find a comfortable position, supported by pillows if needed. Rest your back against a sofa or wall. Place your hands on your beautiful abundant belly. Soften the pelvic floor. Become comfortable with your voice and sing "oooooooooo", "aaaaahhhh" and "mmmmmmmm" aloud. Ohm.

    Practise humming bee breath 5 times.

2. Seated forward bend with bent left knee, sole of the foot to inner right thigh. Soften the pelvic floor. Repeat for the left side.

3. Cradling baby. A deep stretch through the right hip and piriformis muscle. Gentle rock side to side. Both sides.

4. Wide-legged forward fold. Allow your head to fall forwards to experience a little more stretch down the spine and inner thighs. Soften the pelvic floor.

5. Move to all fours. Cow to Cat sequence as many times as you like. Soften the pelvic floor. Make circles or figure of 8 movements to the right, then left, when in all fours.

6. Forward deep lunge. Hands on the floor. Foot turned outwards at 45 degrees. Soften the pelvic floor. Rock forwards, backwards and in small circular motions. Repeat for the other side.

7. Forward deep lunge. Hands on the floor. Foot facing forwards and slightly inwards. Rock forwards, backwards and in small circular motions. Repeat for the other side.

8. Supported wide-legged Child's pose. Rest here as much as you like. Soften the pelvic floor.

9. Move from Child's to all fours. Inhale and lift to Downward Facing Dog. Soften the pelvic floor. Puppy pose as an alternative.

10. Upright lunge. Front foot facing forwards. Sink deep into the posture and allow time for the hip flexor to stretch. Repeat for the other side.

11. Supported Pidgeon pose. From all fours move the right foot forward and to the left under the left shoulder. Outer right ankle on the floor. Have a bolster ready under the right buttock. Exhale and sink the body down, forearms on the floor, head hanging. Breathe into this deep internal and external hip stretch. Exhale, press into the hands. Roll to the right, move to all fours, circle the hips to realign. Repeat for the other side. If this is too strong, do posture 15 as an alternative.

12. Move to a squat with feet facing forwards. Sit on a firm cushion and lean back against a sofa or wall for support if needed. Picture the pelvic floor as a lotus flower which opens as you exhale and soften into the pose.

13. Remain in the squat and turn the feet outwards for 3 breath cycles. Feet outwards assists in the early phase of labour.

14. Supported wide-legged Child's pose. Rest here as much as you like. Soften the pelvic floor.

15. Move to a wall. Put the narrow edge of your mat against the wall. Place your support cushions away from the wall with enough room for your pelvis to rest on the floor. Sit with one side of your body against the wall and back to your mat. Move yourself so your back and head rest on your support and lengthen your legs up the wall. Wiggle to where is most comfortable. Cross your right leg over the left knee. Bend the left knee, with the left sole on the wall to draw the right foot towards you. Repeat for the other side. This is a more gentle option for Pigeon pose.

    Place the soles of your feet together, knees bent and open like butterfly wings. Allow your feet to sink towards the body. Rest here as long as you wish.

16. Legs up the wall. This is a lovely posture to rest tired, swollen legs at the end of the day. Arms out to the side, shoulders soft, body supported, head heavy. Enjoy.

17. Sávāsana. Stay with your legs up the wall or move to a semi-relined or supported side-lying position.

Scan through the body and allow any tightness to soften. Breathe easily. Practise the meadow meditation offered at the end of Ashleigh's chapter, page 122.

Cultural, Herstorical and Political Influences on Late Pregnancy

The hormonal evolution of childbearing has had millions of years to optimise the physiological adaptations that occur in a woman as she becomes a mother. The evolution of westernised medicine has hugely interfered with this hormonal experience, having downstream effects on the mother becoming. As mentioned, sometimes intervention is truly needed to save a woman's life; however, as we discuss with Katie in Chapter 5, this has gone too far.

Impacts of 'his-story' on our birthing herstory

The history of interfering in herstory began with ancient Greek philosophy. The father of modern medicine, Hippocrates (460–370 BCE), left a promising legacy with the Hippocratic Oath, an oath newly qualified doctors swear to practise medicine ethically and honestly and to 'do no harm'.

Despite the oath, 'do no harm' is not being fulfilled across most of our fragmented maternity care. The philosopher Aristotle (384–322 BCE) believed women were secondary, passive and a deformed version of man. In his writings on birthing, he mused: "As to the manner of delivery, various midwives use different ways; some are delivered sitting on a midwife's stool. But, for my own part, I think a bed, girded, and placed near the fire, that the good woman may come on each side, and be more readily assisted, is much the best way."[15]

Here, Aristotle was describing the position favoured in hospital maternity care and how the media represents birthing today: the lithotomy position. The woman lies on her back, legs spread wide, held in place with stirrups, while holding her breath and forcefully straining to birth. The language used infers that the woman is 'deformed', 'delivered' and the passive recipient of others' direction.

Influential 17th century French obstetrician François Mauriceau wrote that the use of upright leaning positions in 'many country villages' was outdated and that it was better to be on a bed to avoid the inconvenience of being carried there. "The widespread adoption of the supine position was perhaps the first instance of 'just in case' obstetrics which was to have such a profound influence on maternity care."[16] Physically, the woman has now rotated through 180 degrees, from an all-fours position – able to move, sway, lunge, squat and upright-kneel – to lying on her back. In this position, her instinct to move, optimising the ability of the pelvis to expand and help the fetus negotiate its way through, is taken away. No other mammal in the world births on its back.

Obstetricians – from the Latin obstare, 'to stand by' – should stand by for when needed; however, the role seems to have absorbed most of pregnancy, labour and birthing into the medical field. Midwife means 'with woman', implying being with her throughout, caring for the physiological and whole aspects of the woman, and referring for obstetric opinion when needed.

Regaining the role of women in women's business has been a long journey and is continuing. Dr Caroline de Costa, in her book *The Women's Doc*, describes her experience of going for an interview at the University of Sydney to train in obstetrics and gynaecology in 1974. She was informed, "We never train women in Sydney," and was shown the door.[17] Her interview with Dr Meg Mulvey, who trained as a doctor during WWII, quotes her: "Women were able to train in Sydney because the men were off to the front. When they came back, the hospitals no longer took women into training."[18] Women were 'allowed' to train in such circumstances only. In 1981, Dr de Costa was one of the fewer than 5% of female obstetricians in Australia.

Today, 50% of obstetricians and gynaecologists are women and have brought with them a more humanising experience of birth. They tend to spend more time with the mother, offer more options, and are less likely to intervene in pregnancy or agree to a caesarean section with no medical reason.[19] However, interventions and the caesarean section rate are still climbing.

I mentioned earlier how research and evidence for best practice is not implemented in a timely manner to benefit women. In 1979, physician Dr Archie Cochrane (for whom the Cochrane database is named, where all evidence is graded on its reliability) awarded obstetrics and gynaecology 'the wooden spoon' for being the medical speciality least informed by scientific evidence. Cochrane observed: "The speciality (obstetrics) missed its first opportunity in the sixties when it failed to randomise the confinement of low-risk pregnant women at home or hospital. Then having filled the emptying beds by getting nearly all pregnant women into hospital, the obstetricians started to introduce a whole series of expensive innovations into the routines of pre- and postnatal care and delivery, without any rigorous evaluation. The list is long but the most important were induction, ultrasound, fetal monitoring and placental function tests."[20]

Interestingly, in the same year, the episiotomy, referred to as a 'little snip', where the perineum is cut, rose to 63% of vaginal births in the USA and 50% in the UK, without evidence of its efficacy.[21]

Routine practices, such as shaving women, giving them an enema before birth and cleaning the vulva with an antiseptic, were imposed with no evidence. These practices intimated that woman and birth are dirty. Thankfully, no longer, but it was not until the 1990s that evidence and guidelines were implemented to prevent variations in care between obstetricians. And yet, practices still oppose the evidence today, and are based on faulty, decades-old data.

Donna Garland, Acting Manager for the Royal Women's Hospital, when interviewed for *Birthtime*, stated: "There are groups who will tell you that the evidence is robust, but while it impacts their businesses, they won't support that evidence."[22]

An example of this is Friedman's curve, which is a one-size-fits-all expectation that women's cervixes will dilate at 1 cm per hour in labour. This is used as a way of monitoring a woman's progress, with no consideration that women labour uniquely and have naturally occurring plateaus (pauses in labour). This measure causes much unnecessary intervention for failure to progress, which we talk more about with Ally. Another example is the number of inductions of labour for post-dates, which is based on the outdated Naegele's rule for estimating birth, as we discussed with Liesja.

Research to improve outcomes for women is not only delayed, but remains second rate. For example, a randomised controlled trial was conducted for a new, simple, low-cost treatment for labour dystocia (where contractions become weaker due to higher acid levels in the muscle of the uterus). Simple, low-cost sodium bicarbonate was taken orally by half the women in the study. With the sodium bicarbonate, spontaneous vaginal birth increased to 84% compared to the control group (no sodium bicarbonate given) at 67%. There were no adverse effects on any fetal outcomes. This simple, low-cost treatment has the potential to improve maternal morbidity and satisfaction worldwide. In 2016 when put forward to the British Medical Research Council, which was offering funding for 'research that would benefit low- and middle-income countries', it was turned down because "it was not a high enough priority".[23]

Caroline Perez, in her book *Invisible Women, Exposing Data Bias in A World Designed for Men*, states: "The evidence that women are being let down by the medical establishment is overwhelming. The bodies, symptoms and diseases that affect half the world's population are being dismissed, disbelieved and ignored."[24]

We noted that women are viewed as a machine and cared for as though going through a factory conveyor belt. The 'obstetric dilemma' is a concept put forward to explain how, as we evolved to become an upright, two-legged walking species, our pelvises became 'inadequate' to cope with the process of birth. The changes mean that the baby has to do movements to rotate through the pelvis and be an active participant in labour and birth. We have had millennia to adapt to this. We developed larger brains. To negotiate the pelvis, the bones of the fetal head are not fused, allowing the head to mould to the shape of the mother's pelvis.

In 'There is no Evolutionary "Obstetric Dilemma"', the work of anthropologist Holly Dunsworth, she clearly states that culture (medicine, colonisation, capitalism, economic inequality, sexism, racism etc.) has helped to construct a childbirth dilemma, then packaged and sold it as a natural evolutionary 'obstetrical dilemma', when there isn't one.[25]

This obstetric dilemma theory places women at a disadvantage – they are seen as a problem to be solved. Often, first-time pregnant women are told their baby is too big for their pelvis, so an induction or caesarean is needed. Nobody can know that without the woman and fetus first having the opportunity to do their thing. In *Birthtime*, Dr Melissa Cheyney, a medical anthropologist and midwife, clearly states: "We didn't get this numerous on the planet because our bodies are so dysfunctional."[26]

Suspected fetal macrosomia (a large baby) is not an indication for caesarean birth. Also, the incidence of birth weight of 5000g or more is rare. Women should be counselled that estimates of fetal weight, particularly in late gestation, are imprecise. Screening ultrasonography done in late pregnancy has been associated with the unintended consequence of increased caesarean delivery with no evidence of neonatal benefit.[27]

Unless there is a very good medical reason, caesarean birth for a suspected 'big baby' should not be offered. Being nudged, through fear tactics, to make choices you don't want is coercive and unethical. There needs to be accountability for this practice, so it stops.

- **Dr Rachel Reed Blog.** 'Big Babies the Risk of Care Provider Fear' https://www.rachelreed.website/blog/big-babies-care-provider-fear
- *Great Birth Rebellion* #141. 'Big Babies – Small Babies' Apple 🎙 Spotify

---

IDECIDE and BRAIN

Remember the IDECIDE tool mentioned with Samantha? Another useful tool for any decision-making process is the BRAIN acronym, where you take a holistic look at your situation. Use it to seek out the following information before making a choice, which can also include doing nothing.

Take time to consider all these factors with any decision at any time:

B – Benefits. R – Risks. A – Alternatives. I – Intuition. N – Nothing.

Inducing labour

When a woman is advised she needs medical intervention by induction, there is so much unknown about how the woman will respond to the process. Assessment via vaginal examination is required to decide what sort of induction method she needs, and how and when to start induction. Assessment is done for the preparedness of her body to labour, the availability of support people, progress, and the time induction might take given the birthing environment. All these things affect the experience of the woman being induced.

How might an induction become positive, empowering and embodied?

With variations of pregnancy, such as pre-eclampsia (a condition unique to pregnancy), where induction may be needed, it is useful to have a mindset of adjustment, using all the mental and physical preparation you have done. The tools, information, practices and ideas you have learned become deeply effective here. The experience can still be yours, with decisions and involvement that optimise your experience. You can use aromatherapy, movement, massage, a yoga warm-up sequence, music, rebozo sifting and acupressure, with breast expressing and nipple stimulation to release oxytocin. Take in nutritious food and fluids for energy. Create a space within the space in the hospital environment. This all helps you be part of the sequence of care, taking part yourself, rather than the induction being something out of your control and 'done to you'.

A closer look into post-dates induction

For induction for post-dates in a healthy pregnancy, rather than for a medical necessity, I will highlight how fixation on a date can cause intervention when it isn't necessary. In *Why Induction Matters*, Dr Rachel Reed discusses the lack of evidence to support the practice of sweeping the membranes to ripen the cervix and get labour started earlier. This is when the caregiver does a vaginal examination, places a finger through the opening of the cervix, puts pressure on the cervix from inside, moving the membranes away from the lower section of the uterus and cervix. It is uncomfortable, often painful, can introduce infection and may be the cause of accidental rupture of membranes, which then leads to a cascade of intervention.[28] If offered, please consider declining.

Drawing from the wisdom and evidence presented in *Why Induction Matters* and *In Your Own Time* by Dr Sara Wickham,[29] let's look into post-dates induction a bit more.

Remember how we chatted about the EDD being an estimate with Liesja? To recap, most pregnancies last longer than 40 weeks – just 35% of women birth in the week around that date. Seventy-five per cent of first-time pregnancies who labour and birth spontaneously do so by 41 weeks and 2 days, and 75% of second and more pregnancies give birth by 41 weeks – the average is around 40 weeks and 2 days. One size does not fit all, but women are being induced at 40 weeks and 1 day for being post-dates when they and their baby are not ready for labour. They are fitted in wherever there is space in the hospital schedule. As such, the EDD can be seen as intervention itself!

Jo Hunter, midwife and co-producer of the documentary *Birthtime*, states: "As a care provider, we're in a very powerful position to be able to coerce women into doing what we want them to do. That's even by saying something like 'you've got double the risk' or 'if you choose to do this, your risk is double'. But we might only be looking at 0.1% to 0.2%. That is double. So, if you say it in a different way, then obviously the women will see it in a different light."[30]

There is a lot of fear instilled about the risk of the baby dying post-dates. However, reframing the 'risk' of stillbirth, when it comes to being post-dates, needs to be made clear.

Here are the statistics for 'low-risk' pregnancies, that is, a pregnancy with one baby, no congenital abnormality and no maternal medical condition. (Data from Muglu et al 2019, cited in Dr Sara Wickham's book).[31]

Gestation	Stillbirth % per 1000 births	Stillbirth Number per 1000 births
39 weeks	0.14/1000	1 in 7,142
40 weeks	0.33/1000	1 in 3,030
41 weeks	0.80/1000	1 in 1,250
42 weeks	0.88/1000	1 in 1,136

Sadly it is not an uncommon experience for expectant parents to turn up at hospital at 41 weeks and 3 days for a post-dates induction and be turned away, because there isn't room for them or not enough midwives. The flood of adrenaline and cortisol, and the rearrangements and sleepless nights aren't conducive to a calm environment, or responsiveness of the woman to induction, when it does happen.

Understanding the statistical possibility of stillbirth after term provides informed choice for decisions about induction. This knowledge may also relieve fear and stress from misinformation. Induction can be an intense experience, and can take days.

- YouTube. Acupressure https://www.youtube.com/watch?v=aef4LT_nxA8
- *Great Birth Rebellion* #116 'Acupuncture and Acupressure' Apple 🎙 Spotify
- The Pregnancy, Birth and Baby website. 'Inducing of Labour' https://www.pregnancybirthbaby.org.au/induced-labour
- *The Midwives' Cauldron* S3 #3 'How western medicine controls the start of labour and why this needs to stop' Apple 🎙 Spotify
- Dr Sarah Buckley Blog. 'Labour Induction: Making Choices' https://sarahbuckley.com/labour-induction-making-choices/
- Australian Birth Stories website. 'How to prepare for a positive induction' https://australianbirthstories.com/birth/how-to-prepare-for-a-positive-induction/

Introducing fetal heart monitoring

External fetal heart monitoring (EFM) still has a huge impact on the experience and outcomes of labouring and birthing women. Your consent is required for continuous EFM. There is no evidence that EFM on admission is beneficial in a healthy pregnancy. At this point in your pregnancy, I invite you to watch the video about EFM with Dr Kirsten Small and listen to her being interviewed on the *Great Birth Rebellion* podcast. As a gentle reminder, you can ask for the fetal heart monitoring machine to be removed from the birth room.

We will discuss the necessity of fetal heart monitoring in assisted labour with Katie in Chapter 5.

- Wishlist 🌿 'External Fetal Heart Monitoring, Dr Kirsten Small' YouTube. https://www.youtube.com/watch?v=aGdknPVOhiw
- *Great Birth Rebellion* #113. 'CTG in labour and birth with Dr Kirsten Small' Apple 🎙 Spotify (A CTG is the printed cardiotocograph of baby's heartbeat and mother's contractions.)

Fear and shame in birthing

The culture of fear around birthing has chipped away at women's belief in their body's strength to birth. An embodied experience of physiological birthing and pain is totally different from the medical interpretation that all pain is pathological. The body produces its own alchemy of hormones to deal with pain in labour. Many women have never heard about what it means to have a physiological, un-disturbed birth. Often, they don't know of the many supportive methods we have discussed that work with the body and its hormones to optimise the birthing experience. Using these methods, wherever and however that may be, is a must – including in hospital and when intervention is required.

With a sense of shame and the need to make sure 'down there' is looking clean, neat and tidy, why do some women feel the need to have a Brazilian wax before entering the birth room? Why do they believe they need to be quiet, so they don't upset support people or those labouring in nearby rooms? Nothing about birthing is clean, neat, soundless or tidy. Birthing is messy, physical, soundful and it is perfectly normal to be so. We are mammals with instincts that are currently being suppressed and interfered with on a large scale.

Labour pain is a normal phenomenon that tells us a woman is birthing. When birthing needs assis-tance, decision-making must remain in her hands. Empowering and supporting her is a prerequisite to her remaining autonomous in the decision-making for procedures, investigations and interventions. She is an active participant rather than a passive recipient. No longer 'done to the woman' but 'doing with the woman'.

Let's take a pause and allow all this information to sink in. Boots and pack off. Chocolate (sugar-free for GD!) and snacks with a lovely cup of tea. You may feel the breath sequence vocalising "Om" will be a good way of releasing some pent-up frustration and disbelief. If it calls you, journal, chat or sink into one of the yoga practices for some self-care and compassion.

Social, Economic and Media Influences on Late Pregnancy

In many countries, postpartum care is a living, breathing, herstorical and honoured social practice. It is embedded within cultures that care revolves entirely around the new mother and baby for 4 to 6 weeks.

In countries of Latin America, postpartum care is the 6 weeks of *cuarentena* or *resguardo* (protection). In the Netherlands, there is a heavily subsidised *kraamzorg*, which is the assistance of a person, most often a woman, who is qualified in postpartum care and breastfeeding support. The kraamzorg helps with light home chores, some cooking and fending off visitors for the first 2 weeks.

In Russia, Greece, Romania and many African and Arabian countries, as well as India, *the 40 days* are observed. In Asia, the *golden month* is practised.

During this time, the recurring themes of rest, good nutrition, support and warmth appear.[23] The new mother isn't responsible for cleaning, laundry, and sourcing, preparing and cooking food. She does not manage the myriad of demands that running a household entails or drive around dropping off and collecting older siblings from school and activities etc. She is encouraged to sleep and rest when the baby does, and is provided with good food and kept warm so that all her energy is focused on recovering from pregnancy, birth and blood loss. She bonds with her new baby and establishes breastfeeding in this time.[32]

Planning for your fourth trimester while in your third!

It is essential that we relearn the culture and practice of postpartum care. We must remember and truly believe that women need this period – emotionally and physically – for natural physiological recovery and adjustment to new mothering. It's about getting to know and falling in love with the newborn baby. Plan to have a period of time that supports, nourishes and promotes rest and sleep as much as possible. At a time of great adjustment and recovery, it's worth preparing to learn the new skills of breastfeeding and mothering in a supported environment.

In Jenny Allison's book, *Golden Month, Caring for the World's Mothers after Childbirth*, she writes, "In Western Culture, independence is regarded as a virtue and something to aspire to in many areas of life. However, if we struggle to become independent too early after childbirth, we risk isolating ourselves from help when we most need it, while our mothers, sisters, friends are waiting (sometimes desperately!) to be involved. Our isolation in turn can feed an illusion of separateness from those around us, which does not help us to flourish".[33]

Remember our changing neuroplasticity, which we mentioned in the physical tree root? This evolved in an environment of support. As Jenny Allison also gently points out: "The Golden Month is an opportunity to strengthen all relationships in the family and the community around it. This happens through the common task of looking after the mother, and from being close to the special loving, oxytocin-laden state of mother and baby... In this situation, we acknowledge our dependence upon one another, our interdependence."[34]

And so, here in late pregnancy, you are celebrating your mother blessing. Gathering your village to celebrate you and preparing to support you after birth. As an idea, maybe ask your village to gift you the book, *The First Forty Days: The Essential Art of Nourishing the New Mother* by Heng Ou, which they take a sneak peek at to prepare to support you![35] Learning from other cultures doesn't mean we have to do exactly the same things, because certain foods and practices will be completely alien to us. We can begin to find new rituals that support our family's needs. Let us integrate practices that value, acknowledge, honour and support the new mother in our westernised culture and society.

The table opposite presents some thought-provoking things to talk about in preparation for your fourth trimester.

> • Wishlist 🌠 *The Midwives' Cauldron* S2 #1. 'The importance of good postnatal care and recovery with Sophie Messager' Apple 🎙 Spotify

Generally talked about and prepared	Wish we had talked about and prepared
Baby shower	Physical and emotional impact of birth
Birth plan	Visitors and boundaries during the 'babymoon'
Birth classes and preparation for birth	Role of partner in daily, nightly support
Baby names	Creating a village we trust
Theme for nursery	Creating a 'feed and support new family group', chores
Cot, car seat and pushchair, baby monitor, colour of clothes	help and a meal train
	Role of grandparents, others – and boundaries
Breastfeeding and buying a breast pump	How to deal with sleep deprivation
Baby announcement cards and photos	Physical, emotional exhaustion
Hospital bag packing, snacks to take	Breastfeeding challenges and the support you may want
Length of maternity leave	Focus on mother versus focus on baby
Partner leave	Mental health
Chore splitting being 50/50	Economic effect of maternity leave, return-to-work
Childcare: who, what, when …	realities
Who we call when labour starts	Pelvic floor health
Our next holiday with the baby	Mother baby social and support groups
Baby will fit into our lives	Dad or parent-partner support groups
Fill the pantry and freezer	Chore splitting and how 50/50 is not reality
	How sex will be affected with a newborn

Money being made from birthing women

There are powerful political influences in late pregnancy. Not least, we currently live in a neoliberal political environment that values individualism, independence and wealth creation. This is intricately linked to the economics that affect how health care is delivered. The neoliberal approach to health care is cost-cutting. It models patients as consumers of health care. However, the 'patient as consumer' model may be a myth, because capitalist consumer models don't fit well into a healthcare structure. A normal consumer has the choice to buy something after investigating the product, how it suits them, the terms and conditions, the warranty of the product etc. The customer sees a transparent, accountable system. This isn't reflected in the choices and experiences women have in the current maternity systems of care.[36]

Nevertheless, there is money being made from birthing women. Economic gain from birthing women, and practitioner comfort and convenience have a long history. From the rise of medical men in the birthing space, who brought their tools to save women in birth, money was to be made. Male midwives and doctors exaggerated complications and the dangers of childbirth to gain more custom, while simultaneously scorning the uneducated care given by female midwives.

Dr Peter Chamberlen invented forceps, a set of metal, hollow spoon shapes that lock together after being placed either side of the fetal head while inside the vagina, to assist with birth. They were kept secret in his family for 3 generations, as they were a means of earning more money when exclusively called to attend complicated births. The Chamberlen family were Huguenots, French Protestants who fled persecution from Catholic-dominant France for England in 1569, where the second and third generations of Chamberlens trained to be doctors. The man-midwife was now fully legitimised and licensed to practice. The family would attend births with the forceps hidden in a velvet-lined box and would ask other attendants to leave the room, hiding themselves under a sheet while they 'delivered' the baby. The Chamberlens made a lucrative living this way.[37]

By the late 1900s, forceps designs were much improved and became an alternative to caesarean section in the hands of well-trained and experienced obstetricians, when used judiciously and respectfully. However, today's medics rarely see forceps because caesarean section is used more widely. With less exposure to their use or training in their use, the skill of using forceps is being lost.[38]

The rise of medical men who made money from birthing women also saw the reduction in women's mobility; they were put on a bed and were lying down for the doctors' convenience of view and access. By the 1900s, "women giving birth in hospital were effectively little more than teaching material for doctors who would go on to deliver upper and middle class women at home for a fat fee".[39]

In US history from the 1920s to the 1940s, American obstetrician Dr Joseph DeLee "recommended routine episiotomy and outlet forceps after sedating patients using ether or schopolomine (methods of sedation). Describing this as the prophylactic forceps operation".[40] Records of the US 1935–36 National Health Survey show that physicians only used forceps in 4.3% of births of families whose income was less than US$450 a year, compared to a higher rate of 14.2% if income was over US$1,859. Caesarean birth rates varied from 1.4% in families on a financial relief scheme, up to 3.7% if income was US$2,000 or more a year. If delivering in hospital, you had a 25% chance of episiotomy if on financial relief, but a 50% chance of episiotomy if earning US$2,000 or more. The wealthier a woman was, the more intervention she received.[41]

The Business of Being Born, a 2008 documentary by Ricki Lake and Abby Epstein on childbirth in the USA, challenges the American healthcare system where the medical fraternity has convinced women they don't know how to give birth. Its obstetric medical model is based on pregnancy and childbirth being pathological rather than physiological, focusing on medicine and intervention. This is a billion-dollar industry in the USA, where profit is valued over what is safest for women and their babies. At the time of broadcasting, the US infant mortality rate was the second highest of industrialised nations; hospitals were an industry with emphasis on filling and turning over rooms quickly to save time.[42] The documentary also showed women having Pitocin (oxytocin) to speed up their labour. In the US, the likelihood of a time-saving 20-minute caesarean is also very high. Again, this is obstetrician-friendly, because it fits their convenience, not the woman's. In Europe and Japan, most births are attended by midwives, but just 10% of women in the US employ midwives.

Australia's own documentary, *Birthtime*, highlights how money speaks in childbirth in this country. Professor Sally Tracy states: "We struggle to try and change anything in our system where money speaks much more strongly than good care, quality care, women's needs, women's choices, and what women want. The money rules, and if there's money to be made in obstetrics, we will have intervention and we'll have our Caesar rate continuing to rise, and we'll have women treated like something on a production line."[43]

As I have mentioned before, not all Australian privately practising obstetricians work in the way of the USA. There are some absolute gems who practise their philosophy of women-centred care and support women's choices and autonomy with integrity and authenticity.

However, obstetricians are not without fear of litigation. This is a huge pressure, as Dr Andrew Bisits states in *Birthtime*: "Care is still dominated by obstetricians. Obstetricians need to make a lot of money. That money is threatened by a whole medico-legal spectrum, which is very substantial. The different thing in Australia is that your status is mainly determined through how you do and perform in private practice. So, if something goes wrong, I think the thought process is, my standing will be threatened, my livelihood will be threatened, my status will be threatened."[44] The fear of being sued over a poor birth outcome leads obstetricians to intervene more in pregnancy and labour.

Media for positivity and feel-good vibes...

Discussion about the media has been rather negative so far, so let's turn that around here and talk about positive media that is nourishing. This is about finding media sites that align with your values, make you feel real, connected and enough, just as you are; media that does not exploit any vulnerability, or is judgy, pushy or advertisey. You'll need to identify people, communities, and online and in-person mothers groups that will truly support you, and where comparisonitis isn't welcome. There is no such thing as the perfect pregnancy, birth, postpartum or mother.

The content and social media resources suggested so far will continue to prepare you with realistic and reliable information. We have been moving away from misinformation and fear about childbirth and mothering. Let's continue to make your experiences of pregnancy informed and positive.

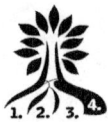

Self-identity, Beliefs and Values, and Spiritual Influences on Late Pregnancy

The language used in birth has a powerful effect on the psychology of a woman, particularly her belief in herself. Some language used in pregnancy and childbirth can be demeaning, negative and undermining. This reduces a woman's confidence in her body, further alienating her from the capacity to birth.

Communication, language and its impact on identity in pregnancy and birth

In *Birthtime*, Dr Rachel Reed states: "One third of women leave their birth experience describing their birth as traumatic. And out of that third of women, two-thirds of them say it is because of care provider actions and interaction – it is what is done and what is said to them during that birth."[45] Dr Sunitha Vimalesvaran and associates, in their article 'Mind your language: respectful language within maternity services', write: "...negative attitudes towards women and childbirth persist. In some socio-political contexts, women may still be treated as baby-making machines ... within a healthcare context, there are reports of mistreatment of women, including disrespect and verbal abuse."[46] Comments from professionals like, "You don't want to put your baby at risk, do you?" could become, "Let's help you have a safe birth". Demeaning language like 'good girl' and 'you're allowed/not allowed' ought to be removed from birthing vocabulary. Current terminology sets up women to identify as a failure, their body broken in some way, needing fixing, not being enough. Communication should be respectful of the autonomy of women too. A 2014 World Health Organization (WHO) statement emphasises the importance of 're-spectful maternity care', where we maintain the 'dignity, privacy and confidentiality' of the woman, and she is free from 'harm and mistreatment'. This emphasises the rights of women to dignified, respectful health care during childbirth.[47] It isn't hard to be kind, considerate and respectful. The Re: Birth initiative of the Royal College of Midwives (UK) set out to discover how language impacts women and the research has led to a pocket guide to change the language used by midwives[48]

This is not yet happening in Australia, but it needs to now – and it needs to happen in the obstetric profession too. Following are some examples of demeaning language and how it can be replaced by conscious language.

Demeaning language	Conscious language
Geriatric pregnancy age >35	Advanced maternal age
Inhospitable uterus	Multiple pregnancy loss
Incompetent cervix	Cervical insufficiency
Failed induction	Induction followed by operative birth
Failure to progress	Slow labour/plateau/pause
Failed homebirth	Homebirth with transfer to hospital
Patient refused	Woman declined
Poor maternal effect	Maternal fatigue
Baby delivered by/I delivered	Woman gives birth

The identity of 'mother' is important

Matrescence and matricentric feminism seek to bring mothers to the forefront of attention, to acknowledge and champion their needs. For birthing individuals who do not identify as a woman nor wish the name 'mother', inclusive language is important. Yet there is a worrying trend that such language may not be beneficial. In a news article, top researchers argue that inclusive language risks dehumanising women. Professor J Gamble has stated: "The trend to erase the use of the term 'woman' or redefine it has started to sweep the world." De-sexed language such as 'bodies with vaginas', 'gestational parent' and 'lactating and postpartum individual' is arguably disembodying, undermining and dehumanising to a woman's/mother's experience of her identity. This language further conceals a woman and mother from sight.[49] The aims of matrescence and matricentric feminism benefit all, no matter their unique identity.

Cultivating self-trust

So far, we have explored values and strengths. Now we're going to explore cultivating self-trust and self-belief, and harnessing them to bind your values and strengths and put them into practice. How can you find this deep well within yourself to draw from, so that it is a foundation for expressing your concerns and feelings? How can you be confident in your heavily pregnant body, identity transition and ability to communicate strongly in birthing and mothering without fear, embarrassment or shame?

To begin, **name** what is upsetting, or worrying you. Talk it out with the person who knows you best. Or if it's private, feel free to journal.

Then, **articulate** it. Having identified your source of stress, worry or uncertainty, ask yourself how these feelings are challenging you.

Next, **acknowledge** any distress this is causing. Take time to work through and accept the changes and feelings. Journal, meditate, cry, yell into a pillow, and allow the frustration, sadness and anger to come through.

Lastly, **find the solution** that will allow you to adapt to your new self-identity and circumstances. Use your values and strengths to cultivate self-trust.

Trust in yourself. It's okay to be nervous, feel emotional and unfamiliar in your very different body, and to have concerns over your identity transition from 'me to we'. It's natural to wonder how your labour, birth and mothering will go, how your life will be impacted by becoming a mother. We all have concerns for the future. Remember, there is no such thing as the 'super mother'. You are good enough just as you are.

Peta Kelly, author, speaker and entrepreneur, states in *Birthtime*: "It's not just the birthing of the baby. It's the birthing of a mother. It's like a transformation of a relationship. What are the possibilities if I really did let myself trust my body and trust Mother Nature and my baby? If we can be in trust, while also being grateful for the back-up care we do have … Then I think more women would be leaving their births with just the most grateful sense of empowerment as well as a beautiful healthy baby."[50]

Area for cultivating self-trust	How might you recognise and do this?
You first Valuing yourself Respecting yourself Self-acceptance Self-worth Self-love Body confidence Self-inquiry Independence balanced with dependence Speaking kindly to yourself Awareness of your triggers Self-confidence Informed, so empowered Identity Wisdom Instinct and intuition Self forgiveness with grace	Surrendering to the natural change of becoming a mother, the process of matrescence Self-forgiveness Knowing you are enough Mindful presence, releasing rumination about past and worry of future Body care/health awareness Authenticity to self, values, strengths Acceptance of support with grace Ensuring the inner vicious voice is not welcome Realistic goals Boundaries No more comparisonitis Self-efficacy and autonomy Inner knowing Patience with yourself as you evolve Self-compassion

- *Birth-Ed* S2, #7. 'Cultivating Self-Trust with Guest Midwife Rachel Reed' Apple 🎙 Spotify

In her book *Circle of Stones*, Judith Duerk describes finding a sense of herself: "A woman must break out of the old mold. She must risk disobeying the given decrees … break out of the role of the good girl … only by prevailing against her guilt and dread can a woman bring her life situations, one by one, under her own jurisdiction and authority. Only by prevailing can she relate to her life through her own wisdom and understanding. As her life comes slowly under her own ken (knowing), a woman comes to her own grounding, a sense of her own substance … A sureness, a steadfastness in herself and her life."[51]

Duerk has described a woman who values herself at last, beyond patriarchal boundaries and cultural constructs. She sees her self-worth in an identity that frees her to nourish all aspects of her existence, with a deep inner knowing that she is invaluable. Valuing ourselves on such a fundamental level and reframing the narrative of mothering places our role as most worthy. Allowing that attitude to shine through action and having others hear, witness and harness our voices, causing a ripple effect, would be a powerful gift to other mothers.

Duerk writes: "How might your life have been different if there had been a place for you? A place for you to go … a place of women, to help you learn the ways of women..?"[52] How powerfully important is that? A safe place to be and learn the ways of women, supporting each other intergenerationally. A place for you.

Celebrate your mother blessing

And so, here, we celebrate you in your mother blessing, bringing your village together to acknowledge your rite of passage as you transition from maiden to mother. As you celebrate, *maitri* is being cultivated. This is active interest in others, friendliness, goodwill, loving kindness and benevolence. Maitri is where we gather and harvest from each other in our relationships and friendships to actively support your matrescence. Living the metta compassion meditation by celebrating you and your shifting identity.

People like to be asked to help. They feel valued when you reach out to them. Just do it.

Practice offering: Self-trust, *Nitya* and golden thread breath

The first practice offering here is about cultivating self-trust and the practice of *nitya*.[53]

Nitya is inhabiting what is innate, native and unique to you. It might be some value, strength or quality deep within you that you relate to instinctively. How might you practise this to support you in your choices, challenges and joys? How can you inhabit this quality as an aspiration for an eternal way of being?

This could be by immersing yourself in your own mantra, word, phrase, visualisation, or small ritual that invites you to inhabit your native state. Ask yourself: "What quality would I love to be permeated by?" Then notice what arises. This may become a source of great strength and comfort to you.

Next, I offer you the golden thread breath. As I mentioned earlier, the most powerful breathing is when we extend the out-breath, lengthen the exhalation to refocus, de-escalate the nervous system and reduce our blood pressure. We slow our breath rate and calm our heart rate. This is your go-to breathing for labour.

Here's how to practise the golden thread breath:

- Find that comfortable position and practise the shoulder and neck roll, spinal stretch, hip wiggle, jaw unclenched.

- Soften through your body, using your senses to notice everything in your present moment. Soft gaze or closed eyes …

- Take a few long, deep inhalations and exhalations to tune into your regular breathing.

- Part your lips very slightly, as though a piece of paper or golden thread is between them.

- Breathe in through your nose, filling your lungs as you did in the 3-part breath.

- Breathe out slowly, deliberately, as if blowing that thread away from you, as a fan blows a ribbon.

- Repeat 5–10 times. This method of breathing is powerful support in labour, so we are practising it early.

To accompany this breathing practice, I also offer this meadow meditation:

- Find your comfortable place, scanning through your body. Supported, heavy, melting, releasing, and softening with easy breathing. No effort.

- Visualise yourself lying on verdant, lush grass filled with delicate wildflowers that gently sway in a light breeze. You are beneath a towering tree, shaded, comfortable.

- Hear the slow drone of bees as they alight from flower to flower, the delicate song of birds above and gentle shushing of leaves. There is a burbling stream to one side of you.

- Smell the clear, fresh meadow air, tinged with wildflower, earth and crushed grass.

- Feel the light breeze tickle across your skin. A soft touch, a caress. Notice the soft yet sturdy ground beneath you and where it holds your body. Cradling you.

- Be here. Dwell in this place. Nourished and held for as long as you wish.

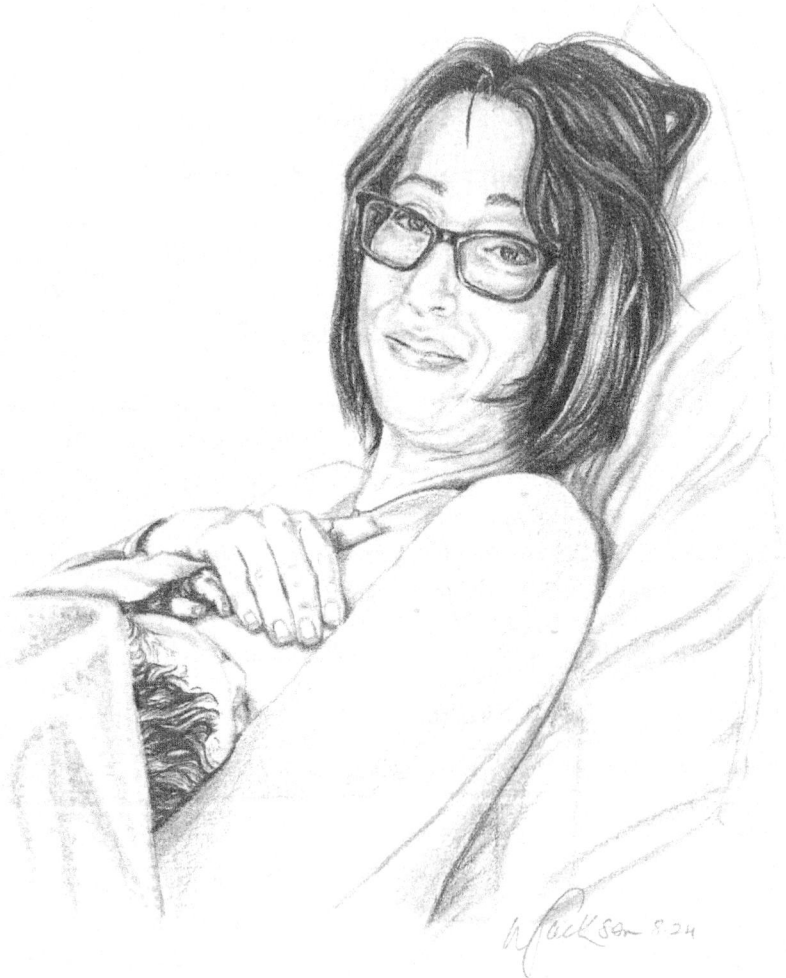

The serenity and peace this image of Ashleigh feeding Rafael evokes is sublime – she is drenched in oxytocin, filled with relief, a sense of wonder and love.

Mother Becoming Insights and Actions in Late Pregnancy

Take a rest on your journey. Backpack off, sore feet resting, have a drink and a snack. You have navigated a lot of knowledge and explored self-inquiry with Ashleigh. How did all this land with you? How do you feel? What do you want to do? Again, take the time for thought experiments, reflections, discussion points with your partner and village of support. Having scribbled notes throughout the chapter, feel free to journal or make a list to make sense of it all.

How might it be for you ...

- If you were confident to say, "Please don't ask me when my baby is due or if I have had it yet"?
- If you were happy to decline unsolicited advice and horror stories?
- If you practised the practice offerings to embody their intricate connectedness?
- If these practices became second nature?
- If you were comfortable with waiting for your labour to start?
- If you mapped possible birth experiences, prepared for variations and felt empowered about your autonomy and confident about being included in decisions.
- If you were prepared for what you'd say if a care provider suggested your baby was too big for your pelvis and offered a caesarean without your being given the chance to labour and birth?
- If you were confident with expectant waiting for labour in your healthy pregnancy.
- If you prepared a space for your separation phase and embraced it, confident in your body, and stayed home for as long as you could?
- If you were comfortable with a date for post-dates induction, fully understanding risk factors if that is what you chose?
- If you felt safe in your birthing experiences, not only physically, but emotionally, culturally and psychologically?
- If we empowered the mother's capacity to birth and her autonomy in the process?
- If, no matter how you chose or needed to birth, you knew you had not failed?
- If you surrounded yourself with positive people and media influences?
- If you requested the bed be pushed to one side in the birthing room, creating a more comfortable environment?
- If you were able to be active and equal in your relationship with your care provider?
- If you prepared as thoroughly for your fourth trimester as your birthing experience?
- If you cultivated your self-trust, keeping your inner voice in check?
- If you built your village and leaned on others, knowing your fourth trimester support is vital for your emotional, physical and psychological wellbeing?
- If your experience of birth were valued more highly than money and institutionalised efficiency?
- If we played neoliberalism and capitalism at its own game, making it work for the paying individuals, ensuring they had an upfront breakdown of costs and transparency of intervention statistics in private care?
- If we could shop around?
- If new terminology were used to replace demeaning language and labels in pregnancy, birthing and mothering?

- If you felt confident to speak up when demeaning or coercive language is used during labour?
- If your birth support could also speak up to this?
- If your identity and the visibility of pregnancy, birthing and mothering were raised, rather than dehumanised and diminished?
- If you had a place to go. A place of intergenerational support and wisdom. A place where mothers feel nourished in mind, body and spirit. A matricentric village.

Late Pregnancy References and Wishlist

1   R Reed, *Reclaiming Childbirth as a Rite of Passage: Weaving ancient wisdom with modern knowledge*, Word Witch. 2021, ISBN 978-0-6450025-1-5

2   R Reed, Childbirth Physiology Course. https://www.rachelreed.website/childbirth-physiology-course

3   K Uvnäs Moberg, *Why Oxytocin Matters*, Pinter and Martin, 2019, p10. ISBN 9781780666051

4   E Hoekzema, E Barba-Müller, C Pozzobon, M Picado, F Lucco, D García-García, JC Soliva, A Tobeña, M Desco, EA Crone, A Ballesteros, S Carmona, O Vilarroya, 'Pregnancy leads to long-lasting changes in human brain structure'. Nat Neurosci. 2017 Feb;20(2):287-296. doi: 10.1038/nn.4458. Epub 2016 Dec 19. PMID: 27991897. https://pubmed.ncbi.nlm.nih.gov/27991897/

5   N Davis, 'Pregnancy causes long-term changes to the brain structure'. Guardian. 20.12.2016. https://www.theguardian.com/science/2016/dec/19/pregnancy-causes-long-term-changes-to-brain-structure-says-study

6   New South Wales Parliament Legislative Council Select Committee on Birth Trauma, Report. 2024. p xvi, xvii. ISBN: 978-1-922960-38-2 https://www.parliament.nsw.gov.au/lcdocs/inquiries/2965/FINAL%20Birth%20Trauma%20Report%20-%2029%20April%202024.PDF

7   Royal College of Obstetrics and Gynaecology. 'Group B Streptococcus'. 2017. https://www.rcog.org.uk/for-the-public/browse-our-patient-information/group-b-streptococcus-gbs-in-pregnancy-and-newborn-babies/

8   KM Levett, CA Smith, A Bensoussan, HG Dahlen, 'Complementary therapies for labour and birth study: a randomised controlled trial of antenatal integrative medicine for pain management in labour'. BMJ Open 2016;6: e010691. doi:10.1136/ bmjopen-2015-010691 https://bmjopen.bmj.com/content/bmjopen/6/7/e010691.full.PDF

9   *Birthtime The Documentary* and *Birthtime The Handbook*, Clark and Mackay, 2021, p111. https://www.birthtime.world/

10   H Keedle , R Lockwood, W Keedle, D Susic, HG Dahlen, 'What women want if they were to have another baby: the Australian Birth Experience Study (BESt) cross-sectional national survey'. BMJ Open 2023;13:e071582. doi:10.1136/ bmjopen-2023-071582 https://bmjopen.bmj.com/content/13/9/e071582

11   *Birthtime The Handbook*, p46.

12   Reed, *Reclaiming Childbirth as a Rite of Passage*, p153.

13   NM Hurst, CJ Valentine, L Renfro, P Burns, 'Skin-to-skin holding in the neonatal intensive care unit influences maternal milk volume'. J Perinatal, (1997). 17(3), 213-217 https://www.researchgate.net/publication/14009525_Skin-to-skin_holding_in_the_neonatal_intensive_care_influences_maternal_milk_volume

14   E Antunes de Campos, N Zanon Narchi, G Moreno, 'Meanings and perceptions of women regarding the practice of yoga in pregnancy: A qualitative study'. Complementary Therapies in Clinical Practice. Vol 39. May 2020, 101099 DOI: 10.1016/j.ctcp.2020.101099

15   M Jowitt, *Dynamic Positions in Birth. A fresh look at how women's bodies work in labour*, Second Edition. Pinter and Martin, 2020, p24. ISBN 9781780666907

16   Jowitt, *Dynamic Positions in Birth*, p31

17   C de Costa. *the women's doc*, Allen and Unwin, 2021, p85. ISBN 9781760529147

18   de Costa, *the women's doc*, p226.

19   C de Costa, *Hail Caesar. Why one in three Australian babies is born by caesarean section*. Boolarong Press, 2008, p 84 ISBN 978192105280

20   Jowitt, Dynamic Positions in Birth, p55.

21   L Enright, *Vagina A Re-Education*,. Allen and Unwin, 2019, p171. ISBN 9781911630029

22   *Birthtime The Handbook*, p78.

23   E Wiberg-Itzel, S Wray, H Åkerud, (2017).'A randomized controlled trial of a new treatment for labor dystocia'. The Journal of Maternal-Fetal & Neonatal Medicine, 31(17), 2237–2244. https://doi.org/10.1 080/14767058.2017.1339268 https://www.tandfonline.com/doi/abs/10.1080/14767058.2017.1339268

24   C Criado Perez, Invisible Women, Exposing Data Bias in A World Designed for Men, Penguin Random House, 2019, p234 ISBN 9781784706289

25   C Tomori, S Han, (Eds), The Routledge Handbook of Anthropology and Reproduction. H Dunsworth. 'There is No Evolutionary "Obstetrical Dilemma". Taylor and Francis, 2021, Chapter 27 https://digital-commons.uri.edu/cgi/viewcontent.cgi?article=1040&context=soc_facpubs

26   *Birthtime The Handbook*, p43.

27   Obstetric Care Consensus: 'Safe Prevention of the Primary Cesarean Delivery. The American College of Obstetricians and Gynaecologists'. Society of Maternal-Fetal Medicine. 2014. https://www.acog.org/-/media/project/acog/acogorg/clinical/files/obstetric-care-consensus/articles/2014/03/safe-preven-tion-of-the-primary-cesarean-delivery.PDF

28   R Reed, Why Induction Matters. Membrane Sweeping. 2018. Pinter and Martin, 2018, p96-7. ISBN 9781780666006

29   S Wickham, *In Your Own Time: How western medicine controls the start of labour and why this needs to stop*, Birthmoon Creations, 2021. ISBN 9781914465024

30   *Birthtime The Handbook*, p82.

31   Wickham, *In Your Own Time*, p98.

32   J Allison, *Golden Month*, Beatnik Publishing; 2016; p17. ISBN 9780992264840

33   J Allison, *Golden Month*, p95.

34   J Allison, *Golden Month*, p17.

35   Heng Ou. *The First Forty Days: The Art of Nourishing the New mother*. Abrams The Art of books; 2016. ISBN 9781617691836

36   E Horton, 'Neoliberalism and the Australian Healthcare System (Factory)'. In Shaw, R (Ed.) Proceedings of the 2007 Conference of the Philosophy of Education Society of Australasia. Philosophy of Education Society of Australasia. p1-7. https://pesa.org.au/images/papers/2007-papers/horton2007.PDF https://www.semanticscholar.org/paper/Neoliberalism-and-the-Australian-Healthcare-System-Horton/a11fffdc-756c458df81036352ecb6aa21e0182ca

37   Jowitt, Dynamic Positions in Birth, p33.

38   de Costa, the women's doc, p173.

39   Jowitt, Dynamic Positions in Birth, p35.

40   M Thomasson, J Treber. 'From home to hospital: The evolution of childbirth in the United States 1928–1940'. 2008. Explorations in Economic History.Volume 45, Issue 1, January 2008, Pages 76-99. https://doi.org/10.1016/j.eeh.2007.07.001

41   M Thomasson, J Treber. 'From home to hospital' p80.

42   R Lake, A Epstein, Business of Being Born. Documentary. https://vimeo.com/ondemand/thebusines-sofbeingborn2#:~:text=Watch%20The%20Business%20of%20Being%20Born%20Online%20%7C%20Vimeo%20On%20Demand%20on%20Vimeo

43   *Birthtime The Handbook*, p77.

44   *Birthtime The Handbook*, p77, 78.

45   *Birthtime The Handbook*, p33.

46   S Vimalesvaran, J Ireland, M Kashu, 'Mind your language: respectful language within maternity services' The Lancet. March 06, 2021. Volume 397, Issue 10277, P859-861. https://www.thelancet.com/journals/lancet/article/PIIS0140-6736(21)00031-3/fulltext

47   WHO. 'Prevention and elimination of disrespect and abuse during childcare'. 2014. https://apps.who.int/iris/bitstream/handle/10665/134588/WHO_RHR_14.23_eng.PDF

48   The Royal College of Midwives Re:Birth https://rcm.org.uk/wp-content/uploads/2024/03/rcm-re-birth-report.PDF

49   W Tuohy, 'Inclusive language risks 'dehumanising women', top researchers argue'. Sydney Morning Herald. January 29, 2022 https://www.smh.com.au/national/inclusive-language-risks-dehumanising-women-top-researchers-argue-20220126-p59red.html

50   *Birthtime The Handbook*, p142, 143

51   J Duerk, *Circle of Stones. Woman's Journey to Herself*, New World Library, p80. ISBN 9781880913635

52   J Duerk, *Circle of Stones. Woman's Journey to Herself*, New World Library, p32

53   Lorin Roche. *The Radiance Sutras*. Verse 109 of Yuki Practice. Sounds True; 2014. p 338. ISBN 978-1-60407-659-2

Wishlist

1. Dr Sarah Buckley 'Ecstatic Birth. Nature's Hormonal Blueprint for labour' https://sarahbuckley.com/newsletter/

2. Dr Sarah Buckley Blog Oxytocin https://sarahbuckley.com/pitocin-side-effects-part1/

3. *Great Birth Rebellion* #140 'Baby Brain' with Neuroscientist Dr Sarah McKay. Apple Spotify

4. YouTube Video series. R Reed. 'Occipito-posterior position (back-to-back) in labour'. https://www.youtube.com/watch?v=ZLUW85oiXeU&t=10s

5. YouTube Video. M O'Brien: 'Learning to birth with biomechanics, are we getting right'? https://www.youtube.com/watch?v=7cX58bXeEQ8&t=1046s

6. Kirsten Small, You Tube Video. Electronic Fetal Heart Monitoring. (EFM): Effective, Fruitful, Mandatory? https://www.youtube.com/watch?v=aGdknPVOhiw

7. *The Midwives' Cauldron* S2 #1. 'The importance of good postnatal care and recovery with Sophie Messager' Apple Spotify

Chapter 4
Undisturbed Physiological Birthing with Ally

Meeting Ally

Ally and I met at a beginners Ashtanga yoga course and were delighted to discover we were on the same Hatha Vinyasa teacher training. We bonded over coffee and our passion for talking about all things pregnancy and birth, new mothering and yoga.

I remember Ally's animation as she described her utter euphoria and immense sense of achievement and pride in herself in birthing her first baby, Audrey, at home with her midwife and doula. She said she had never felt so powerful. Her experiences led her down a life-altering path of perceptions and ways of living with her husband, Mick. Soon after birthing Norah, Ally moved back to her home in Nova Scotia.

To me, Ally embodies Mother Earth. Her passions for nature and nurture, family and belief in the strength of birthing women have shaped her life in ever-evolving circles. Witnessing her journey and growing family is an ongoing joy. I witness her nurture all things birthing and life, from her own babies, to nurturing yeast for sourdough, seeds into food and trees, her family, Blossom the cow in calving, the pigs with piglets, the cat with kittens, bees and honey and so much more. These illustrate the essence of Ally.

Mama of Audrey, Norah, Edith and Vance, here is Ally's letter to you.

"My experience of birth"

Dear Mama,

If, when I was younger, someone had said that I would be the mother to 4 children as an adult, I'm not sure I would have believed them. And here we are. Four children, a large family by today's standards.

My impression and understanding of pregnancy and birth, as I grew up, was loosely based on those I had watched in *Gilmore Girls* and *Friends* and the ones you read about in health class at school. It was something that you 'got through' and perhaps scheduled so you could return to work earlier. I didn't dream of how many children I might have. There was no plan in terms of when or how many. My life was to unfold. I trusted that things would fall into place if becoming a mother was the path for me. According to my mother, when I was quite young, I insisted I was never going to have children and never move out!

As it does, life unfolded and flowed and I found myself – somewhat excitedly and a bit unexpectedly – pregnant with my long-term partner and soon-to-be husband, Mick. We were in the midst of planning our wedding, and buying and renovating a house. We had talked about children and decided after the wedding and honeymoon would be the time we would start a family. Our first child, Audrey, had other plans.

I found out I was pregnant on the day we were moving out of our rental house, which was due to be demolished as soon as we packed up and made our way off the porch. I hardly knew anyone who was pregnant, let alone people close to us who had children. I was in a state of shock and fear about everything pregnant mothers are told to worry about – like lifting things that are too heavy, sleeping the wrong way, eating the wrong food and the list goes on. I took it all to heart and it bubbled inside me. I was too worried to tell anyone, for fear that something would be wrong, so we spent the first few weeks in a state of quiet limbo. I was anxious and felt like I was behind where I wanted to be in terms of research and delving into the world of pregnancy, birth and motherhood.

I had a dating scan to determine how far along I was and then the 12-week scan to ensure, medically, that everything was okay. In the society that I followed at that time, after 12 weeks, it was deemed an appropriate time to spread the news that I was pregnant. The anxiety, fear and confusion seemed to lessen with this news being released and I settled into pregnancy with a little more ease. During this period, I worked in the construction industry, which was a very male-dominated energy. Although I felt as if I didn't know as much as I would have liked about the transition of maiden to mother through pregnancy, I made the decision that my work environment was not conducive to the pregnancy I was beginning to envision. So, I gave my notice and instead put my energy into helping my Mick build his new business.

That being said, I made one of the most important, life-changing connections through my work. The owner of the company and his wife had recently welcomed a child and they had hired a doula to attend the birth. After I revealed my pregnancy, he suggested I might call her, if it were something I would be interested in. The concept of a doula was relatively new to me, but as my reading progressed on topics of pregnancy, birthing and motherhood, it seemed to be the logical next step to have an additional person to support me as I traversed this new-to-me land.

An awareness had grown, in my husband and me, through the years leading up to becoming pregnant. We started to question where our food was coming from. We began a slow overhaul of our consumption of external gratification and turned the focus of our minds and therefore our actions towards nourishment for the whole body. Reflecting, it seems a natural progression towards a reconnection to ourselves, which, although not always linear or simple, is always for the better. The farmers markets were a consistent favourite for countless weekend mornings. We both grew up leading active lifestyles and this continued as we began the transition into a family.

I connected with the doula my boss had suggested and we had an instant and beautiful reciprocity. She was softly spoken, with a confidence that comes from an innate knowing and a true passion for her very important work. Her warmth and reassurance were overwhelming in the best of ways. I decided alongside her that, yes, she would be the woman to walk alongside me in this momentous transition. My life has forever shifted since knowing and learning from her. She was the stepping stone to everything that I have come to strive and navigate towards in my life –

living simply but intentionally with grace and love. A wise woman, healer, listener, teacher. Speak too much about her in front of her and she will humbly wave her hand with a sweet grin.

As my first pregnancy progressed, I called the local midwives with the intention of a homebirth, supported by my husband and doula. My experiences with the midwives in the various antenatal appointments were positive and seamless. It appealed to me, the comfort of having someone, an expert, help me along in my changing body. As a child, a check-up at the doctor's office was bourgeois, so going to the midwives felt like an extension of this. It was reassuring to know someone was crossing all the T's and dotting all the I's and that the responsibility of making sure everything was okay was not in my hands.

My belly slowly grew and swelled. We finished the renovations on the house, hosted family from afar, got married and settled into life as a married couple. The visits and chats with my doula were cherished and I left each encounter feeling more at home in my body, my mind going over everything she had said. I often felt a sense of returning, of remembering, as if she were reminding me of knowledge within me. There was such trust, from her, in me. For my body, for my baby, for all women. Being near her reawakened this trust within me. A resonance that has mirrored through my life ever since.

I continued exploring pregnancy, birth and early motherhood through books recommended by my doula and others. I still felt a sense of anxiety and unknowingness for the early days. At the same time, as I approached the end of my pregnancy, I felt stable and grounded, knowing my body and that birth was a natural process it innately knew.

My due date came and went. I felt full and vibrant. It was early February in Australia, and it was hot! I spent many hours walking, in the early mornings and late afternoons. We would visit the beach in the evening, my belly expressing to the world that our baby was almost ready. I didn't feel any urgency. I knew it would unfold as it was meant to. The voice of my doula was always there, with her gentle reassurance and trust.

I remember the day of the birth with such clarity. My mother was staying with us and had been there since our wedding. We were sitting down to lunch – toast with cheese and tomato – and as I sat down, something felt different. I knew this was the beginning. I called Mick and let him know that he might want to take the afternoon off. I texted our doula and let her know that it seemed as if things were starting. She said to continue on through the afternoon and keep her updated. Mick came home and we excitedly spent the time chatting and connecting.

My surges flowed, gently increasing. By dinnertime, they were getting stronger. Mick made a beautiful salmon pasta for dinner. I was rocking on a yoga ball, and he would come and hold my hand through each surge before returning to stir or chop in the kitchen. As the evening progressed, so did my labour. It was a gradual, smooth escalation of sensations I had never experienced. I knew from the very beginning that I was not interested in a water birth, so we were swaying and rocking in the front lounge room. Personally, the idea of birthing in water created feelings of isolation for me. I didn't want to have that separation – even the thin walls of a pool – from Mick. My mum was in charge of our small dog in the den. I didn't want too much commotion, or too many people in the birthing space. I'm thankful for her understanding and acceptance to await the birth in a separate area.

Our doula arrived, then shortly after, our midwife as well. I had nourishing snacks and electrolyte drinks. It was all very relaxed with the tinge of excitement and awe. As the intensity grew, my clothes had no place on my body. My awareness for the human body, nudity, freedom has grown tremendously over the past decade, but at that point and time, my nakedness was not something I felt overly comfortable with. However, birth erased all capacity for my thinking mind to negotiate with my subconscious mind. Off came the clothes.

Birth surged forward; I sank in deeper. It was after midnight and the second midwife was called. The house was dark and calm. I remember her coming in, and for a split second, my mind turned on; I was worried I was going to 'lose my place' in the birth, but it all continued along with a steadfast seamlessness. The energy was held captive. I was held captive. Birth ensued.

For most of the labour, I was squatting through the surges. When it was time, I birthed our baby, on hands and knees, leaning over the arm of our blue couch. Mick held my hand with embodied calm. We had requested quiet and no lights upon the baby's arrival. Our midwife passed our newborn through my legs as I awkwardly, but intuitively, turned myself around and put her on my belly. A girl. Our own girl. We named her Audrey.

At that moment, we became a family. Happy tears and smiles and a feeling of elation. Me, a mother. The sanctity of birth; we revelled in its embrace. Touching tiny pink fingers and ears, remarking on the beautifulness that we had created, introducing our daughter to my mum. Both our doula and the midwife later described our birth as 'textbook' and 'extraordinarily normal'.

Audrey latched on with ease and I birthed my placenta within the hour, completing the birth of my first child. We looked over the extraordinary organ with gratitude before cutting the cord. I had arranged to have my placenta encapsulated, so our doula tenderly prepared it to be collected. The midwives filled in their forms and paperwork, weighed and measured our baby, tidied up the space and were on their way. Our doula stayed a little while longer and then made her way home. Both she and the midwife called in the morning to see how things were going. Mick and I were ready for bed. We had a little hanging baby hammock, which I had researched and researched. It was meant to rock if the baby stirred and mimic movement of the womb. We placed Audrey in her new hammock and crawled into bed. I was on an emotional high, but was asleep in minutes.

The days that followed were a joy and a whirr. It was all so new, but luckily we had each other to fumble through it. The first night after the birth, Audrey was crying, and we couldn't figure out what it was. She was fed, warm and changed. Our backs were sore from leaning over the bed, checking and re-checking her nappy. Maybe she didn't want to sleep because it was a little wet. So we changed it. Still crying. We'd check again. Oh! Maybe it was still a little wet. Again we'd change it. On and on. In hindsight, all she wanted was closeness to me. Had I just brought her into bed and nursed, this would have comforted her. I had such a fear that she just wouldn't be a 'good sleeper' and I didn't want to encourage 'bad habits'. This learned fear – after much experience, reading and remembering – was eventually replaced with the knowing that babies are meant to be with us, on us, sleep with us. They need their mothers, like they need to breathe. We regulate each other. Babies are not separate from us, even after birth.

My unlearning began and the anxieties I held surrounding sleep and schedules were slowly mended with listening, and compassion towards myself and my baby. I came from the era and world where 'cry it out' had been encouraged. This wasn't something we wanted to try, but we thought we needed something to 'make' her sleep. Instead of really digging deeply and listening to my innate knowing, I turned to books that outlined schedules and tips.

I had arranged for postpartum suppers and a few snacks. This was such a blessing. The worry of cooking and thinking about such an important staple was taken care of. The wonderful lady made organic, nourishing, hearty dishes that kept all of us satisfied. Oxtail stews, broths with rice and beef, ratatouille, baked custards. I had also prepared and frozen lots of meals, so in the first few months, we were able to focus on our new roles. My mum took care of washing the nappies. She was amazed that the hot Australian sun whitened and dried them in an instant. I took the days slowly as we began our journey as mother and child, as a new family.

We went through all the previously unknown feelings, emotions that come with the responsibility of a baby, the responsibility of becoming parents. I felt a deep support from my husband as well as the community we were slowly building. Our doula lovingly encouraged meetups with other new mothers and mothers groups, and her visits remained an anchor.

Giving birth changed me as a woman. As a girl, it wasn't my 'plan' to have 4 home-birthed children and live in a farmhouse in the country. But this is what I am meant to do. Birth was some of my most important work. Raising children, raising a family, with awe and awareness for the natural world, is some of my greatest work. My births shifted generations of fear and lack of connection that was felt through my mother's generation, my grandmother's generation and beyond. My children will not carry that forward as the only history anymore. It's still there, it is still part of them, but their births are a bigger part of them. A return to remembering and listening to the body. An instinctiveness, that with support, openness and trust, is available to them. I am forever grateful for my children, who chose me to be their mother.

Ally

Dear Mother Becoming,

With Ally, we are chatting about labour and birth with no intervention – supporting and witnessing a woman as her body sings its own song, moving in tandem with her baby in a time-honoured dance of undisturbed physiological birth.

The journey so far has been challenging at times, with anger, frustration and sadness. Yet at the same time, there has been a gaining of new knowledge, wisdom, awe and recognition of your own immense capacity. Let's celebrate and acknowledge this for a moment. You are awesome!

We continue exploring the phases of labour here with Ally. This chapter looks at the deep absorption into self of the liminal phase of late labour. We then explore the emergence phase of birthing (known as the second stage) and the extraordinary magical happenings of the integration phase (the third stage). These are offered with the understanding of how labour progresses as a rite of passage without the constraints of time and medical management.[1] In undisturbed birthing, we are supporting women with low-risk pregnancy to spontaneously labour physiologically with no induction, augmentation or medical pain relief. This means vaginal birth with no instruments, no episiotomy, or complications such as a third-degree tear of the perineum (where the anal sphincter is involved) or postpartum haemorrhage.

Undisturbed birthing is also where delayed cord-clamping occurs and the baby remains skin to skin with the mother until after the first breastfeed, supporting a magical myriad of happenings during

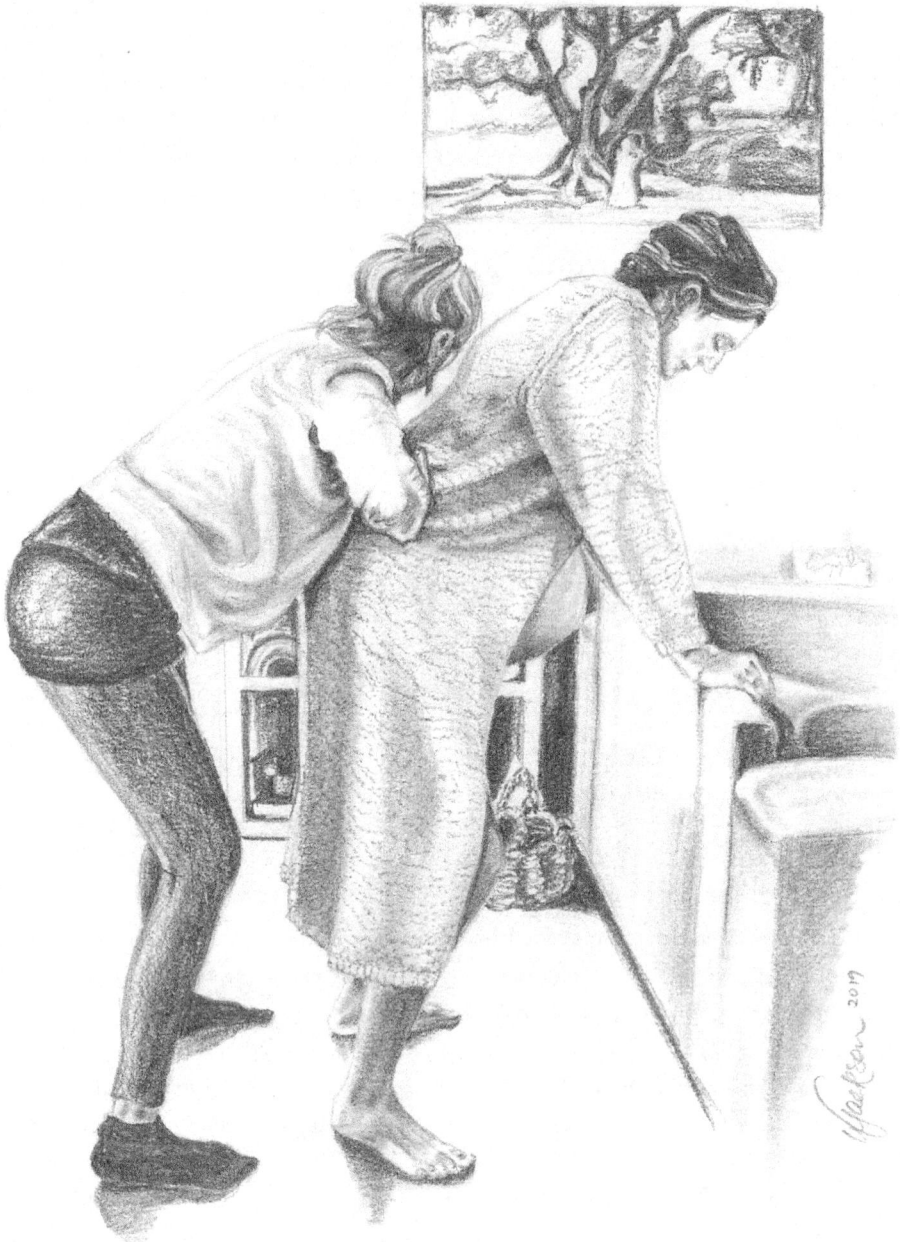

Ally, at home with her doula during the night, leaning comfortably forwards, knees apart, slight bend, feet outward, as firm, stable, continuous pressure is applied, pressing inwards from either side of the pelvis, providing reassuring trusted touch and pain relief. Ally's doula gently rocks side to side with her movements, responding to Ally's needs as her body moves instinctively in the dance between mother and baby as labour occurs.

integration. This is where feeling safe is of paramount importance, and the mother emerges from birth feeling emotionally and physically healthy, all made more possible with midwifery continuity of care.

In *Birthtime*, Dr Rachel Reed states: "We often talk about the gold standard being continuity of care, which is a woman having a relationship with her midwife and the midwife actually being with the woman, as in following the woman on her journey whatever her journey is. For some women, that will be hospital birth; for some, homebirth; for some women, it will be an elective caesarean section."[2]

Undisturbed physiological birth is exactly that – undisturbed. It's a woman following her own needs and instincts to move. Midwives and birth support watch, wait and pause for a while to fully assess the labouring woman before they offer suggestions for alternative positions, or make a hands-on adjustment for assisting the baby to move and for the mother's comfort. This considered pause is to make sure they are not interfering unnecessarily. It may seem as though they are not doing much; however, their experience, intuition and knowledge through observation, listening, supportive touch, words of encouragement, presence, maintaining the environment for oxytocin and endorphins to flow, and where time isn't a limiting notion, is value beyond words.

As obstetrician Dr Kirsten Small says in *Birthtime*, "We don't go around asking people, 'What's a physiological bowel motion?' 'What's a physiological erection?' No, we just accept that the rest of our bodily functions work really well. But somehow, we're not allowed to give birth in a way that's physiological."[3] In the same way as we don't call a neurosurgeon for a headache, we don't need an obstetrician in physiological birthing. This is the midwife's speciality.

Vanessa Olorenshaw writes: "The physical and emotional experience of birth is something extremely precious and the strength and power of a woman's body and mind when she gives birth are wonderous. The vast majority of healthy women with healthy pregnancies are capable of something extremely physical and raw – and they can do it. We don't hear that enough. We can do it."[4]

You have read Ally's story of undisturbed physiological birth at home. If you are interested in exploring home birthing more, here are some resources.

- *Birth-Ed* S1 #13. 'Home Birth with Guest, Midwife Kemi Johnson' Apple 🎙Spotify
- Natalie Medding's *Why Home Birth Matters*. Book[4]
- *Birth-Ed* S2 #1. 'Doulas and understanding the labour process' provides a foundational understanding of undisturbed birthing. Apple 🎙 Spotify
- Dr Sara Wickham website. 'Is homebirth safe?'
  https://www.sarawickham.com/research-updates/is_home_birth_safe/

Your village will be activated here too and much excitement starts bubbling over …

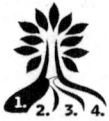

The Physical, Hormonal and Emotional Influences on Undisturbed Physiological Birthing

The crescendo of hormones in labour

The intermingling notes of all the hormones that have been introduced so far are expressed in the symphony of labour and birthing. Remember, anything that disrupts the conductor and musicians means the music will be out of tune or not in sync. A birthing woman needs to feel safe enough to drop into the limbic system, part of our earliest mammalian brain development, allowing the neocortex or 'thinking brain' to shut off. So, the hormones, brain and body need to be in a supportive environment, where external incoming messages of calm, quiet, low light, touch, love and safety are harmonious and can flow together.[5]

Prolactin levels increase 10 to 20 times during pregnancy. Apart from producing milk, prolactin also has a deeply calming effect, working in harmony with oxytocin and oestrogen to promote maternal behaviours. It becomes much louder as birth nears, stimulating oxytocin release, and contributing to the crescendo of oxytocin peaks in late labour and birth. The sucking of a baby on the nipple strongly stimulates Prolactin to be reproduced again and again. Prolactin also increases in male partners during their partner's pregnancy.

Oxytocin flows into the bloodstream in pulses, causing rhythmic uterine contractions. In late labour, this musician peaks, supported by high levels of prolactin to assist with the emergence phase. This peaking and the baby's head pressing on the almost fully open cervix promotes the Ferguson reflex, which is a large surge in oxytocin. This reflex is the instinctive urge to bear down in unison with the uterine expulsive contractions. Oxytocin is coordinating the neuroendocrine response in labour. This is the nervous system making and releasing hormones into the bloodstream. The psychological and physiological aspects of labour and birth need to be nurtured in an environment where oxytocin thrives. Oxytocin has natural pain-relieving and anti-stress effects, promoting labour with love, bonding, and decreased pain, fear and stress. Continuity of known carer facilitates this amazing process, even when birth interventions are required.

At birth, the baby has a lot of oxytocin flooding their body too, which promotes bonding, healing and growth, and lowers stress and inflammation. Remember, melatonin and oxytocin work in harmony in a dusk-like, quieter, non-busy atmosphere. Oxytocin effects on the maternal brain during birth prepare the woman for mothering, increasing social skills, lowering anxiety and having amnesic effects (not remembering). It also prompts the pleasure centre of the brain to release dopamine (a chemical transmitter), increasing experiences of reward.

Beta-endorphin is our body's natural opium. This hormone sings through your body, adding a seriously feel-good sway to the rhythm of labour's song. Labour is an extended, physically challenging period of time, and this hormone plays a massive role in responding to normally occurring physiological pain sensation, especially when it is supported in the right environment.

Dr Sarah Buckley, in *Birthtime*, says: "At the same time that oxytocin is causing these rhythmic contractions of labour, it's also switching on intrinsic pain-relieving mechanisms for the mother. It's turning on instinctive mothering behaviours."[6] As a natural opioid, it also supports immune function, physical activity and psychological wellbeing, all necessary in birthing and recovery. When fear is put aside and beta-endorphins are free to sing, the mother looks totally stoned between contractions. She may even sometimes fall asleep, dropping into liminality. Physiological pain during childbirth may be considered positive because it signals to the body that labour is happening.

Beta-endorphin communicates with the labouring woman, telling her to move, while providing relief as surges in intensity increase, and indicating the impending arrival of the baby. Rhythmic contractions (surges) thin and open the cervix, and thicken the top of the uterus to push the baby down and outwards. In undisturbed physiological birthing, intense, purposeful contractions are manageable with intuitive support and non-pharmacological methods of pain relief.

Physiological labour pain can be held in an environment of positive, powerful, joyful empathy, and belief in the labouring woman, from her support and carer. This is what is needed, rather than an attitude of sadness, sympathy and suffering, which is undermining to her confidence. Pathological pain is something quite different. It is a warning to the body of inflammation, heavy bruising, infection or broken bones that need medical intervention and treatment.

We continue here with adrenaline. It plays in the body at the start of labour, providing a surge of awareness and activity alongside cortisol to assist in preparing for birth, before retreating to a safe space. Preparations mean activating the village for childcare, calling the midwife and doula, and doing whatever is needed before withdrawing from the usual activities of life.

Adrenaline serves another purpose in labour. If a woman feels fearful, surprised, intruded upon, unsafe, unprotected or confused, or if she experiences excessive external stimuli, this inhibits oxytocin. Labour will slow or completely stop. This response has kept women safe for millennia. It's a primal response.

Sinking into the liminal phase

The birth room and space is to be held with reverence and respect. Treated as a sanctuary. What is happening here is miraculous, transformative. Indeed, there is a high flow of oxytocin within all the people present. Would we storm into a sacred place or revered ancient site – with loud noise, voices demanding attention and bright lights – to interrupt a hymn, a prayer, a chant, meditation or peaceful ambiance? No, we would not. Any intrusion into that space needs to be considered and consensual. The birthing woman should be treated with the utmost respect: undisturbed, using hushed tones and dim lighting. Stimuli should be unobtrusive, so she feels safe and adrenaline isn't stimulated. The mother becoming song can be sung.

To support and nourish a woman into this liminal state of being and transition, the wisdom of Rhea Dempsey is profound. In her article, 'Understanding Pain Dynamics in Normal Birth', Dempsey explains the concept of working with pain. This means embracing its intensity while understanding it as functional, engaging with pain as a friend with the ability to release beta-endorphins and turn inwards. She talks about riding the intensity of childbirth and how every woman reaches a point of 'crisis of confidence', usually lasting about 20 minutes. This is a pivotal moment that needs intense support. Birth supporters need to witness a woman's potency rather than pitying her, empathising with belief, rather than undermining a woman's strength and capacity.[7]

Interviewed in *Birthtime*, Dempsey describes oxytocin: "The oxytocin is driving the contractions, those big, beautiful, strong contractions. Oxytocin is a fantastic, multitasking, wonderful, brilliant goddess of a hormone that's opening our hearts as well as opening our bodies."[8] She encourages mothers to understand the dynamics of pain in normal labour and birth in a different way. To recognise it as: "Pain is my friend. Pain is my friend."

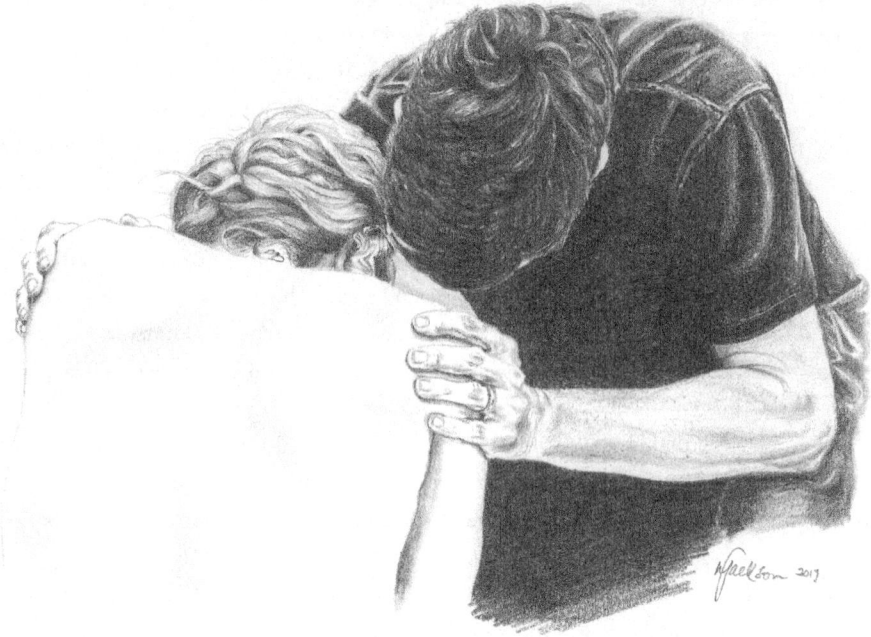

Held with love, Mick's hands say it all. Holding Ally with such tenderness, yet also strong in his powerful belief in her. Ally leans into that belief, love, strength and support with such trust in her ability to sink into openhearted vulnerability and express her labour in safety.

Dempsey further describes how pain is affected by the wider circles of culture, family, friends, birth-place culture, known support and attitudes towards pain. Working with a pain relief paradigm of trusting the body, lack of fear and the presence of a trusted midwife vastly increase the ability to sink into liminality.[9] Please have a listen to Rhea Dempsey on pain, oxytocin and attachment. Your birth partner will find her particularly informative; she will change their perception of pain as suffering, and show them how they can be supportive in this unique situation.

You may have heard of marathon runners passing through a 'pain barrier' to carry on. Here, your partner, midwife and doula – in their wisdom, trust and belief in your capacity – bring their expertise to support you. As Professor Hannah Dahlen says in *Birthtime* of the relationship between midwives and the women they care for: "There's trust, there's a relationship, there's the building of trust in their own bodies over nine months. Then there is keeping them off beds, keeping them mobile, massaging them, acupuncture, aromatherapy, and water."[10] She also describes: "One of the big issues around intervention and birth and what we know begins a cascade – and they're often things like an epidural – is we need to get much better at helping women work with pain."[11]

From the perspective of the professional attitude and philosophy of working with pain, Professor Nicky Leap, a midwife, states in *Birthtime*: "A lot of doctors and nurses and midwives come from a culture of providing adequate pain relief. That's their job when people are sick and injured. But now that whole culture of adequate pain relief has been brought into the childbirth arena."[12]

None of this is to make you feel guilty for choosing an epidural (more about those with Katie in Chapter 5), particularly with medical induction. However, fear of labour has been so ingrained by the media and it need not be so. The following resources may be supportive and comforting, if fear of pain in labour is very real for you.

Birthing women are unique individuals and they experience pain differently for different reasons, including previous physical trauma, abuse, differing pain thresholds, cultural perceptions and some complications of childbirth that are more intense. Other methods of pain relief may be needed. It's okay. It's not a failing to have medical pain relief.

Some complications of childbirth do need support and monitoring. However, all of these offered insights, knowledge and practices of support to create a peaceful environment can be used in other situations. For example, you can incorporate them to optimise the experience of induction for a medical indication.

- *Great Birth Rebellion* #47. 'Managing labour pain without medicine' Apple 🎙 Spotify
- *Great Birth Rebellion* #20. 'Sterile water injections' Apple🎙Spotify

Pauses in labour are normal

Labour can have pauses, known as *physiological plateaus*, at any stage or phase. They are not predictable and can occur at any time during labour and birth. These are natural pauses, part of a self-regulation of the mother and baby working together. After a natural pause the woman resumes her labour.

Transferring to hospital can cause a pause because external stimulation and questions on admission re-activate the thinking brain. The liminal phase is interrupted, the flow of oxytocin decreases and adrenaline increases. We spoke about creating a space in the hospital to help women drop back into liminality.

Some hospital guidelines require a vaginal examination on admission to assess the progress of labour. There is no evidence to back up this routine practice and you can be prepared to decline if you wish. The single assessment of dilation of the cervix is not a reliable indication of labour progress and this will be discussed in Tree Root 2.

In the hospital environment, these pauses are often misinterpreted as 'a failure to progress'. Artificial rupture of membranes is encouraged and a drip of Syntocinon (synthetic oxytocin) often advised. It's hard to negotiate or advocate for yourself and decline such intervention when you're in an environment of pressure. You could request a sign on the door that says: 'Please do not disturb. My midwife will come to you. If entering, keep the lights low and talk in hushed tones. Thank you for maintaining my oxytocin.' You can also ask for time to self-regulate, create your environment, take in nourishment and fluids, and use the following practice offerings.

Here are some suggestions to tailor to your own needs.

Assisting labour to flow

Environment

- Visualisation and meditations
- Music breathing, hypnobirthing or sound
- Massage, aromatherapy, acupressure
- Augmenting yourself by nipple stimulation to reflood your body with oxytocin.

Body health and fuel

- Rest, snacks, drinks
- Repeat.

Mindful health

- Gentle encouragement from your support
- Affirmations
- Loving murmurings
- Visualisation meditations from this book
- Self-belief, love, worth, trust, strength
- Breathing practices to calm the nervous system.

Physical practices

There are no time constraints or order in which you might like to do these. Use these 4 elements to support your comfort and progress of labour.

1. Slight lean forwards, knees apart, opening the pelvis as baby's head descends into the pelvic bowl. Includes sitting postures, like on a birth ball
2. Upright, using gravity for downward movement of the baby
3. Using your instinctive sway to encourage your baby's rotation in the pelvis
4. Knees in, calves out (KICO) to open the pelvic outlet. (Video in goody box.)

- Yoga flow for pelvic warm-up, softening and releasing
- Walking feet apart, penguin waddle, add sway
- Belly dance figure of 8
- Squatting rock, gently onto your hands and back again, side to side
- Upright kneeling, with pelvic pressure from partner
- Sitting forward on a birthing ball and rock, pelvic pressure
- Sitting forward, facing the back of the toilet with a pillow to rest your arms and head on
- Standing sway, leaning on wall, raised bed or held by partner
- Shower and sway
- All fours and rocking with open leg lunge, with pelvic pressure from partner
- One leg up on a stool or chair, rocking, changing sides
- Hopscotch app
- Birthing, KICO, wherever you are in the emergence phase.

Additional support from your team

Midwives and doulas have a deep understanding of how labour progresses. With this they may suggest some options to help your baby negotiate your pelvis and at the same time provide more comfort for you. This is offered to support you, rather than to interfere in your individual experience of labour. Midwives may suggest some of the following, especially when they suspect the baby's head is at an odd angle entering the pelvis. (This is demonstrated in the optimal birth video with Ashleigh). It's ultimately up to you what you want to do. Always. Your choice.

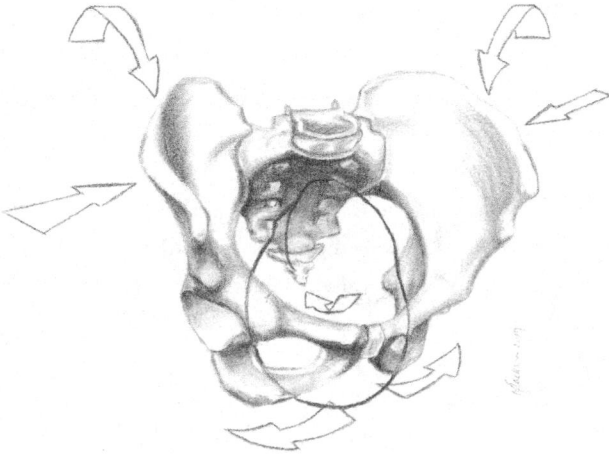

Illustration C. The straight arrows inwards indicate where to place the hands for pressure either side of the iliac crest to ease sensation in labour. Curved arrows indicate the hand position to press inwards and downwards to assist the opening of the sacrum and symphysis pubis. This is also deeply comforting in the liminal phase of labour.

- Refer to illustration C for where to place hands and apply pressure to provide comfort and assist with opening the pelvis
- Rebozo 'sifting' against the wall
- All fours with rebozo 'shaking the apples'
- Side-lying release
- Downward dog and inversion.

The intensity of labour and birth isn't to be undermined. The work a woman's body does is huge, while the baby actively participates in the process by adapting to the pelvic bowl. The baby is descending, rotating, head shape moulding, all the while gently nudging the cervix to encourage its opening and helping to stimulate contractions. The movements of both woman and baby are an intricate dance. Instinctive. Working together. This liminal phase is hard work. It isn't called labour for nothing. However, as Ally expressed, the self-empowerment and fulfillment of potential is a phenomenally euphoric experience.

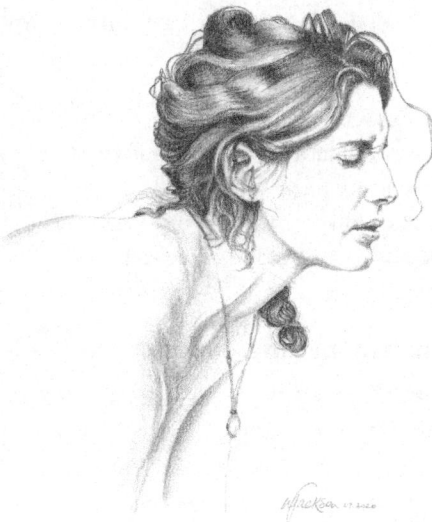

Mother becoming ... Ally, sinking deeply into her liminality, trusting in herself, her body and her baby. Her expression has that slight frown, eyes closed, lips parted, breathing through her contractions, or *surges* as she names them. The hormones of birth play in harmony as this song of labour, so incredible to witness, is free to flow.

The emergence phase

The liminal phase becomes the emergence phase when the baby descends and puts pressure through the pelvic floor nerves and on the rectum. The woman's vocal expression becomes deeper in sound: grunting, throaty and powerful. Alongside this, the muscles of the diaphragm, abdominal wall and uterine contractions change, becoming expulsive. Urges to bear down happen.

As mentioned before, adrenaline is heard loudly at this time, not negatively jarring, but re-activating the thinking brain, ensuring it is safe for birth to happen. Rousing the mother in readiness to move with the instinct to push. Women in undisturbed birth don't need vocal direction by birth attendees on how to push. They do so instinctively at the height of contractions. Again, because this phase is unique to each woman, the energy and pushing differs in duration.

The baby is still an active participant, because along with the pressing sensation on the cervix, the tissues in the pelvis are slowly stretched with each forward and rotating movement in tandem with contractions. The baby retreats backwards slightly and rests in between. As the vagina is stretched and the baby's head presses firmly downwards, the resistance of the soft tissues of the pelvis allows for rotation and descent of the baby's head. This stimulates even more oxytocin to provide stronger, longer contractions.

The bladder moves up as the urethra stretches out of the way over the baby's head. With the head pressing on the rectum and pelvic floor, the pelvic bowl is filled, and the sacrum moves outwards. This process becomes externally visible. (Refer to illustration A in Chapter 2.) There is no room for poo in the rectum before the baby is born. Poo at birth is normal and nothing to be anxious about. There is no space in the woman for inhibition now. Midwives and doulas have seen, heard and are comfortable with the expressive rawness of this phase. The mother becoming releases, softens, makes space through the pelvic floor between contractions and allows this opening to happen as the urge to bear down overcomes her.

- *Great Birth Rebellion* #11. 'The Labour Process' Apple 🎤 Spotify

- KICO 'Knees in calves out' YouTube. https://www.facebook.com/watch/?v=143530261072624

- **Wishlist** 🌾 Dr Rachel Reed YouTube. 'Transformation of the Uterus During Labour' https://www.youtube.com/watch?v=fF7HcH30u7o&list=PLzk4kScwvULLizGTz3kqevIK5QYnEpf25

- *The Midwives' Cauldron* S1 #3. 'Pushing and Cervixes' Apple 🎤 Spotify

- **Wishlist** Beautiful Birth Club YouTube. 'Push' assesses the man's 'progress' in making love to his partner in a birthing room, all under the watchful eye of midwives and doctors. Hilarious, yet poignant. The environment we need to make love, orgasm and create a baby in is the same environment a woman needs to birth in. https://www.youtube.com/watch?v=XdiUiC9iUP0&list=PL6n-MQ99SxK6lJj1OA9jF-8y77ntdgk5J&index=12

The clitoris, urge to push and the perinium in the emergence phase

During the emergence phase, the baby's head is being compressed inside the vagina within the pelvic bowl. During contractions, it moulds to shape. The bones of the baby's head are not solid, but consist of plates that can move and slide around the cushioned brain so that they shape to fit the internal structures of the mother's pelvis. This compression on the baby's head stimulates their vagal nerve.

Alongside vagal stimulation of the baby, the placenta is being compressed in this phase, causing interruption in the flow of blood to the baby. This naturally drops the baby's heart rate. The heart rate recovers when compression is reduced at the end of each contraction. This periodic reduction in oxygen releases a healthy stress response in the baby, preparing them for life outside the womb, prioritising the heart, lungs and brain. This healthy eustress activates stored fat, priming them for alertness and energy to initiate instinctive breastfeeding behaviour.

Oxytocin and beta-endorphins produced in the baby during labour prime the baby for birth and bonding. These hormones help them cope with the stress of being warm, squashed and fed by mum's blood one moment, and being out there in a cold, bright, hyper-stimulatory environment the next.

With expulsive contractions, the baby experiences added pressure on their bottom and they make small movements in between to help the process of being born. The baby is active in the dance with mum, rather than a passive body being forced out. As the baby moves down, reaches and stimulates the pelvic floor, the back of the baby's head travels down the inner aspect of the maternal *symphysis pubis* (front of the pelvis). Here, the baby presses on the stretched urethra and, most importantly, massages the inner aspect of the clitoris before and while the head emerges under the pubic arch. Birth researcher and author Margaret Jowitt's article, 'The clitoris in labour', describes this in detail, highlighting how stimulation in this way triggers the Ferguson reflex. This sends increased pulsed oxytocin to the uterus, in turn triggering the *fetus ejection reflex*, increasing the urge to bear down.[13]

The clitoris, being linked to the *levator ani* muscles, contracts, in turn enlarging the opening through the pelvic floor. This stimulation of the clitoris leads to engorgement of the *vestibular bulbs* that wrap around the vagina and the *crura* lining the pelvic arch. These all function to protect the back of the baby's head when being born, especially if the mother is in a forward-leaning position.

It wasn't until 2005 that an Australian urologist, Helen O'Connell, and her colleagues mapped the clitoris through MRI. It shows the external clitoris as the tip of an iceberg. The clitoris is so much more than a 'button' at the top of the vulva. Hidden under the vulva, it extends either side all the way down to the vagina, and in female arousal engorges as a penis does.[14] Use the goody box resources to inform yourself about your clitoris, because we are not taught about this essential part of our anatomy and its function in our sex education in school.

As the baby's head becomes visible, it stretches the tissues of the perineum and lower pelvis. You can minimise trauma to these tissues by adjusting the posture to KICO. This creates space in the lower pelvis and allows you to moderate the speed of birthing. A slow birthing minimises trauma, allowing time for stretching without any outside pressure on the perineum (such as a bed). Free to move her legs, the woman can slow the birthing process. As Rachel Reed says in her book, *Reclaiming Childbirth as Rite of Passage*: "A spotlight is shone onto the stage of the woman's perineum; everyone focuses on the performance of her birthing vagina. Watching the perineum does not reduce the chance of tearing, and instead may disrupt the woman's sense of privacy and physiology."[15]

A huge surge of adrenaline spikes in the mother as the baby's head *crowns* (the maximum diameter at the outlet of the vagina). Her sound becomes higher, with shorter, lighter breaths, to take pushing pressure upwards rather than downwards. She also moves her legs together to slow the progress of the birthing head. When left to guide themselves in physiological birthing, birthing women can often be seen moving from open-legged squatting to upright kneeling, allowing for the natural motion of KICO, along with a slightly forward tilting movement of the pelvis.

As the emerging head is born, there is a pause. The baby's body is being thoroughly compressed in the pelvis, squeezing fluids and mucus from the lungs and airways. At the same time, the shoulders drop into the pelvic bowl and a sideways rotation (*restitution*) action takes place. Again, the baby actively moves, pressing their feet against the top of the uterus. With the next surging contraction, the baby is fully born. Emergence is complete.

It is not unusual for some tearing of the perineum to occur. First-degree tears involve the skin only. Second-degree tears involve some degree of the muscle of the pelvic floor. These can often heal by themselves and recent research suggests surgical glue is a better solution than having stitches (*suturing*). Listen to the *Great Birth Rebellion* podcast on 'Perineal suturing' for detail and reassurance. Perineal tears and repairs are discussed with Katie in Chapter 5 and Alysia in Chapter 7.

- 'Discovering the anatomy of the clitoris' ABC news video https://www.abc.net.au/news/2024-06-06/discovering-the-anatomy-of-the-clitoris/103948278
- *The Midwives' Cauldron* S3 #12. 'Talking all things clitoris' Apple 🎙 Spotify
- *Great Birth Rebellion* #14. 'Pushing out your baby' Apple 🎙 Spotify
- Dr Rachel Reed Blog. Perineal 'Bundles' (OASI) and Midwifery' https://www.rachelreed.website/blog/perineal-bundles-oasi
- Wishlist 🌿 *Great Birth Rebellion* #21. 'Perineal suturing' Apple 🎙 Spotify
- Supporting the physiology of labour and birth at home or the hospital. Animated video. From 'The Practising Midwife Journal' https://www.facebook.com/reel/859956072338035

Dad's hands are ready, open to receive his daughter, as Ally moves instinctively into position to assist her baby's birthing. Here, leaning forward with hands on the sofa, her right leg is up and out to the side, foot firmly planted on the floor to make space for the baby's shoulders. Time is suspended, as Norah's head, shoulders and body are born.

The integration phase

The magical myriad of happenings continues in this next phase of integration as the baby adapts physiologically to life outside of mum. The cord is still pulsating. Mum still provides oxygenated blood while the baby takes time to breathe for themself. Eye-gazing between mother and baby combines with the immense high of euphoria and achievement. There is a flood of oxytocin in all those present at the birth, providing an atmosphere of love, connection and bonding as this new life integrates into the family.

As the mother holds, touches, strokes, investigates and talks to her baby, with the added stimulation of cool, light and noise, the baby will breathe on their own. Medical terminology for the period of time between the baby's birth and the birth of the placenta is called *the third stage*. It's important to delay clamping the cord as there is still a third of the volume of the baby's blood in the placenta and cord. The gentle pulsing is passing the blood into the baby. This usually takes about 2 minutes, but may be longer.

The Cochrane Review on cord-clamping advocates for the practice of delayed cord-clamping, which particularly benefits premature babies and decreases neonatal and infant anaemia.[2] When planning for delayed cord-clamping during caesarean section, the provision of sterile towels to keep the baby warm while cord blood flows to them may help. It is important to be aware that due to having an incision in the uterus, if there is heavy bleeding, the cord will be cut sooner. Indeed, if at any time there is a medical complication or the baby needs urgent medical attention, the cord will need to be cut.[16]

Placental birth in the emergence phase

Mother and baby are skin to skin, warm and comfortable. A myriad of amazing things is still happening all at once. In undisturbed physiological birth of the placenta, the umbilical cord remains uncut, keeping mother and baby together. There is time for the cord to stop pulsing and for the placenta to detach on its own from the inside of the uterus due to further oxytocin release and contractions (often associated with the baby's first breastfeed). Those attending the birth can adopt a 'wait and watch' approach, which is hands-off.

With further contractions, a heaviness and urge to bear down occurs after the placenta has separated from the uterus. There is a trickle of fresh blood seen at the entrance to the vagina and a lengthening of the cord as the placenta drops down to sit at the now almost closed cervix. The mother usually moves to an upright position to allow gravity to assist the birth of the placenta and membranes. This usually takes around 30–60 minutes.

Some women choose to have a *lotus birth*, a term first used in the US in the 1970s, when Clare Lotus Day asked her obstetrician not to cut the cord. She kept the placenta and cord attached to her baby until it dried and fell off naturally.[17] The practice of lotus birth usually involves covering the placenta in herbs. It detaches in its own time, usually at about day 3 after birth.

The placenta belongs to you, the mother. It can be taken home to be buried in the garden or on cultural homeland, the place marked with a plant, tree or ornament, sometimes with a ceremony. The placenta may be dried and put in capsules to be ingested by the mother.

In the book, *Placenta: the Forgotten Chakra*, Robin Lim describes how the Maori women of New Zealand have regained the practice of burying the placenta and cord on tribal land, confirming the sacred link with the Earth Mother. In Australia, the practice of burying the placenta on Country for Indigenous mothers is hugely significant. In Bali, a boy's placenta is buried on the right side of the entrance to the family home; a girl's is buried on the left side, with Sanskrit prayers and wishes for both. Then a stone is placed over the placenta and it is ritually celebrated each day with offerings of flowers and rice.[18]

The medical management of placental birth is called an *active third stage*. An injection of Syntocinon is given into the mother's thigh at the birth of the baby's body to speed up the process of the third stage and to prevent mum 'losing too much blood'. This is very common and not needed in undisturbed birth. Delayed injection of Syntocinon and delayed cord-clamping are still possible in medically managed birth and Syntocinon does not cross the placenta to the baby. The delivery of the placenta by *controlled cord traction* occurs when there are signs of separation of the placenta from the uterus, as already described.

During this entire transitory phase from life in the womb to life outside and integration, another magical occurrence might be happening: the breast crawl. In Chapter 6 with Alysia we will explore the breast crawl and baby-led attachment during the first golden hours of being skin to skin.

- **Wishlist** Dr Rachel Reed YouTube. 'Placental Transfusion of the Baby After Birth' https://www.youtube.com/watch?v=y3w_uiP95IM
- Dr Rachel Reed Blog. 'The placenta, essential resuscitation equipment' https://www.rachelreed.website/blog/placenta-resuscitation
- *The Midwives' Cauldron* S3 #5. 'Placentas and Cord Blood' Apple Spotify
- Dr Rachel Reed YouTube. 'Birthing the Placenta' https://www.youtube.com/watch?v=fl9M91dk2sk
- *Birth-Ed* S1 #15. 'The first 24 Hours with Marie Louise'. Apple Spotify

Water for labour and birth

More women are choosing to labour and birth in water for comfort, and there has been debate about the safety of this. Ethel Burns et al, in 'Systematic review and meta-analysis to examine intrapartum interventions, and maternal and neonatal outcomes following immersion in water during labour and waterbirth', confirms that water immersion significantly reduced the use of epidurals, injected opioids and overall maternal pain. There was also a reduction in episiotomy and postpartum haemorrhage. Waterbirth increased women's satisfaction in their birth experience and the chance of an intact perineum.

However, waterbirth was associated with increased odds of *cord avulsion* (where there is a tear in the umbilical cord). The risks of this occurring were still low. There were no differences in any identified neonatal outcomes, providing "clear benefits resulting from intrapartum water immersion for healthy women and their newborns."[19]

Babies have a dive reflex up to 6 months of age; this means that the baby will not breathe until they are in air, because the trigeminal nerve in the face is not stimulated in water. If at any point, while the head is being born, a woman lifts herself free of the water exposing the baby's head to cold air, she is encouraged to leave the water for the rest of the birth.

The *Great Birth Rebellion* discussion about 'Waterbirth' gives detail about the dynamics, positive effects, research outcomes and safety in water-birthing. If you are interested, listen in. Further to this, typing 'waterbirth' into a search engine will provide many videos of births in water. The *Australian Birth Stories* podcast contains over 40 such waterbirth experiences for your listening. Yumi was one of the mothers interviewed on *Birthtime*. Her story of waterbirth after a traumatic first birth is intense, but ends so affirmingly.

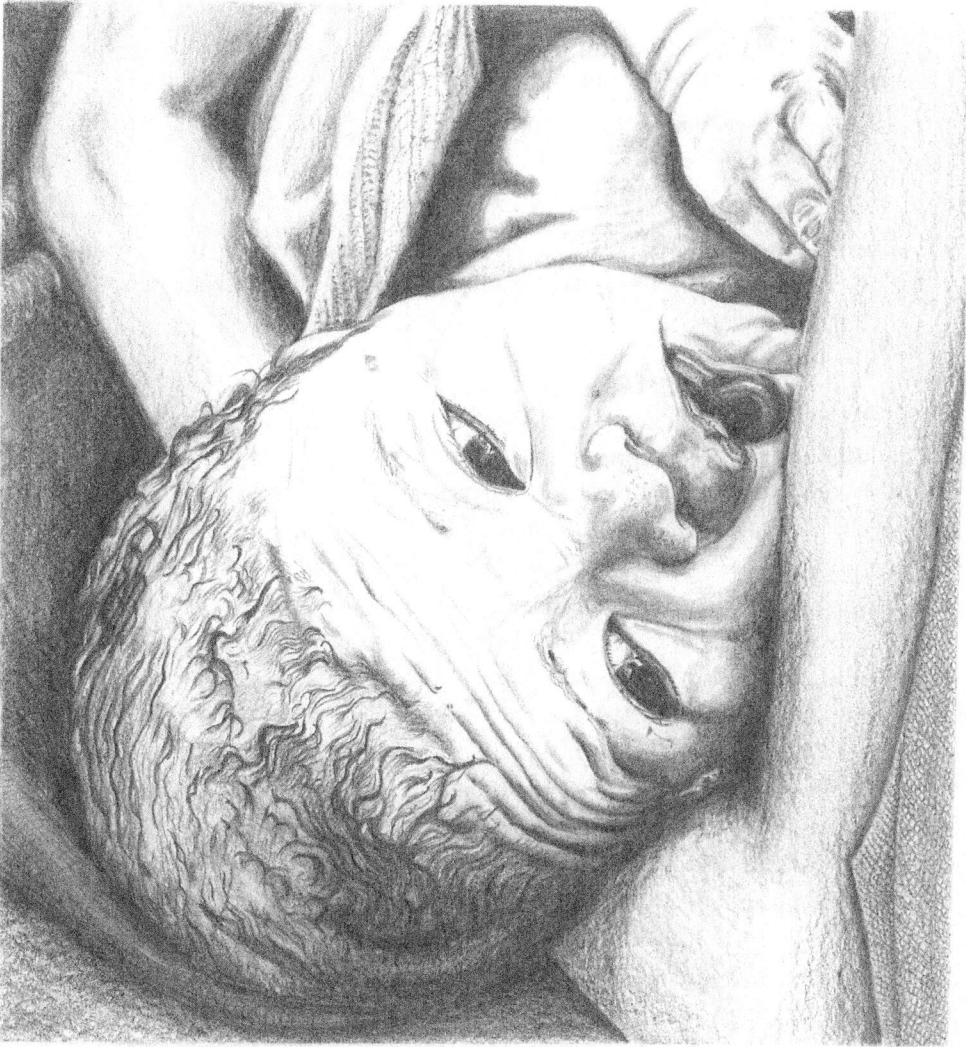

Norah   *WJackson*

Here, Norah is alert, looking towards her dad's voice. She has just had her first feed and is still attached to mum via the umbilical cord, which has long since stopped pulsating. She has received all her blood from the placenta. Ally is birthing the placenta as this photo was taken.

The NSW inquiry into birth trauma Recommendation 25 states that maternity wards be co-designed with consumers to provide a birthing environment that meets the needs of birthing women and their support, and ensure that water immersion is available.[20]

- *Great Birth Rebellion* #17. 'Waterbirth' Apple 🎙Spotify
- **Dr Sara Wickham website.** 'The benefits of waterbirth' https://www.sarawickham.com/research-updates/more-benefits-of-water-for-birth/
- *Australian Birth Stories* #223. 'Yumi' Apple 🎙Spotify
- **Pregnancy, Birth and Baby website.** 'Waterbirth' https://www.pregnancybirthbaby.org.au/water-birth#:~:text=Water%20immersion%20during%20labour%20and,your%20labour%20is%20progressing%20normally

---

Breech birthing

As a normal variation, 3–4% of babies present their bottoms into the pelvis. Obstetrician Dr Bisits advocates for first-time mothers to birth a breech vaginally. A mother who has birthed vaginally before is more likely to be supported in a vaginal breech birth. A first-time mother should be given the same support. This is in order to have the opportunity to experience the unique journey of labour and the physiological flood of oxytocin and other hormones, even if a caesarean birth happens.

Breech presentation may be due to a placenta praevia, or an anomaly of the uterus or baby, but most of the time we don't know. After investigations to discover why the baby might be breech, an *external cephalic version* (ECV) is offered. This is where the obstetrician manually attempts to turn the baby to head down. ECV is not always successful.

A breech baby has a few different ways of presenting its bottom into the pelvis. A *complete* breech is when both of the baby's knees are bent and the feet and bottom are closest to the birth canal – almost like a sitting, folded Buddha. A *frank* breech is when the baby's legs are extended upwards beside the head and the bottom is closest to the birth canal. These 2 presentations can birth vaginally.

An *incomplete* breech is when one of the baby's knees is bent and so a foot and bottom or both feet are closest to the birth canal. Incomplete breech is also known as a *footling* breech. This isn't a safe choice for the baby to birth vaginally; so, in this circumstance, a caesarean birth is offered.

With pressure on the woman from family and friends not to birth vaginally, even when the position of the baby makes it possible, it's hard on the woman emotionally when she wants to labour and birth vaginally. There is also pressure on obstetricians because of the culture of fear in medical practice around breech birth. Talking about the risks and benefits of breech birthing empowers women in making their decision and may help you in yours.

Remember Liesja's letter to you about her first birth, with Freya appearing into the world bottom first? Liesja felt held and supported to birth Freyja vaginally, with no preconceived ideas of fear around it. Supporting a woman's choice with confident language and a positive mindset is so important. Please listen to the *Great Birth Rebellion* chat with Dr Bisits about all things breech.

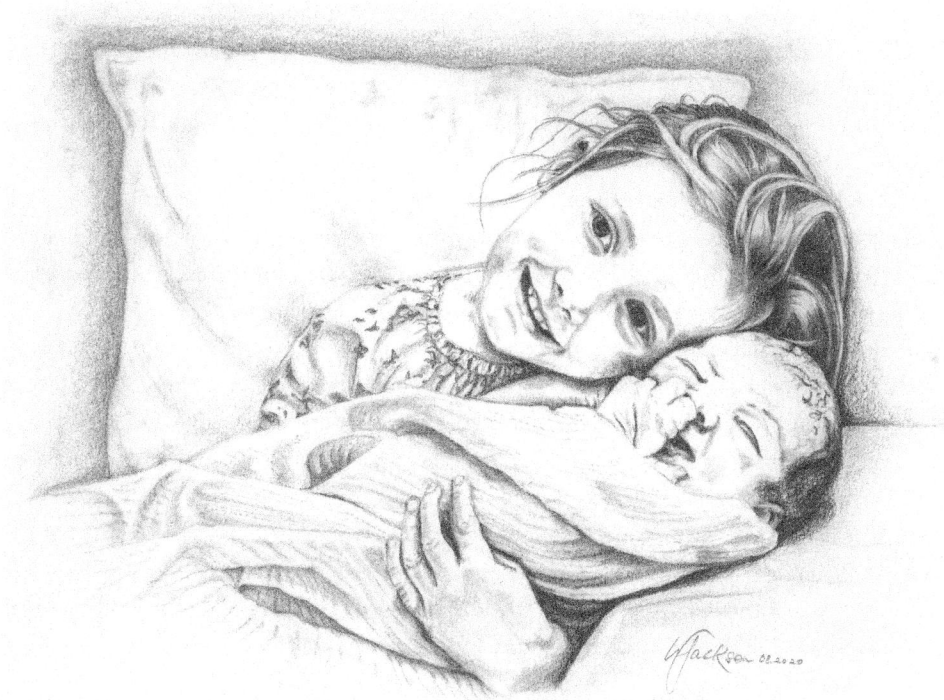

Norah being held by her big sister, Audrey. The joy and love on Audrey's face is too precious for words.

- *Great Birth Rebellion* #26. 'Breech' Apple 🎙 Spotify
- Breech Without Borders '10 mechanisms of upright breech birth' YouTube. https://www.youtube.com/watch?v=DXXwzdnmy9U&list=PLqoVCUc3-TDR1r6Hf-Q0hC-KG4NzGsYVb

Freebirthing. What and why?

Freebirth is not the same as homebirth. Freebirthing and planned homebirths might sound similar, but the risks are very different, as Professor Hannah Dahlen explains in a recent article: "Planned home births involve care from midwives, who are registered experts in childbirth, in a woman's home. These registered midwives work privately, or are part of around 20 publicly funded home birth programs nationally that are attached to hospitals."[21]

Freebirth is without a health professional like a midwife being present. The woman might employ an unregistered birth worker (usually a doula, lay-midwife, childbirth educator or ex-registered midwife) to support her without understanding all the risks involved. The numbers of freebirths are not known, but they did rise alongside home birthing with a midwife during the COVID-19 pandemic.[22]

Also known as *unassisted* or *wild pregnancy and birth*, women choose freebirth because they have been born and raised in a culture of not having health professional involvement. Some women choose to educate themselves as fully as they can through books, community and online groups. They plan to freebirth because they believe in and trust their bodies after previous professionally supported home birthing experiences.

Some women want a homebirth, but a midwife is not available or they don't fit the health service's current policy definition of 'low risk'. If they are unable to access a privately practising midwife, they choose to go it alone.

For more than a decade, there has been extensive research into why women choose to freebirth. In the book *Birthing Outside the System: The Canary in the Coal Mine*, midwife Melanie Jackson (host of the *Great Birth Rebellion* podcast) writes a chapter about 'Freebirth and high-risk homebirth, giving birth outside the system in Australia'. There, she explores why women make this choice. The research found that one in 10 women has experienced disrespectful or abusive care, previous trauma or coercion in the current hospital birthing environment. Fearing a recurrence – and when they are not heard, valued, or supported to find a different care pathway to prevent recurrence – they choose to go it alone. In short, many women are choosing freebirth because they are not supported in their choices within the models of care currently available in Australia. Some fear intervention and may not feel emotionally or culturally safe. And some are choosing it because there is not enough access to home birthing services, particularly in rural areas.[23]

There is a rise in the number of doulas and birth-keepers advertising themselves for services outside the system. This is a growing industry that has no regulation. Indeed, the Australian Doula College has a code of conduct that advocates against doulas attending freebirths. The possible risks and benefits of this choice are explored in an ABC article 'The Price of Freebirth'.[24] This is explored in the *Great Birth Rebellion* chat 'Freebirth in the Media with Charlotte King, ABC Reporter'.

As ever, there is no place for judgement here. We haven't walked in the shoes of women who make these choices for themselves.

Recommendation 26 of the NSW inquiry into birth trauma is to "investigate expanding publicly funded homebirth services".[25] Again, this is needed countrywide.

- *Great Birth Rebellion* #70. 'Freebirth in the Media with Charlotte King, ABC Reporter' Apple 🎙 Spotify

---

Practice offering: *Dhyana*, with a lotus and bee meditation

In preparation for more structured meditation, the concentrated yogic meditation practice of *dharana*, which is drawing the senses inwards, can be likened to the separation phase. This then leads into *dhyana*, the meditative withdrawal into the self and releasing of outward perceptions. When witnessed in a woman in labour, this withdrawal into her liminal phase is a potent sight to behold.

This visualisation of the lotus and the bees is used for intensity in labour and birthing.

- Imagine you are a lotus flower with your petals opening out towards the sun. Each petal has a goddess as a bee who flies out, gathering nectar and pollen, and comes back to the heart of the lotus flower to nourish you. The bees bring the sweetness of nectar warmed from the sun for energy and with love. These goddess bees rest within each petal as it closes for the night, absorbing the nectar and warmth.

- An analogy for you: send your goddess bees out into the world while you are experiencing a contraction. You open to the sun, absorbing its warmth and sustaining light. Then, in the space between contractions, you close to rest. Replenish yourself from the nectar your bees gathered in readiness for the activity of the next surging wave of contraction.

- Incorporate the breath as prana, that of lifeforce, along with nectar, gathering and using the energy with every inhalation … Then use your voice as you exhale … hummmmmmm in harmony with the bees. This is a primal, instinctive and embodied experience.

- Your hum may be quiet, heard only in your mind to begin with, becoming outwardly expressed, louder as you need. Hum.

- Visualise softening, and actively soften the pelvic floor, opening, like the lotus flower. Picture seeing the descent of your baby's head, the widening of your cervix, the top of the womb thickening and pressing downwards.

- Rest in between, breathing for yourself and your baby, using the nectar …

- OOOOHHHH AHHHHHHHH HMMMMMMMMM.

With increased awareness of your body and belief in it, you may say to yourself as a chant, an affirmation or a meditation … "I now release and allow my values, strengths and self-trust in my preparation and in my birth support to guide me." Make up your own.

Practice offering: Yoga flow for undisturbed birthing

The postures in this offering are for comfort in labour and birth in any environment.

This flow is offered with yoga postures altered for comfort in labour. Use what works for you in any order. There is no one-size-fits-all flow or schedule. Everything you have learned and practised when preparing your body for labour is harnessed here.

Privacy, movement, fluids, snacks, touch, massage, sound, smell, soft lighting and your trusted birth support enhance oxytocin and beta-endorphin.

1. Supported wide-legged Child's pose. Rest here as much as you like. Soften the pelvic floor. Imagine yourself in the lotus flower meditation. Sound out "Ooooooo", "aaaahhhh", "mmmmmmmm". Long exhalations of golden thread breath. Rest in between each surging contraction. Sink into your oxytocin-rich body. Listen to it. Move as you need to.

   Your birth support places their hands either side of your pelvis, providing inward pressure to provide relief as explained in Illustration C, page 139.

2. Lean over a birthing ball, a sofa or table, or against a wall, or arms wrapped around your birth support. Do the Cow to Cat sequence as many times as you like. Soften the pelvic floor. Make circles or figure of 8 to the right, then left. Your birth support provides pelvic pressure, if wanted. Use the ocean meditation of floating over waves if it resonates with you.

3. Forward lunge. Foot turned outwards at 45 degrees. Soften the pelvic floor. Rock forwards, backwards and in small circular motions. Repeat for the other side. Pelvic pressure.

4. Sit in a high squat on a birthing ball with your feet facing outwards. Rock side to side and make circular movements. For support, lean forwards, arms crossed on a pillow on a table or bed. Pelvic pressure.

5. Lean against a wall or your partner. Make figure of 8 circles with a slight right knee bend and your foot facing outwards at 45 degrees. Then with your foot facing inwards, make the same movements to fully release the ligaments and muscles around the right hip. Repeat on the other side. Pelvic pressure. Use the tree meditation if it supports you in the depth of labour.

6. Upright kneeling, with something soft under your knees, supported by your partner. Or your upper body supported on a sofa or bed. Feet outwards in the first phases of labour and inwards near to the time when your baby is to be born. KICO. Pelvic pressure.

7. Seated back to front on a chair or on a toilet. Head and arms supported by a pillow on the top of the chair or cistern. Pelvic pressure. Long strokes down the back or massage in between contractions.

8. Sit sideways on a sofa or bed with the right leg bent at the knee and your foot dangling off the edge. Place the hands on the sofa or bed, left foreleg or foot on the floor. Lean forwards into the hands and gradually lower your body forwards to feel the outside of the right hip stretch. Repeat on the other side.

9. Supported side-lying posture for rest on the floor, sofa or bed as you need. Place firm cushions or a bolster between the knees. Golden thread breath with "ooooooo", "aaaahhhh", "mmmmmmmm" as you feel the need to. Choose a meditation that feels right for you in this moment. Lotus, meadow, ocean, tree or your own. Move into any posture your body tells you to birth in. Hold your mind, body and soul with love, wonder and appreciation. You are extraordinary.

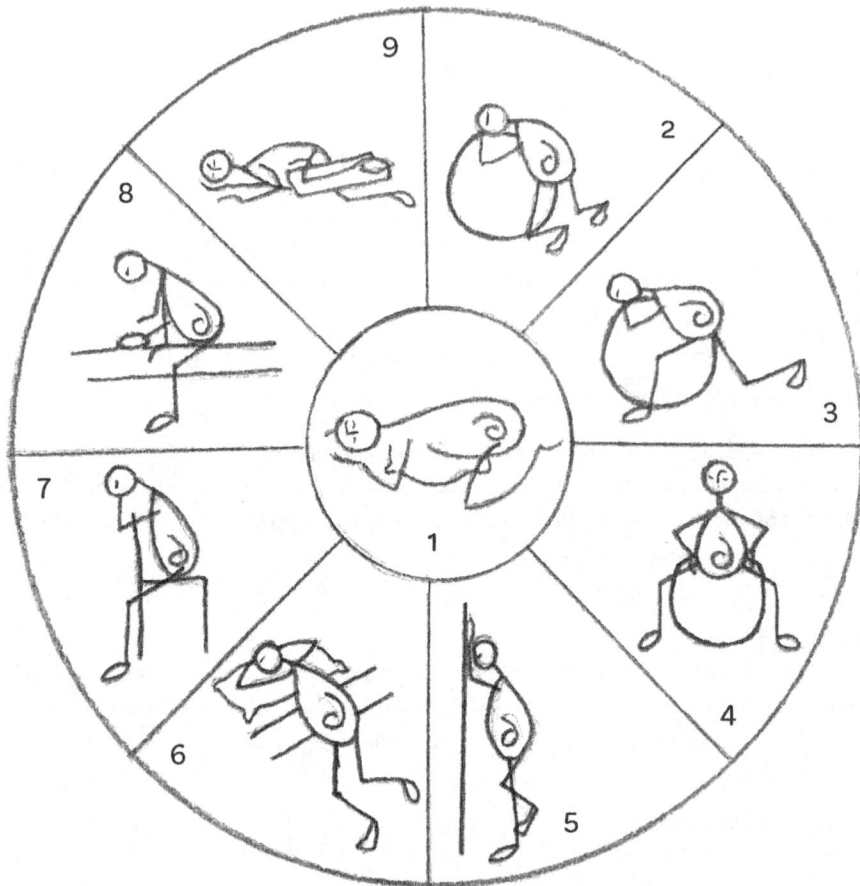

Cultural, Herstorical and Political Influences on Undisturbed Physiological Birthing

Here we go again. More history. "Please no!" I hear you say. Before you throw the book at the wall again, dear Mother Becoming, know that we are still on the journey of learning and understanding the 'why' for how maternity care looks today. This knowledge supports your authority and autonomy when you labour and birth.

I've mentioned the delay in implementing evidence and best practice in obstetric care. This flows directly into our next discussion, which is about how labour progress is monitored and assessed using inaccurate methods such as Friedman's curve. Here is the background to our herstory.

Assessing labour progress

In 1955 Dr Emmanuel Friedman plotted on a graph (*partogram*) the cervical dilatation rates of 500 white women in hospital. He determined that birthing women 'should' dilate at 1 cm every hour in labour. This graph, Friedman's curve, which we have mentioned before, monitors progress once labour is established at 3 cm. However, the curve is a one-size-fits-all method of 'assessment of progress in labour'. For starters, some women walk around with a 3 cm dilated cervix and are not in labour.

This tool of assessment was made when sedation was common practice and women were restricted to the bed. The women were aged between 17 and 43 and were a combination of first-, second- and third-time births. There were 74.5% spontaneous vaginal births, 20.2% forceps, 2.4% assisted breech births and 0.8% caesareans.[26] (Notice how low the caesarean rate was then!)

The research does not consider spontaneous, unmedicated physiological labour progress or differing cultural heritage.

Using this graph, in 1969 Dr Kieran O'Driscoll devised active management of labour as a method of reducing 'prolonged' labours.[27] O'Driscoll is instrumental in developing the use of Syntocinon during labour to shorten it. His 1973 paper states: "Active management of labour has been developed to the extent that an assurance is given to every woman who attends this hospital that her first baby will be born within 12 hours."[28]

His patriarchal approach, although well-meaning, to prevent prolonged labour, meant Friedman's expectation of 1 cm dilation per hour became deeply entrenched and rapidly widespread around the world. Dr O'Driscoll had huge respect for midwives and advocated strongly for one-to-one intensive midwifery care (although he did not believe that husbands should be present). However, his ideal put a very big nail in the coffin of physiological labour, and this deskilled midwives in physiological birthing.

This tool of assessment mandates regular vaginal examinations of the cervix as the main way to assess progress of dilation and therefore labour. When it comes to vaginal examinations, assessment differs between health professionals. Also, babies' heads are different sizes, not a standard 10 cm, which is deemed to be a fully dilated cervix.

Each examination only informs the carer of what is happening at that particular time. It does not consider each woman's unique way of labouring or all the other parameters of non-invasive assessment of progress that are employed by midwives. It places time limitations, and often labels such as 'labour dystocia' or 'failure to progress', on the mother. It allows for interventions to commence, and it became a convenient method of making labour fit into an institutional timetable, making it run in an efficient, timely, controlled manner.

The Obstetric Care Consensus: 2014–2016 recommended that Friedman's curve should no longer be used.[29] As I write this, it is 2025 and the assumption that women should dilate at 1 cm an hour in labour still heavily influences assessment.

In 2020 the World Health Organization published the *Labour Care Guide: User's Manual*, which provides a visual of a partogram with explanation for its use. It is an excellent resource for professionals worldwide. The partogram was originally designed for remote areas to allow time for transfer if complications arose, not for low-risk labour. It states: "In active first stage, plot 'X' to record cervical dilatation. Alert triggered when lag time for current cervical dilatation is exceeded with no progress."[30] The partogram is useful as part of holistic assessment in managed labour like an induction.

The partogram is still a linear representation of assessment of labour. When used for low-risk women, where both mother and baby are well, it does not allow for the effects of midwifery COC or physiological plateaus. The WHO states that "digital vaginal examination at intervals of four hours is recommended for routine assessment of active first stage of labour in low-risk women".[31] This is not based in sound evidence, nor does it consider other methods of non-invasive observational physiological assessments by the midwife.

One of these non-invasive ways of knowing the progress of labour is the 'purple line', which appears and extends from the anus upwards to the *natal cleft* (base of the sacrum) and is visible in about 75% of women. This may be argued by medical clinicians as unreliable; however, the unique progress of cervical dilation does not happen in isolation, as a myriad of other physiological and emotional events are happening at the same time.[32]

> • Dr Sara Wickham website. 'Evidence for the purple line' https://www.sarawickham.com/questions-and-answers/evidence-for-the-purple-line/

Physiological plateaus (pauses) in labour are normal

Physiological plateaus are common, and occur at any stage throughout the phases of labour and birthing. These are rest periods, where self-regulation of the mother and baby working together results in good birth outcomes for them both. The woman self-resumes her labouring.[33] Awareness and understanding of this natural phenomenon needs to become part of midwifery and obstetric training.

'Failure to progress' and augmentation

During childbirth, one of the most common diagnoses of pathology is failure to progress. An intervention called augmentation is suggested to speed up labour. This intervention involves having the waters broken (artificial rupture of membranes (ARM); *membranes* are the *amniotic sac*), usually followed by a drip of intravenous synthetic oxytocin.

As many as one in 3 women is augmented in spontaneous labour. In Australia, the numbers are 41% of first-time birthing women and 21% of women who have had one or more births. Rising rates of labour augmentation with oxytocin have been reported internationally, in some countries reaching an incidence of nearly 80%.[34]

ARM is not recommended at any time in physiological labour. The amniotic sac is there for a reason: to equalise the pressure around the uterus, cushion the baby and placenta, and provide equal distribution of pressure on the opening cervix as it is drawn up over the baby's head. In naturally occurring labour, there is no evidence to back up the cultural belief that breaking the waters will speed up labour.

ARM is associated with increased pain, and some babies become distressed due to cord or placental compression. Sometimes the cord is flushed over the baby's head into the vagina, which is called a *cord prolapse*. This requires emergency caesarean birth. The Cochrane Review states that "the evidence showed no shortening of the length of the first stage of labour and a possible increase in caesarean section. Routine amniotomy is not recommended for normally progressing labours or in labours which have become prolonged".[35]

In addition, Dr Kerstin Uvnäs Moberg demonstrates that in measuring plasma (blood) oxytocin levels, a maximum of 3 peaks in 10 minutes occurs during normal vaginal birth. There is a giant peak in oxytocin called the Ferguson reflex. A Syntocinon intravenous infusion is a continuous dose rather than intermittent. Blood plasma levels of oxytocin may become 3 to 4 times higher than in spontaneous labour. When offered after an ARM to speed up labour, the overall reduction in time is about 2 hours; however, the incidence of forceps and caesarean births is not reduced.[36]

As Dr Sara Wickham's website article 'What is a labour plateau?' explains, "The timespan of labour is individual, non-linear and essentially unpredictable. The discomfort that some people have with these notions, however, should not mean that a particular labour pattern is deemed pathological just because it doesn't fit a curve that wasn't evidence-based in the first place and that doesn't account for individuality."[37]

What if these pauses were recognised as just that – a pause? How might labour and birth be revolutionised in the medical institutional care provider approach? Midwives have a holistic philosophy, which is suited to continuity of care and has a positive impact on birth outcomes for mothers and babies. Knowledge and experience of physiological birth, faith in women, and physical and mindful support practices are needed in our current culture of hospitalised birthing. Midwives often find themselves in a position of philosophical difference in the hospital environment; they see physiological plateaus being misinterpreted as pathological failure to progress.

Part of the ICM position statement on the appropriate use of interventions for midwives is to "take measures to avoid unnecessary interference in the progress of normal labour and birth". This means supporting the woman in her informed decision after she has been given complete information about any proposed use of technology and interventions and she understands the implications of their use.[38] Coupled with the ICM Bill of Rights for Women and Midwives statement that "every woman has the right to receive care in childbirth from an autonomous and competent midwife",[39] we can see how a midwife working in a hospital environment under the strictures of the partogram may be undermined in that very autonomy.

As hospitals are currently the main place of birth in Australia, placing women within the domain of midwife-led care on a labour ward – with guidelines that reflect childbirth physiology and holistic philosophy – would help women feel safer to birth in hospital.

It's okay to decline medical intervention in a well mother and baby

Given that vaginal examination in a well mother to 'diagnose progress' and ARM to 'speed up labour' are not supported by evidence, declining is absolutely okay. Labour does not fit a scheduled timeline. It will be unique to you. There is no need to interfere in this physiological process in a well woman and baby. As we evolved, we didn't put sticks up our vaginas to pop the sac. Remember the BRAIN and IDECIDE mnemonics. They are there to support you.

Before augmentation, the following manoeuvres should be considered for incorporation into care for suspected labour dystocia:

- rebozo 'sifting' against the wall
- all fours with rebozo 'shaking the apples'
- side-lying with release
- Downward Dog and inversion (if possible).

In *Men, Love and Birth*, Mark Harris states, "We live in a society in which doctors try to convince us we need them in order to give birth. What we've seen over the years is a medicalisation of the birthing process, and if we want to get a little bit political, it's driven predominantly by the male gender, or 'male energy' if you like."[40] He goes on to describe how men are goal-fixated and have invented stages of labour. He adds, "The male way of fixing stuff is to count and quantify," and how "gadgets and men have tended to go together when it comes to birth."[41] He likens us to Stone Age men and women living in the fast lane. In an evolutionary sense, we have had such a short time to adjust to fast-paced, technological living, and this doesn't fit with the unpredictability of the dance of labour and birth.

Friedman assessed 500 women. What if the data and holistic assessments of 500 women who laboured and birthed physiologically were used as a baseline instead? We would have a vastly different framework. Labour isn't about how dilated a woman is. She can walk around 5 cm dilated for months before labour starts. She can be at 4 cm in labour and an hour later have her baby in her arms. Or she can be at 3 cm for 5 hours, while other changes take place, like the baby descending and rotating, plateauing and cervix thinning. That is the kind of research that needs to be done, research that takes the experiences and satisfaction of the women into consideration too.

How might it be if all medical and midwifery students had to witness physiological births – at least one of them at home – as a mandatory part of their training so that they understand the power of birthing?

- · WHO Labour Care Guide User's Manual. https://iris.who.int/bitstream/handle/10665/337693/9789240017566-eng.pdf?sequence=1
- · Wishlist 🌿 'Pauses and slow times in labour are normal' Facebook video. https://www.facebook.com/dr.marina.weckend/videos/903404747908784
- · Dr Rachel Reed Blog. 'In defence of the amniotic sac' https://www.rachelreed.website/blog/amnioticsaclabour
- · *The Midwives' Cauldron* S5 #3. 'Labour Pauses–Failure to Progress or Just Normal?' Apple 🎙 Spotify
- · Wishlist 🌿 Dr Rachel Reed Blog. 'Understanding and assessing labour progress' https://www.rachelreed.website/blog/understanding-labour-progress

---

Vaginal examinations

Currently, vaginal examination for assessment is done with the access, convenience and comfort of the practitioner in mind, not of the birthing woman. For example, examination may take place before induction to decide the best method, to administer medication for induction, to break the waters and to assess progress. The woman – often on her back, feet drawn up towards the bottom and knees out to the side – is in a very exposing position. Examination is uncomfortable, often painful, particularly in labour during a contraction, because it restricts the nutation (outward movement) of the sacrum, which is compressed when on her back. In labour, if a woman is upright kneeling or on all fours and a vaginal assessment is required, there is no need to put her on her back on the bed. It can be done where she is most comfortable – after her consent.

What if all midwifery and medical students were trained to do vaginal examinations with the woman on her left hand side, in more comfort and dignity than on her back? Particularly to assess for type of induction, administering medication for induction, or in labour, if needed. If instrumental birth is required to expedite the birth of a baby, then the lithotomy position on the back, semi-sitting with legs supported in stirrups, is probably the most sensible. However, when setting up for this, the birthing woman can be kept comfortable until the last possible moment; she maintains her dignity, and care providers speak with utmost respect and kindness, and explain continuously. The hospital birthing environment today is not designed around female physiology and emotional safety, but to fulfil the needs of care providers, time management and invasive procedures.

Talking about assessing the cervix, 'Vaginal examinations' will be a helpful listen at this point, as it will help you understand what you may expect of your care when in labour. Thankfully, there are lots of giggles to lighten the mood of such an intimate topic.

- *The Midwives' Cauldron* S4 #10. 'Vaginal examinations' Apple 🎙 Spotify

Birthing on Country: an Australian herstory and what we can relearn

Our herstory in Australia goes back thousands of years before colonisation with Birthing on Country. Grandmothers' Law was taught by Elders to new generations of traditional midwives for attending to pregnancy, birth and postpartum, and was 'women's business'. Traditional knowledge of Birth Law was held in ritual, initiation, ceremony, spirit, singing, cultural obligation, traditional medicine and taboo. It was handed down from generation to generation to support women in their communities. What we can learn from the rich cultural history of First Nations women is of great value.

European settlers, missionary dormitories and colonial policy had a devastating effect on Grandmothers' Law. Indigenous women were restricted or prohibited from practising traditional birthing culture by the segregation and separation of families and communities. White colonists removed a generation of children from their families. This has caused untold harm, not only to families, but also to Grandmothers' Law. The loss of such rich knowledge has deeply affected spirituality, intrinsic cultural identity and belonging for the 500 unique First Nations that existed before colonisation.

By the 1920s, the Queensland government decreed that the practice of Birthing on Country was to stop. Indigenous women had to travel hundreds of kilometres away from all they knew to birth in western, culturally unfamiliar hospitals. This was instigated without any consultation with Elders. The intention was to provide safety for mother and baby, and provision of what was then deemed to be the best medical care possible, but with unparalleled ignorance and lack of respect for Grandmothers' Law. Without the familiarity of cultural birthing practices or matriarchal support, Indigenous women were labouring and birthing in an alien environment, with language barriers and racist attitudes.

The move to birthing in hospitals wasn't just for Indigenous women, but for all women. Untrained independent midwives had been caring for women at home, in lying-in homes and small maternity hospitals until the 1920s. The wholesale removal of birthing to hospital under the guise of safety, less injury during birth and fewer maternal deaths affected all women in Australia.[42]

Birthing on Country is an international movement returning maternity services to First Nations communities for improved health and wellbeing. Each First Nations people had their own rich cultural heritage and practices of bush medicine with traditional midwives. While much has been lost, the strong common theme of abiding by Grandmothers' Law holds.

Indigenous women laboured and birthed in culturally significant and sacred places. Some of these were with 'birthing trees', often near water. The trees were shaped to have hollows as hand holds. The significant practice of ritually burying the placenta on Country to form a spiritual link between the child and that Country cannot be overstated. This culturally significant practice can easily be supported by ensuring that the mother leaves the place of birthing with her placenta. Birthing on Country isn't exclusive to birthing on specific Indigenous land. It is about being culturally aware, respectful and supportive – listening to what is significant and important to the mothers, and respecting choices and the inherent wisdom of Grandmothers' Law.[43]

Westernised culture can learn from the wisdom of Grandmothers' Law too, and can absorb the wisdom into COC practices for all women.

The TMCC's Call to Action on Birthing on Country highlights how Indigenous mothers and babies in resourced westernised countries have an increased risk of adverse outcomes due to social situation, poverty, racism and intergenerational trauma. For Indigenous women in a relationship-based Birthing on Country COC model – where they feel culturally and spiritually safe, and their social and family situation and inclusion is taken seriously – they are more likely to engage with maternity care. They feel safe to disclose sensitive information and make healthcare changes to contribute to their own and baby's improved health outcomes.[44]

"The role and practice of Indigenous doulas offers a promising approach to redressing the colonisation of Indigenous childbirth while contributing to improving Indigenous maternal and infant outcomes. Indigenous doula practice shares many best-practice characteristics with Indigenous Healing Programs and as such is also likely to promote intergenerational healing."[45] Recommendations 33 and 34 of the NSW inquiry into birth trauma suggest that we "ensure culturally safe care is accessible for all First Nations mothers and babies" and that we "acknowledge and address the diverse needs of various demographics in the maternity care system". This includes "refugees, First Nations, LGBTQIA+, rural and remote regions, and persons with pre-existing conditions or disability".[46]

Interviewed by *Birthtime*, midwife Melanie Briggs says, "Our women feel that when they're in there (hospital) and being cared for by midwives, that they're great midwives, they're so amazing, but their connection to our culture is not there. We're just trying to change the way our women are treated. They just want dignity. They just want to be treated as a human being. They don't want to be judged. They don't want to come out feeling traumatised. They want to come out feeling empowered and feeling like: 'Look what I've just done. I've just created a human being!'"[47]

We can relearn, regain and return to ritual, initiation, ceremony and embodied practices from First Nations women worldwide. With utmost respect and without cultural appropriation, there is much wisdom and knowledge to rediscover that has been lost to women raised in a westernised culture. Vanessa Olorenshaw captures this perfectly as she writes: "Feminism must recognise the importance of the female birthing experience. It is not, of itself, a burden; we must celebrate and protect that experience. There is something so truly humbling about the birth of a mother (note 'mother' here, not 'baby') that it is a betrayal that this is a topic which fails often to receive the veneration it deserves."[48] We will explore this more in the spiritual element.

Phew! Time for another break. Put the kettle on. That was another heap of information to take in. In this pause, sit with what really stood out for you and think for a while, chat to a friend or journal to find some clarity. Do whatever works for you. It may take a few days to seep in. Using your values and strengths, begin to cultivate self-trust in how you wish to approach your birthing. Hold within yourself the essences of self-worth and compassion while processing your thoughts.

And always remember to breathe.

Social, Economic and Media Influences on Undisturbed Physiological Birthing

You retreat from the world as your labour begins and you give birth, physically removing yourself from the hustle and bustle of everyday life, removed also from social media and emotional connections that keep your attention outwards. In your own secure social bubble with your intimate trusted support, these few days are precious and the experiences are forever remembered. Your village is activated, taking care of children, pets or any other dependents, cooking up a storm.

Continued preparation for your fourth trimester

Building your village and connection is vital for the entire family and community. Asking for help is normal, a huge strength of character – not a failing. Your village is going to provide for you and your family in the weeks to come. Hopefully your favourite recipes and snacks will be made for you. Yum!

Visitors can be exhausting, so having some pre-arranged boundaries for your fourth trimester is ideal and could save your sanity. Let visitors know they might not get to hold the baby and should wait until the parents are ready to hand them over. You can even encourage them to leave a meal at the door without disturbing the family. Visitors become helpers. When people do arrive, they are to bring prepared food, snacks or some shopping. *They* make the tea, not Mum or Dad. They do small chores like tidy the kitchen, give the loo a clean, put laundry on, hang out the washing etc. Up to you.

Create a 'feed and support the new family' group, where you put in messages and requests, and communicate when visits would be okay. It's for others to work out who, what, when and how to fulfil requests. Having a 'Do not disturb; mum and baby resting' sign on the front door is another must.

Disengaging from social media and the world news for a while and turning your phone notifications off creates a more peaceful environment to promote rest.

- **Wishlist** *Birth-Ed* S1 #8. 'A Mindful Fourth Trimester' with Sophie Burch Apple Spotify
- **'Gender wars and household chores'.** An animated comic demonstrates behaviour patterns and experiences in couples when a baby arrives. https://www.theguardian.com/world/2017/may/26/gender-wars-household-chores-comic?fbclid=IwAR3WteLfVJeMFY_WeMJeh_ZTrHp6Q5FhPhz1a2NzQ9Q

Money to be made from birthing ... continued

How is pregnancy and birth funded in Australia? The Transforming Maternity Care Collaborative highlights how public and private maternity care is *activity-base funded*. So, services and hospitals are funded for the activity they do. Hospitals receive more money for a woman who has more complex care activity and more interventions. Hospital care activity attracts higher funding than outpatient and community-based care.

In its article 'Private Obstetric Care Increases Risk of Unplanned Caesarean for Low-Risk Women', the TMCC explains: "In the private maternity system, there are financial incentives to intervene in normal physiological processes, without a clinical indication." Unlike public hospitals, private hospitals receive more money for a caesarean than vaginal birth from private health insurers. The most recent figures indicate that a caesarean birth in a private hospital is $11,500 compared to a vaginal birth at $8,500. Private obstetricians charge fee-for-service antenatally, which is unregulated. Public obstetricians work set hours for a set salary, so are not incentivised by financial gain through interventions.[49]

In the TMCC blog, they ask, "What if all low-risk women planned to birth in a birth centre or at home?" They highlighted that, when COVID-19 hit, many women chose to give birth at home due to being separated from their birth support. Hospital savings from fewer caesarean births and bed hours for all low-risk women who birthed at home or in a birth centre were significant.

As an indicator of how much money can be saved, "... a USA analysis has determined an annual saving of $US 11 billion if 10% of all births occurred at home or in a freestanding birth centre".[50] Wow, that's a lot! "Significant health resource savings could occur by shifting low-risk births from hospitals to home birth and birth centre services. Greater examination of Australian women's preferences for home birth and birth centre birth models of care is needed."[51] Women's choices to birth at home and in birth centres need to be taken seriously, not just because it saves money, but because it is what they want.

The TMCC wishes women to understand the implications of their advised or chosen model of care and to have access to alternatives, like midwifery continuity of care, birth centres and home birth. Its article 'Health services lack incentive to be cost effective' came from a study about cost and the benefits of maternity care up to 12 months after birth. It found public midwifery group practice care costs 22% less than other models of maternity care, with a cost-saving of approximately $5,000 per woman to hospital funders, due to shorter inpatient hospital stays.[52]

I went through the advocacy section of Maternity Choices Australia and noted that their proposals to increase midwifery-led care from 8% to 75% in every state and territory could lead to an economic saving to the taxpayer of $1.262 billion. I'm only talking about the dollar cost here. The emotional and physical costs will be discussed with Katie in Chapter 5.

If funding followed the woman, focused on outcomes rather than output, and reduced costs due to less motivation for intervention, how might that affect the culture of birthing? A value-based approach could move us away from the focus on output towards outcomes. Solutions that deliver efficient high-quality, patient-centred care minimise 'perverse incentives' for intervention. In value-based care programs, care providers are held more accountable for improving patient outcomes.[53] How might value-based care improve maternity services?

The TMCC suggests a Learning Health System (LHS), as "High value maternity care will produce the highest level of benefit for women at a given cost, and deliver what matters the most to women."[54]

What women value should be at the heart of value-based maternal and newborn care funding. Previous history shows that when all services come from one budget, high technological care takes priority over continuity. Funding for COC models and out-of-hospital services needs to be allocated separately from acute hospital services. Funding for remote and regional care needs to be thoroughly evaluated so that the care provided for women and newborns achieves the best outcomes with the available resources.[55]

Self-identity, Beliefs and Values, and Spiritual Influences in Undisturbed Physiological Birthing

Transformation

The hormones we have chatted about create a transformation in you. You are never going to be the woman you were. You are more. Like the butterfly emerging from its chrysalis, you are changed. You may not feel as beautiful as that butterfly after birthing, but the rite of passage you have just experienced has influenced the entirety of your being in a profound way.

It's okay to inhabit the deep femininity of mothering. It's okay to embrace it, welcome it, revel in it, and celebrate this extraordinary pinnacle of feminine creation and ability. It's okay to surrender and sink into the mess of physical change, emotions and feelings. To inhabit a world where you are supported to rest, heal, feed, hold, smell, touch, kiss, stroke, and fall in love with your baby.

Shakti. Feminine energy and power

Within yogic philosophy, *shakti* is the feminine energy of the active power of the divine. The *pranashakti* is lifeforce, expressing herself as a flow of energy for and within the body. Shakti is Mother Nature. She is the power of generation and creativity, the power of words, the energy of mantras, and the creative power of imagination, ability, strength, effort, capability and effectiveness.

Shakti captures the essence of a labouring and birthing woman so beautifully, recognising feminine strength and power.[56] "When women can take their power from their birth, they can do anything. That's how we change the world. We change childbirth and we have women who are powerful, who can take the lead … know their strengths and they can work within their communities." These were the words of Professor Pat Brodie when interviewed on *Birthtime*.[57]

Combine these with the words of midwife and author Jane Hardwicke Collings, also interviewed on *Birthtime*: "Birth is women's business. We're pretending it's not, but it is. When women understand themselves and claim their power, everything will change."[58] Vanessa Olorenshaw adds: "From a feminist perspective, the way we are conditioned to see nothing enormous and significant in the work of women in birthing their babies is just one of the ways the strength of women is undermined. Just think back to the countless times you have heard the phrase 'doctor delivers baby' or 'father delivers baby' or 'taxi-driver delivers baby'. Erm, no. Mother delivers baby. Anybody else just catches a baby. End of chat."[59]

It is extraordinary to witness the power of liminality, emergence and integration through the rite of passage of birthing, into a new identity. This power of transition from conception to pregnancy to labour to birth to mother is an astonishing spiritual journey to be acknowledged and celebrated.

> • *Happy Mama Movement #149.* 'The Yoga of Birth' talks about the gentle philosophy of yoga practice in pregnancy, birth and mothering in a beautiful, soulful way. Apple 🎙 Spotify

Creating rituals, a spiritual practice of acknowledgment

Women supporting women is the key to finding what has been broken and lost in ritual and ceremony. It is essential to rebuild community with matricentric values, and provide systems of support that value birthing and mothering. A non-judgemental community to find intergenerational spiritual connection and friendship.

Possibilities for creating new traditions through ceremony and rituals:

- the mother wears the bead bracelet from her mother blessing ceremony during labour and birthing. As she labours, she knows their love, support, belief and strength are with her

- creating a sacred space for birthing, with affirmations, tokens, photographs, music, scent, whatever is meaningful to you

- in emergence, baby is caught by mother, partner or both

- uninterrupted skin-to-skin time

- words of welcome to your newborn child, like a poem or song

- partner cuts cord or lotus birth

- placental ritual, encapsulation or burial

- creating handprints and footprints of the baby

- mother nourished with energy-rich foods after birth

- honouring the practice of rest, quiet, warmth and nourishment

- a familymoon, with restrictions on visitors and time spent with you

- naming ceremony, welcome into the family, community.

As part of identity

I wish to honour the work of Ruth Skilbeck by acknowledging the over 100,000 Indigenous babies removed from their mothers between 1909 and 1969. Adopted or fostered, their true heritage of identity and Country was denied them as part of the White Australia Policy of assimilation. Skilbeck's mother was one of the Stolen Generations. Ruth's search to find her real family took place in the year before her mother died.

Ruth's writing is emotive and confronting. It illustrates the challenges faced by the Stolen Generations and their offspring, because the identity of her mother's mother had been concealed. Skilbeck writes of the overarching attitude that mothers don't matter in our society and culture, and asks: "What about women's histories? The hidden histories? The stories of identities that were forbidden to be told? Of women's existence not allowed to be mentioned?"[60]

Although her journey has been hard, she graciously expresses: "This story is told as grief and healing, like a prayer or listening to music, an emotional catharsis."[61]

Practice offering: Tree meditation for labour

This tree meditation is offered to you as an alternative for labour.

- As you have been practising already, do a body scan. Releasing, softening, lengthening.

- Breathe as you find your most comfortable positions as your labour phases unfold, harnessing what you have practised.

- See yourself, where you are, standing, seated, kneeling, side-lying. Picture roots, tendrils, light lines leaving your body and reaching the earth.

- Ground your body, heavy, held, supported, and stabilised by the roots you created, held fast and firm in earth.

- Reach deep ... As you breathe in, draw energy, light, strength, purpose, nourishment, resolve, whatever descriptive words work for you ... from the earth beneath.

- Absorb this into the trunk of your body... the trunk of a strong, stable tree.

- As you release the breath, allow it to flow out of you completely, as though branches extend into unfolded leaves, and exhale in the air around you ... surrendering your breath.

- Through each cycle of long breath in, long humming breath out, be rooted deeply. Nourished and powerful, deeply grounded, allow the energy to dissipate throughout your body, used in harmony with motion, then released back into the atmosphere.

Mother Becoming Insights and Actions in Undisturbed Physiological Birth

Here we are again, near the end of another chapter, with Ally's words and images having guided you through. Replenish yourself. Gather yourself. What has come up for you? Your birthing partner has probably heard you say, "Hey! Read this bit! Watch this! Listen to this! What do you think?"

After reading this, revisit your scribbles, notes and doodles. Put it all together and clarify your thoughts. Note your questions, any enlightening and frustrating moments. With all you have been exposed to so far, the information is there to help you ask your healthcare provider questions, and find your own answers too. Yes, it has been a lot to take in. All that, while you prepare, prepare, prepare for your fourth trimester.

How might it be for you ...

- If your internal narrative around birth were positive and self-affirming?

- If your cultivation of self-trust empowered your labour and birthing experience, no matter how it happens?

- If you knew you were enough, and released fear?

- If you knew you had not failed, no matter your birthing experience?

- If homebirths and birth centre births were offered as first choices, without all the unnecessary fear attached to them?

- If Recommendation 26 of the NSW inquiry into birth trauma truly led to the expansion of publicly funded homebirth services?

- If all medical and midwifery students had to witness physiological birth and home birth before qualifying?

- If your birthing space were respected as a sacred environment?

- If the space were set up to support you; moving the bed, ensuring privacy in a hospital birth room?

- If midwifery COC were made available to all women irrespective of complications, were present in private practice, and filled care with normality and closed the spiritual gap?

- If all medical professionals were trained to learn vaginal examinations (when really needed) with the woman on her left side and with comfort and dignity in mind?

- If textbook images were rotated through 90 degrees and we saw illustrations of left lateral positions for vaginal examination?

- If physiological plateaus in all stages of labour with a well woman and baby were honoured as time for the woman's body to restart when ready?

- If physiological birthing were included in the training curriculums and textbooks for all health professionals?

- If value-based care funding through an LHS gave women a choice of high-value models of care, like midwifery COC?

- If midwifery COC, which would save the government and the taxpayer millions of dollars, were taken seriously and acted on?

- If hospital care, when necessary, were still provided with your group or team of midwives?

- If private practice interventions and caesarean rates were published transparently?

- If institutional practices were audited and made accountable, so that convenience and money made from birthing were not a driving force?

- If Recommendations 33 and 34 of the NSW inquiry into birth trauma were put in place countrywide for culturally safe care for all First Nations mothers and babies?

- If we acknowledged and addressed the diverse needs of refugees, First Nations peoples, LGBTQIA+, and persons with pre-existing conditions and disability?

Undisturbed Physiological Birthing References and Wishlist

1   R Reed, *Reclaiming Childbirth as a Rite of Passage: Weaving ancient wisdom with modern knowledge*, Word Witch, 2021, p211. ISBN 978-0-6450025-1-5

2   *Birthtime The Documentary* and *Birthtime The Handbook*, Clark and Mackay, 2021, p103. https://www.birthtime.world/

3   *Birthtime The Handbook*, p51.

4   V Olorenshaw, *Liberating Motherhood: birthing the Purple Stocking Movement*, Womancraft Publishing, 2016, p64. ISBN 978-910559-192

5   R Reed, 'Childbirth Physiology Course'. https://www.rachelreed.website/childbirth-physiology-course

6   *Birthtime The Handbook*, p 50.

7   R Dempsey, 'Understanding Pain Dynamics in Normal Birth'. Pdf Birthing Wisdom. https://www.birthingwisdom.com.au/wp-content/uploads/Article-PainIsMyFriend-RheaDempsey.pdf

8   *Birthtime The Handbook*, p50.

9   Dempsey, 'Understanding Pain Dynamics in Normal Birth', p66-7

10   *Birthtime The Handbook*, p46.

11   *Birthtime The Handbook*, p45.

12   *Birthtime The Handbook*, p45.

13   M Jowitt, 'The clitoris in labour'. Midwifery Today, 2008, 127:24-25. p24.
https://www.researchgate.net/publication/336848170_The_Clitoris_in_Labor

14   Jowitt, 'The clitoris in labour', p 24.

15   Reed, *Reclaiming Childbirth as a Rite of Passage*, p 211.

16   Cochrane Database of Systematic Reviews. 'Cord-Clamping'. http://www.cochrane.org/CD004074/PREG_effect-timing-umbilical-cord-clamping-term-infants-mother-and-baby-outcomes

17   10. LA Zinsser, 'Lotus birth, a holistic approach on physiological cord-clamping'. Women Birth. 2018 Apr;31(2):e73-e76. https://pubmed.ncbi.nlm.nih.gov/28882580/

18   R Lim, *Placenta the Forgotten Chakra*, Half Angel Press; 2010 ISBN 0976290774

19   E Burns, C Feeley, PJ Hall, J Vanderlaan.' Systematic review and meta-analysis to examine intrapartum interventions, and maternal and neonatal outcomes following immersion in water during labour and water-birth'. BMJ Open. 2022 Jul 5;12(7):e056517. https://pubmed.ncbi.nlm.nih.gov/35790327/

20   New South Wales Parliament Legislative Council Select Committee on Birth Trauma, Report. 2024. p xvii, ISBN: 978-1-922960-38-2 https://www.parliament.nsw.gov.au/lcdocs/inquiries/2965/FINAL%20Birth%20Trauma%20Report%20-%2029%20April%202024.PDF

21   H Dahlen, 'Free birthing and planned home births might sound similar, but the risks are very different'. *The Conversation*. February 20, 2024. https://theconversation.com/free-birthing-and-planned-home-births-might-sound-similar-but-the-risks-are-very-different-223852?fbclid=IwAR3qEjCitSFAWGBv2HOB6n-ZA8DvYwq-6uF3LhE9bf0bJlPoTWp1Nj5FlNq8

22   Dahlen, 'Free birthing and planned home births might sound similar, but the risks are very different'

23   H Dahlen, B Kumar-Hazard, V Schmeid, Editors. *Birthing Outside the System; The Canary in the Coalmine*. Routledge Press, 2020, p59-79. ISBN 978036750660516.

24   C King, A Burns, 'The price of Freebirth. ABC Regional Investigations'. 24.2.24. https://www.abc.net.au/news/2024-02-24/women-and-doulas-shun-medical-system-in-freebirth-revolution/103430942

25   New South Wales Parliament Legislative Council Select Committee on Birth Trauma, Report. p xvii.

26   E Friedman, Labor in Multiparas. A Graphicostatistical analysis. Obstetrics & Gynecology 8(6):p 691-703, December 1956. https://journals.lww.com/greenjournal/Citation/1956/12000/A_graphicostatistical_analysis.7.aspx

27   K O'Driscoll, RJA, Jackson, JT Gallagher, 'Prevention of Prolonged Labour'. Br Med J 1969;2:477. p 135. doi: https://doi.org/10.1136/bmj.2.5655.477

28   K O'Driscoll, J M Strong, M Minogue, 'Active Management of Labour British Medical journal', 1973, 3, 135-137 https://www.ncbi.nlm.nih.gov/pmc/articles/PMC1586344/PDF/brmedj01567-0029.PDF

29   Obstetric Care Consensus: 'Safe Prevention of the Primary Cesarean Delivery'. The American College of Obstetricians and Gynaecologists. Society of Maternal-Fetal Medicine. 2014. https://www.acog.org/-/media/project/acog/acogorg/clinical/files/obstetric-care-consensus/articles/2014/03/safe-prevention-of-the-primary-cesarean-delivery.PDF

30   WHO, 'Labour Care Guide User's Manual'. 2020. p22. https://www.who.int/publications/i/item/9789240017566

31   WHO, 'Labour Care Guide User's Manual', p28.

32   A Shepherd, H Cheyne, S Kennedy, C McIntosh., M Styles, C Niven, 'The purple line as a measure of labour progress: a longitudinal study'. BMC Pregnancy and Childbirth, 2010, 10(54). DOI:10.1186/1471-2393-10-54

33   M Weckend, K McCullough, C Duffield, S Bayes, C Davison, 'Failure to progress or just normal? A constructivist grounded theory of physiological plateaus during childbirth'. Women and Birth Volume 37, Issue 1, February 2024, Pages 229-239 https://doi.org/10.1016/j.wombi.2023.10.003

34   Weckend, Failure to progress or just normal? p230.

35   Cochrane Review. 'Amniotomy for shortening the length of labour'. 2013 https://www.cochrane.org/CD006167/PREG_amniotomy-for-shortening-spontaneous-labour

36   K Uvnäs Moberg, Why Oxytocin Matters, Pinter and Martin, 2019. ISBN 9781780666051

37   S Wickham, 'What is a labour plateau'? https://www.sarawickham.com/articles-2/what-is-a-labour-plateau/

38   International Confederation of Midwives (ICM) Position statement on the appropriate use of interventions for midwives. https://internationalmidwives.org/resources/appropriate-use-of-intervention-in-childbirth/

39   ICM Bill of Rights for Women and Midwives Statement. 2024. https://internationalmidwives.org/resources/bill-of-rights-for-women-and-midwives/

40   M Harris, Men, Love and Birth, Pinter and Martin, 2015, p75. ISBN 9781870662251

41   Harris, Men, Love and Birth, p 76.

42   O Best, B Fredericks, Editorss. Yatdjuligin. Aboriginal and Torres Strait Islander Nursing and Midwifery Care. Third ED. Cambridge University Press; 2021. p142-3. ISBN 9781108794695

43   Birthing On Country. The Molly Wardugga Research Centre. 'https://www.birthingoncountry.com/

44   TMCC. 'Call to Action on Birthing on Country'. https://www.transformingmaternity.org.au/2021/09/heed-the-call-to-action-for-birthing-on-country/

45   S Ireland, R Montgomery-Anderson, S Geraghty, 'Indigenous Doulas: A literature review exploring their role and practice in western maternity care'. Midwifery. Volume 75, August 2019, Pages 52-58 https://doi.org/10.1016/j.midw.2019.04.005

46   New South Wales Parliament Legislative Council Select Committee on Birth Trauma, Report, p xviii.

47   Birthtime The Handbook, p61.

48   V Olorenshaw, Liberating Motherhood, p 64.

49   TMCC. 'Private Obstetric Care Increases Risk of Unplanned Caesarean for Low-Risk Women'. https://www.transformingmaternity.org.au/2022/03/private-obstetric-care-increases-risk-of-unplanned-caesarean-for-low-risk-women/

50   TMCC. 'Place of Birth. What if all low-risk women planned to be in a birth centre or at home'. https://www.transformingmaternity.org.au/2021/09/what-if-all-low-risk-women-planned-to-birth-in-a-birth-centre-or-at-home/

51   EJ Callander, C Bull, R McInnes, J Toohill. 'The opportunity costs of birth in Australia: Hospital resource savings for a post-COVID-19 era'. Birth. 2021 Jun;48(2):274-282. doi: 10.1111/birt.12538. Epub 2021 Feb 12. PMID: 33580537; PMCID: PMC8014177. https://www.ncbi.nlm.nih.gov/pmc/articles/PMC8014177/

52   TMCC. 'Health Services Lack Incentive to be Cost Effective'. 2021. https://www.transformingmaternity.org.au/2021/06/health-services-lack-incentive-to-be-cost-effective/

53   E Teisberg, S Wallace, S O'Hara, 'Defining and Implementing Value-Based Healthcare: A Strategic Framework'. Acad Med. 2020 May;95(5):682-685. doi: 10.1097/ACM.0000000000003122. PMID: 31833857; PMCID: PMC7185050. https://www.ncbi.nlm.nih.gov/pmc/articles/PMC7185050/

54   TMCC. 'The Learning Health system to achieve better value'. https://www.transformingmaternity.org.au/2022/04/the-learning-health-system-to-achieve-better-value/

55   A De Jonge, S Downe, L Page, D Devane, H Lindgren, J Klinkert, M Gray, A Jani. 'Value-based maternal and newborn care requires alignment of adequate resources with high value activities'. BMC Pregnancy Childbirth 19, 428 (2019). https://doi.org/10.1186/s12884-019-2512-3. https://bmcpregnancychildbirth.biomedcentral.com/articles/10.1186/s12884-019-2512-3

56   Lorin Roche, The Radiance Sutras Sounds True, 2014, p184. ISBN 978-1-60407-659-2

57   Birthtime The Handbook, p 141.

58 *Birthtime The Handbook*, p 58.

59 Olorenshaw, *Liberating Motherhood*, p 63.

60 R Skilbeck, (2013). Remembering Australia's Forgotten Mothers: Reclaiming Lost Identity in Colonial History. *Journal of the Motherhood Initiative for Research and Community Involvement*, 3(2). Retrieved from https://jarm.journals.yorku.ca/index.php/jarm/article/view/36315 p167-177. p163. https://jarm.journals.yorku.ca/index.php/jarm/article/view/36315/33033

61 Skilbeck, Remembering Australia's Forgotten Mothers, p175.

Wishlist

1. R Reed. YouTube 'Transformation of the Uterus During Labour'. https://www.youtube.com/watch?v=fF7H-cH30u7o&list=PLzk4kScwvULLizGTz3kqevIK5QYnEpf25

2. YouTube Video. 'Push,' A satire short film. Beautiful Birth Club'. https://www.youtube.com/watch?v=XdiUi-C9iUP0&list=PL6n-MQ99SxK6IJj1OA9jF-8y77ntdgk5J&index=10

3. *Great Birth Rebellion* #21 'Perineal Suturing' Apple Spotify

4. R Reed. YouTube Video. 'Placental Transfusion of the Baby After Birth'. https://www.youtube.com/watch?v=y3w_uiP95IM&t=5s

5. Facebook video 'Physiological Plateaus Research'. https://www.facebook.com/dr.marina.weekend/videos/903404747908784

6. Dr Rachel Reed Blog. 'Understanding and assessing labour progress'. https://www.rachelreed.website/blog/understanding-labour-progress

7. *Birth-Ed* S1 E8 'A Mindful Fourth Trimester' with Sophie Burch. Apple Spotify

Chapter 5

Assisted Birthing with Katie

Meeting Katie

Katie and I met the day she came to hospital to be induced at 40 weeks for her second child. I remember meeting her so clearly. Her vitality and friendliness filled the assessment room. As we walked into the birth suite, I remember saying, "Ignore the bed. We won't be using that." And I remember her surprise at this. Then she asked, "Can I go to the toilet when I need to?" I was shocked that this strong woman felt she needed my permission to go to the bathroom. When you read her letter you understand why she asked me that.

It was beautiful to be part of Katie's birthing experience, with her openness to be fully involved in her induction by harnessing mobility, nipple stimulation, mindfulness and meditation, aromatherapy, massage, upright forward-leaning positions and listening to her body. During each surging contraction, she dropped deeply into herself, using her senses to take herself to her favourite place, the beach. Responding with belief in her body, she created a completely different mindset and experience from her first birth.

While upright kneeling, Mason was passed to Katie through her legs, and they gazed at each other before he took his first breath. Witnessing that moment of 'I know you' between them was precious beyond words. When they joined postpartum yoga with Samantha and Clémentine, my heart was full.

Mum to Jake and Mason, here is Katie's letter to you

"Like night and day"

Hello to the person reading this,

It is after much procrastination that I began to write about my journey of pregnancy, births and beyond. It took me 3 years to complete. I am a mum to 2 great boys. Their births were like night and day by comparison. One was full of fear and not having any control of the situation. The other was full of comfort, support and trust for my body, my midwife and the process of birth.

During both of my pregnancies, I developed gestational diabetes. This determined that my labour would be induced on my due date. My first pregnancy was under the care of a private obstetric GP, and the second an obstetric GP through the public care system. I only saw one midwife for my pre-admission check with my first pregnancy.

I didn't go into labour before 40 weeks, despite 2 stretch and sweeps being done. My GP was away on holidays, so about a week before my expected due date, I was introduced to his offsider, another male GP, before my final appointment. They hoped I would go into labour before my due date to avoid an induction. No luck there.

On 25 April 2013, I presented myself at the hospital as instructed around 8:00 pm. I was hooked up to fetal monitoring and a midwife administered a gel to ripen my cervix. My obstetric GP had also prescribed a sedative to make sure that I slept. I fell into an uncomfortable, but deep, sleep and awoke hours later feeling like I'd been hit by a truck. My whole body was sore. As it turned out, the gel had started my labour and I'd been contracting all night as I slept. I was happy that my contractions had begun and thought they would let my labour progress naturally from there, but boy, was I wrong.

My husband, Wayne, and I were taken into a birthing suite around 9:00 am. I was still having contractions that were fairly regular, but was only dilated to around 3 cm. I was again attached to fetal monitoring and a canula was put into the back of my hand. A midwife explained that my doctor had written up a plan for me that the midwives would follow, and that I would be given Syntocinon to increase my contractions until my baby was born. While attached to the drip, I was free to move around, sit on a fit ball and do my best to relax. I did the best I could to get comfortable. My Syntocinon was increased every half hour, and the contractions got stronger and closer together as a result. It was very hard to move around attached to a drip and fetal monitoring.

Throughout the day, my mum, Wayne's mum and Wayne were all in the birthing suite with me. At one point, I looked over at the mums who were happily eating and drinking on the sofa, and Wayne was sitting in a chair beside them. They were all sitting and looking at me, but not interacting with me. I felt like an animal in the zoo.

After 12:00 midday, the contractions were strong and close together. I had hoped that they would leave the Syntocinon at this level because it was intense already. I had asked my midwife if it could be left at that level, and I was told no. My doctor's plan meant it was to be increased yet again. I didn't feel ready for stronger contractions. In fact, I felt worried and frightened. By 1:00 pm, I was experiencing what I would describe as rolling contractions, where one contraction ended and another started almost immediately with no relief to even take a full breath in between. I felt sore and exhausted. I struggled to breathe. I noticed that my Syntocinon was to be increased yet again. I remember feeling terrified as tears rolled down my face.

I needed relief. I couldn't keep going this way. I was only 4 cm dilated. Between rolling contractions and lack of full breaths, I asked my midwife what type of pain relief I could have. She recommended 'the gas'. I sucked down on the mouthpiece, but after just a few breaths I felt so nauseated I couldn't continue. I was still in so much pain and asked if there were any other options available to me. She said I could have an epidural. I had originally been against epidurals, but in the moment, I needed something – anything – so I agreed. I waited while still enduring rolling contractions and struggling to breathe. It felt like a never-ending contraction at this point.

It took almost an hour for the anaesthetist to get to me, as I endured more rolling contractions. All the paperwork was filled, and he got my husband to sit in front of me and hold my hands while I hunched myself over my beach ball of a belly. It felt impossible, but eventually my epidural was administered. My left leg went completely numb, and my contractions stopped completely. *Huh?* I thought.

I remember how relieved I felt once the pain had subsided. I was so exhausted. The midwife told me that they would need to increase my Syntocinon dose to get my contractions going again. The worry must have been obvious on my face because she reassured me that I wouldn't feel the contractions now. The next couple of hours were a blur. I passed out and was in and out of consciousness. I do remember agreeing to let a midwifery student do an internal exam. I remember saying, "She has to learn somehow. I can't feel a thing. Go for it." And not much else.

When I eventually came to, I was confined to the bed, watching my tummy dance around with contractions, but not feeling any of them. My left leg was still numb and completely immobile. I tried to move it many times with no luck. I lay there, with my dancing belly, my husband in a chair by the bedside, and my mother and mother-in-law sitting on the couch in the birthing suite, chatting away to each other and not really doing much else.

The rest of the afternoon was just contractions I couldn't feel, and dilation checks regularly. I needed to go to the toilet for a wee. Wayne and the midwife helped me into the bathroom. A short while later I felt the need to go to the toilet again and asked the midwife if I could go. She asked if it was for a wee or a poo. I told her that I needed to go poo. I was checked and told that I had dilated to 10 cm, and I didn't in fact need to poo, but would need to prepare myself to push. I said to her that I was sure I just needed a poo. She explained to me that the feeling of the baby coming down and ready to be born can feel like needing a bowel movement. I was petrified that I would poop myself during labour. I was now certain that it would happen and braced myself for the inevitable.

My epidural was stopped to allow me to feel the contractions and be able to push. My midwife was a bit sad because she would always be there for the lead up, then there would be a shift change and she would miss the actual birth. I told her that I was determined to have the baby before she left.

I had diligently been giving myself perineal massage prior to giving birth, every day since reading somewhere that it could help. I asked the midwife to get warm washcloths so that they could be applied to my perineum during birth. My obstetric GP arrived just in time for the main event.

Because I was attached to so much stuff (drip, epidural and monitoring) and I didn't have full feeling back in my left leg, I was advised that I would not be allowed to move into a more comfortable position and would have to deliver lying on my back. My heart sank. I didn't ever dream of delivering on my back. I had a midwife on either side grab a leg and hike up my legs, with my doctor between my legs while I was instructed to push. My mum and mother-in-law left the room when it came time for me to push and went to the waiting room. I never recognised an urge to push, but was told to push, so I did as I was told. Wayne held my hand and helped me get into position.

The midwives had originally used the warm compresses to see if they would help, but it didn't help. I was told that I needed an episiotomy. I didn't question it and my obstetrician proceeded with it. As I pushed, the inevitable happened and I felt myself poop. The midwives cleaned me up, one whispering, "It just keeps coming," as they continued to clean me. I remember telling them that I had told the midwife that I needed to go.

I pushed over and over again until my baby was crowning. I felt a pop or a rip that I would describe as like a rubber band snapping. I knew immediately that I had torn despite the episiotomy. The stinging sensation that accompanied it was undeniable. I told the doctor that I was aware that I had just torn.

One last push and my child was born, a beautiful baby boy. It was just after 7:00 pm on 26 April. He was tidied up a little and he squeaked before being placed on my chest and the cord being clamped and cut. At the time, I assumed it was cut by my husband, but I had no idea. I do not recollect trying to feed immediately, as my son was sleepy and lethargic. I was told it was common after an epidural. I don't remember delivering the placenta, but I recall being told to push the epidural for one last dose so that I would be numb while I was stitched up. I asked my doctor how many stitches. "Just one long continuous stitch," he told me. The doctor congratulated me on the birth of my son and took his leave.

Following the epidural wearing off and being allowed to get cleaned up, I was moved into a private hospital room. I had a few quick visits from family who had been in the waiting room, then was instructed on how to feed my child by an older midwife. She said, "Hold your boob like you would hold a hamburger and bring your child to the nipple." I was surprised that it worked. Although I was convinced that he got nothing, his first feed was amazing, and I was filled with a sense of accomplishment and euphoria.

We decided to name him Jake. It was hard to sleep in the maternity ward with noises constantly floating down the halls. I couldn't wait to go home. I was sore and uncomfortable. It had always been said that you 'check your dignity at the door' and that was just how it was done. The whole process made me question why anyone would ever want to do that again. The upside was that I had a beautiful baby boy. We went home the following afternoon. Two nights in hospital was enough.

The next day, I was overwhelmed by people coming and going all afternoon. I was busy making tea and coffee while my child was passed around from person to person between feedings. I wished I had just stayed in hospital. All I wanted was to rest. I felt invisible now that my child had been born.

My mother-in-law stayed with us for the first week, helping with laundry and cooking dinners while I attended to our child and recovered from birth. My husband had a week off also, but that whole week was a blur. The midwives visited me every other day to check my stitches and check Jake's weight, which steadily increased for the first week.

But Jake didn't sleep for very long and was constantly hungry. He would often fall asleep on the breast, which felt like he was constantly feeding. I struggled to sleep during the day, so the advice of 'sleep when baby sleeps' didn't work for me. He would only go 45 minutes at most. If I tried to sleep, I would be nodding off as he was waking again. When my milk came in, I felt like a glorified dairy cow. My boobs were so terribly sore and hard that my son struggled to latch. My letdown was so strong that it was like I was shooting my child in the face as I tried to attach him to my nipple. He would end up gagging, soaked and wearing more than he drank. My opposite breast would also expel its contents at the exact same time so I would also end up soaked, and with little milk left for him to consume. I was sure that he cried because he was still hungry. I was determined to breastfeed, but I was so sleep deprived and exhausted.

Once Wayne went back to work, I spent most days alone with a small screeching baby. Jake would only sleep on my chest, so I would set myself up on our double chaise sofa surrounded by pillows just in case I fell asleep while holding him. I struggled to feed myself properly and take care of myself. I would often cry with exhaustion while all alone. My father noticed that I wasn't doing too great and started to bring me lunch as often as he could. He would sit holding Jake so that I could go for a shower, which helped me feel a bit more human. Wayne and I struggled along for the first few weeks. The lack of sleep was getting to both of us, and we were both exhausted and struggling.

After a while, Jake's weight at appointments wasn't increasing as much as the child health nurse wanted. He was also a very colicky baby. My letdown reflex had not improved, and Jake would only get one breast full of milk when he would be wanting more, which I couldn't figure out how to give him. I tried shuffling him back and forth between breasts that were pretty much empty, so he would cry because he was still hungry. I felt like a failure, but I was still determined to keep breastfeeding.

By now, I was getting depressed. I tried to get some fresh air and took a walk with Jake in the pram to improve my mood. My mood did improve, but I had no milk for hours afterward as my energy stores were very low. During my pregnancy, I had not put weight on, so baby had gained weight as my body lost it, while being on a very strict eating plan for my GD. At this point, I looked like a skeleton. Breastfeeding was drawing whatever energy stores my body had left. The child health nurse thought that my body had no fat stores to draw from, so maybe that meant my milk did not have the calories my baby required, leading to his low weight gain.

I was spiralling. I was failing. I struggled to look after the house, keep up with washing and take care of my child. I barely took proper care of myself. Most days I lived on the couch. I had many thoughts that my child would just be better off if I was dead. I thought of ways that I could take my own life and give him a better chance without me. I had so much love for my child, but I was struggling to go on. Sleep deprived and so exhausted. Stuck in a haze of crying (my own and Jake's), feeding, diaper changes and laundry. I grieved for the life I had left behind to have a child. I felt sub-human.

One day, my husband told me that I had passed out. Jake was crying for hours wanting to be fed and he just had to hold a screaming baby for hours because whatever he tried I would not wake up. I woke up a few hours later, unaware that I had been asleep for that long, then went on as usual, still struggling. I'm sure Wayne was also struggling with depression at this point.

Every time I would do the depression questionnaire with the child health nurse, I would tell her what she wanted to hear so that I would not be made to take medication. Despite this, I was still at the top end of the scale. I assured her I probably just needed some sleep. She told me there was a reason sleep deprivation was used as a form of torture and to hang in there. I would probably feel much better once I got a decent night's sleep. I didn't see it happening any time soon. I was the one my child relied on, the only one to feed him, the one who spent all day and most of the night up with him, the one who cleaned each wet and messy nappy. It was all super overwhelming. I knew I couldn't survive like this for much longer. I was at the end of my rope.

Breastfeeding continued to be a challenge and I struggled with my severe letdown. I tried to pump to increase my supply between feeds and was consuming breastfeeding cookies, which seemed to help a little. I still couldn't exercise to improve my mental health because my milk would stop producing for a few hours when I did. I tried to pump milk when Jake had a slightly longer sleep to improve my milk supply but to no avail.

More than once, I attempted to express milk and even catch the milk from the opposite breast while feeding to use if Jake was still hungry or later the same day. But even with refrigeration, my milk would sour and be useless. Jake would refuse to drink it and would then cry because he was hungry. I didn't understand why my milk would smell sour so soon after pumping it. Much later, I found out that some mums produce an enzyme in their milk that sours it if not pasteurised almost immediately.

Again, I felt like a failure. I couldn't figure out a way to give myself the time out I needed to stay sane. I was still depressed, although not having as many suicidal thoughts. I was still determined to persevere with breastfeeding. My husband and I were beginning to talk about my health being more important than breastfeeding. Jake was still gaining weight far too slowly.

My child health nurse and I chatted about Jake's lack of weight increase. I was doing everything to give him as much milk as I could manage, but she spoke to me about supplementing him with formula. When I got home, I cried, then had another conversation with my hubby about formula. At 10 weeks, I started giving him one or 2 feeds a day of formula. I liked getting Wayne to give him the formula feeds so that I could get other things done around the house. Around the same time, Jake started having longer sleeps after the formula feeds, so we would make his bedtime feed with formula. He slept longer. I got more sleep too. I felt more human, less zombie, and less suicidal.

Over the next few weeks, I increased Jake's formula feeds. We all got more sleep and were less irritable. I still struggled to adapt to being a new mum with the constant change, but I managed to make time to go walking and get some exercise. It was hard fitting things in between feeds and nap times. I found myself feeding Jake and settling him down in the pram before going for a stroll. The fresh air, change of scenery and movement improved my mood slowly. I started to feel more like my old self and could take care of myself more consistently. I would get dressed in actual clothing in the morning so that getting out of the house became easier.

At the prompting of my child health nurse, I joined a mothers group. I felt less alone, less like I was going to be crushed by the overwhelming feelings. The weekly catch-ups gave me something to look forward to. Eleven years later, a few of the mums I met there are some of my closest friends. We still catch up whenever we can. They are my people. They have helped me keep my chin up when things get rough and been some of my biggest supporters. At the time, it felt like the group saved me from myself. As our children grew together, they also formed bonds of their own. I'm grateful for those women and their families. I am also thankful for the child health nurse who prompted me to join.

It took Wayne and me 3 years to feel like we might be able to try again for our second child. I was scared and apprehensive, but didn't want my first child to grow up in the world lonely. I always wanted 2 children. Once we felt ready, trying to fall pregnant didn't take too long. I had kept track of dates, then one day I noticed myself gagging when brushing my teeth. Sure enough, I had another bun in the oven. I went to see my doctor to get things organised for my antenatal care.

I was sent for a dating ultrasound. I knew when my husband and I had been intimate and estimated that I was around 3 weeks pregnant. The lady doing the ultrasound estimated 5 weeks gestation, so my doctor said that we had to go with the results given and that it would be noted on my chart that I was at 5 weeks gestation. I didn't like the idea and kept on letting my healthcare workers know that I was 2 weeks behind the dates given at appointments.

As I had GD again, I did not see a midwife for my antenatal care. I was assigned an obstetric GP who worked in the antenatal clinic at the hospital. At 39 weeks, I was given a stretch and sweep. He hoped it would bring on my labour and help me avoid an induction. It was sooooo uncomfortable and didn't work.

On 9 October 2017, Wayne and I made our way to the maternity ward at the hospital for my scheduled induction. Around 9:00 am, we were introduced to Wendy, who would be my midwife. (Yes, that's the Wendy writing this book.) She showed us through into a birthing suite and must have noticed the concern on my face. She told me not to worry, that I would be well looked after. Once she had me settled, I told her that this was not my first induction; that the last one had been awful. I asked her if it was normal to have rolling contractions with the Syntocinon. She said the Syntocinon is to get the contractions started, but didn't need to be increased if I was having steady, strong contractions. I was relieved.

Then Wendy asked how I felt about lavender essential oil, which I do like. She proceeded to swan around the room putting lavender essential oil all over different things around me! The linen, the pillow, everywhere, until the calming scent of lavender surrounded me. It was a comforting, familiar smell. She guided me to do breathing exercises to help me calm down.

When it came time to break my waters, Wendy got herself ready with the little finger hook. She struggled to get my membrane to rupture, saying that it was quite tough. Out gushed the amniotic fluid. It looked like my baby was in its own Olympic-sized swimming pool. I told her that I'd not felt much kicking over the past few weeks. She advised me that my contractions would get more intense from now on, but assured me that they wouldn't get anywhere as bad as the Syntocinon contractions from my first birth.

I started Syntocinon on a low dose. With the fetal monitoring, I was encouraged to move around, bounce gently and rock my hips on the fit ball, and just get comfortable. If I could get my contractions going naturally, Wendy told me, I would need less Syntocinon. She explained that if I stimulated my nipples, it could get me releasing my oxytocin and contracting well enough on my own. I was willing to try anything! It felt awkward, but I trusted her advice. Soon enough, I was contracting fairly well on my own, and not requiring the Syntocinon to be increased, or at all. I was so relieved I almost cried.

When I couldn't tolerate Wayne trying to rub my back, Wendy asked me if I would like to try meditating through my contractions. She asked me about where I would prefer to be if I wasn't here, a place that made me feel calm. I told her it was the beach. So, the meditation went like this:

> Close your eyes and imagine you are sitting on the beach. Can you feel the sand beneath your feet? Listen to the waves crashing onto the sand, the seagulls in the distance. Feel the warmth of the sun on your skin, and a breeze gently brushing your skin. Smell the salt air in your nostrils. Now how do you feel?

I told her I felt good, so she suggested I take myself back there in my mind whenever a strong contraction came. This was like 'checking out' and visiting my favourite place. I could tell that I was having a contraction, but the pain didn't bother me. I remained calm and breathed through each one. I would bring myself back to the room between contractions, and everyone else around me was calm.

I had asked Wendy if I was allowed to go to the bathroom because I felt like I needed to poo. She said definitely and I asked if she had to check how dilated I was first. She said no, and that it was probably a good idea to go to the bathroom before I got to pushing because it would come out before the baby if it was in there. I told her that I had not been allowed to go poop before pushing during my first delivery and had then pooped myself. She told me it was important to go to the bathroom if I needed.

Once I'd been to the bathroom, I was checked and was at around 8 cm dilated. Wendy told me that she was going to have a quick lunch break. There was another midwife coming in, who would stay with me. If I felt the urge to push, I was to let that midwife know and Wendy would be called back in. I didn't know how to tell because I'd not felt the urge the first time, but Wendy told me to trust my body and that I would know when my body was ready.

I started to feel a sensation I'd never felt before. Wendy had only been gone around 10 minutes, and it wasn't very strong, so I just wasn't sure. The sensation got stronger. I was surprised that instinctively I felt like I needed to push. I told the midwife looking after me and she sent for Wendy straight away. When she came back, Wendy said she thought it would happen quickly once she left the room. She advised me to get into a good position to let gravity help bring the baby down with the contractions, so I kneeled on the bed and put my arms up on the top of the raised backrest section. As the contractions came, I pushed. It didn't take long at all to deliver my baby boy. We called him Mason.

I turned over to sit and my son was put straight into my arms and skin to skin with me. He was covered in vernix and goop, but he was perfect. Another midwife commented that he was definitely not 40 weeks gestation, because vernix like this wouldn't be found on full-term babies. I told her about the incorrect gestation on my records after my dating scan. She said it made sense. I delivered the placenta with no issues. Mason was cleaned up a little and I was advised to try to feed him immediately as it would help my uterus contract. He latched straight away. I felt like this was how birthing should be. Wendy was like my angel, a fated introduction into my life when I was terrified of what could have been. I was covered with a blanket, and we covered Mason under the blanket too.

I felt a warm sensation at my vagina, so I put my hand down to check what it was. When I brought my hand up, it was covered in blood. I was haemorrhaging. The doctor was called in immediately and she ended up fishing out a clot that weighed around 400g. With my total blood loss, they said I was lucky not to require a blood transfusion. I had a catheter inserted with a bag to collect my urine, was given something to help my uterus contract and put on an antibiotic drip.

Wendy checked if I was okay before telling me she had to go pick up her son, who had been waiting at the train station for some time while I gave birth. I hugged her tightly. I also told her that she was amazing and thanked her for all she did for me. She told me that I did the amazing thing with the right support and guidance.

I was shown to a room at the back of the maternity ward, in the area furthest from the birthing suites so that I might be able to get some rest. I was introduced to the midwife who would be looking after me overnight. Her name was Alysia (the same Alysia who writes to you in the next chapter). I had a couple of family visitors pop in to meet our new arrival and we took some photos. Jake beamed as he got to meet his baby brother.

I asked Wayne what he thought of me naming our son in honour of Wendy for his middle name. I checked with Alysia what Wendy's surname was and told her why I needed to know. She thought it was a lovely idea and told me that Wendy's surname was Jackson. So, Mason became Mason Jackson. Sure that Wendy would be thrilled, Alysia told her the next time she saw her.

Yet again, I was determined to breastfeed. Again, I struggled. I had baked multitudes of breastfeeding cookies and muffins in preparation for our new arrival. I was lucky enough that Jake was on school holidays when Mason was born. I didn't have the luxury of sitting around this time though. I had another child to look after and a house to manage. In less than a week, Jake had to be taken to school and picked up in the afternoon. I walked him to school, with Mason in the pram. This reanimated the problem of my milk not producing during exercise. Wayne noticed that I was starting to spiral down the rabbit hole again. I was exhausted and depressed. He reminded me that my health was more important than persisting with breastfeeding, and that Mason would be fine as long as he was fed. I had to agree. Mason wasn't even 3 weeks old when we switched him to formula. I cried with deep aching sobs that yet again I had failed to breastfeed.

Still, I was determined to get out of my depressive state, so I started trying to do yoga when Mason was asleep and Jake was at school. I would walk as much as I could, but struggled with pain in my pelvis. Six months postpartum, my GP recommended that I see a chiropractor. I had a standing X-ray, and on my second appointment I had my pelvis realigned. The crunch of it going back into place was audible; the pain relief, instant.

Wendy had told me about her postpartum yoga class, and eventually I got up the courage and enough money to join her mum and bub yoga class. It helped me feel better and keep my body more flexible. Wendy loved seeing Mason and me. We have kept in touch ever since and have grown to be great friends. Both my boys adore her.

My 2 pregnancy journeys were so different, as were my births and postnatal periods. I am grateful to everyone who helped me, held me up when things got rough and allowed me to do the same for them. I am also grateful for the opportunity to share my story with others, so they know they are not alone. Many other women go through birthing experiences that leave them traumatised. So many suffer from postpartum depression.

I must thank you, dear reader, for bearing with me as I get this information out. If my story helps even one woman to advocate for themself or others, it will be worth it.

Kind regards,

Katie

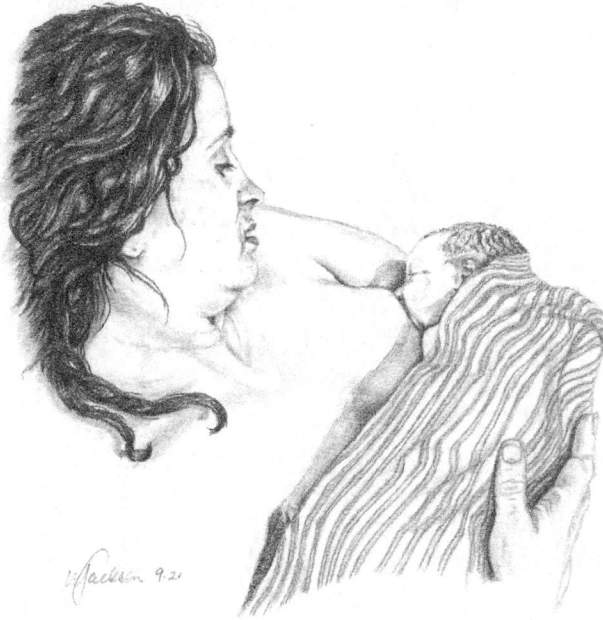

Katie gazing at Mason as he has his first feed in the golden hour after birth. Katie's sense of wonder at her achievement of birthing the way she had dreamed of, never thinking she would be supported to do so, was incredible to witness. Her determination and raw power filled the room with focused energy that left Wayne and me emotional and filled with awe.

Dear Mother Becoming,

This is a hard chapter to write, and a long introduction. You have just read Katie's experiences and how her first birth left her traumatised, and how she struggled with breastfeeding and PND after both births. Writing her story 10 years afterwards was stressful and filled with tears, because the memories are as clear for her as if they happened yesterday.

It is my intention to approach our conversation here with as much sensitivity and compassion as possible. This book is about reducing fear and anxiety about birthing. We learned about cultivating ahimsa with Liesja, holding an attitude of non-violence and peacefulness in mind and body. We will need that peaceful state of being because we are going to be talking about obstetric violence, human rights in childbirth and birth trauma here with Katie.

This book has never been about my story, yet I experienced traumatic births, suffered PTSD and severe PND. My experiences have led to deep empathy, knowledge and heartfelt understanding. This provides a foundation upon which to talk about difficult and often-neglected subjects from a position of strength, all towards fulfilling my dearest wish: to prevent birth trauma, PTSD and PND in birthing women and mothers today. I aim to support those of you who have this experience.

I have a strong hope that this chapter will give you confidence and autonomy, dear Mother Becoming, in preparation for birth and the transition to motherhood. It's a place for all mothers who have experienced birth trauma to find acknowledgment, insight and understanding. If any of this chapter rings true, I hope to assist you in beginning to process your story.

Naming this chapter 'Assisted Birthing with Katie' acknowledges that complications arise during pregnancy, birth and postpartum, and that assistance is needed. It does not mean a woman has failed in any way or is somehow less. There is no place for the label 'failed' here. Women's needs and experiences are unique when there are birthing complications. Often, they come with feelings of a loss of control over their hopes for birth. This chapter offers ways to maintain your sense of control during changes in your birth experience.

With Katie, we will be discovering ways of supporting physiological processes within medical birthing – such as promoting oxytocin, prolactin and beta-endorphin production to assist with an empowering experience of labour, birth, bonding and breastfeeding to promote feelings of maternal satisfaction and wellbeing. A positive birth doesn't mean a 'hallowed, unmedicated, pop the baby out and onto the boob, no worries' kind of experience. A positive birth is very much how you are treated, engaged with and respected by care providers. A positive birth can also be a complicated, unexpected, exhausting, mind-boggling experience, yet with your involvement, and respect for your autonomy by care providers, it can be empowering. You can make it your own by:

- creating the environment you want and need
- having support for positive experiences with embodied mindful presence
- being part of the informed decision-making process in medically managed birthing.

Rather than 'done to you', you are engaged and confident in your experience.

At the end of this chapter, you will know more of what to expect in assisted birthing care, what should not be happening, and how to negotiate this while maintaining oxytocin levels, and minimising adrenaline and cortisol responses.

There is a reason why we have much lower maternal and neonatal deaths and injury rates in countries where there is access to midwifery and medical care when truly needed. Here in Australia, this access is a blessing. However, maternity care has become over-medicalised, with too much induction of labour, and too many elective and questionable 'emergency' caesarean sections. This will all be explored further in this chapter.

It is my hope that you take what you learn in this book into the hospital environment. Complications and assistance do not make a traumatic experience inevitable. Working within the maternity care currently available, you can have a mindful experience, especially when you need to alter the pathways of your map if complications arise. Ultimately, you have sovereignty over your own body and the authority to agree or disagree to any suggested care, investigations and interventions. I aim to help you be confident in your own autonomy, informed choices, able to communicate your desires, and comfortable accepting or declining offered care. Consent needs to be given freely and acknowledged with dignity. Your decisions should be respected, then maintained at all times. This influences how you feel about your birthing experience.

As we now discuss obstetric violence, human rights in childbirth and birth trauma, please hold ahimsa with you. Feelings of disbelief and anger will arise. Acknowledge them, but please don't let them grip you, because sitting in anger isn't healthy. If this is too much for you right now, come back to it. If this will be triggering for you, read it with someone beside you. Please know that I am with you – heart, mind, and spirit. We are connected through the stories of so many, all towards making change. Have a cuppa and your journal with you to reflect on how these words land. Write how these pages make you feel, so your feelings aren't bottled up. And as always, chocolate or your favourite treat is definitely required.

Big breath, here goes …

Human rights in childbirth

Every woman should be free to make her own choices in pregnancy and childbirth, even if the care provider does not agree. Every woman also has a right to equality and freedom from discrimination. However, findings from across the world show degrading and dehumanising treatment – maternity care has been a breeding ground of abuse of women's human rights. While this may sound shocking, when we review the literature, it's hard to sugarcoat it as anything else.

In 'Why Human Rights in Childbirth Matter', Rebecca Schiller talks about the right to receive safe and appropriate care that respects a woman's fundamental human dignity, with the right to privacy and confidentiality. Schiller states: "Failure to provide adequate maternity care, lack of respect for women's dignity, invasions of privacy, procedures carried out without consent, failure to provide adequate pain relief without medical contraindication, giving pain relief where it is not requested, unnecessary or unexplained medical interventions, and lack of respect for women's choices about where and how a birth takes place, may all violate human rights and can lead to women feeling degraded and dehumanized."[1]

That obstetric violence is the name for what happens to women in childbirth leaves a sense of disbelief that such a thing could occur. But it is real. By Dr Amali Lokugamage's definition, "Obstetric violence is the act of disregarding the authority and autonomy that women have over their own sexuality, their bodies, their babies and in their birth experiences. It is also the act of disregarding the spontaneity, the positions, the rhythm, and the times the labour requires in order to progress normally when there is no need for intervention. It is also the act of disregarding the emotional needs of mother and baby throughout the whole (childbearing) process."[2] Ultimately, it is about disregarding a woman's human rights.

In *Birthtime*, Dr Rachel Reed talks about her Australian research findings in this regard: "In the research that we conducted, it was around coercion, so women feeling that they were being coerced into making decisions or having things done to them through coercion – all the way through to actual violation, women being held down while somebody conducts a vaginal examination."[3] On obstetric care: "It's more medicalised, more abusive, more disempowering, and that's what I've witnessed just over the last decade."[4]

Vanessa Olorenshaw adds to the picture, when she writes: "When women are treated as less than, as incidental to, as incompetent in making decisions about their own bodies (particularly in context of pregnancy and birth), it speaks to the very core of our values. We can start to see that our status as mother – our power to create and birth life – can be used against us: we can be held hostage, and our rights can be suspended at will."[5]

The picture of a broken maternity system doesn't stop there. This is an international issue, as well as an Australian one.

In the UK, systematic mistreatment of women in childbearing led to the White Ribbon Alliance developing its 2011 'Respectful Maternity Care Charter: The Universal Rights of Childbearing Women'. The WHO issued a position statement in 2014 calling for prevention and elimination of disrespect and abuse in facility-based childbirth. Then in 2019, the United Nations (UN) reported that the "mistreatment of childbearing women by maternity services during pregnancy, labour and childbirth is so normalised that it is often overlooked and not recognised as violence against women, including within Australia".[6]

The worldwide organisation Human Rights in Childbirth (HRiC) advocates for change and the protection of women: "Women's rights are human rights, because women are human too. The last century has seen a long struggle, around the world, for legal recognition of that basic fact."[7]

The submission to the Australian Rights Commission by Human Rights in Childbirth highlights how a culture of disrespect and abuse in maternity care impacts the health of women physically and psychologically. This is coinciding with the rise of maternal and infant morbidities. Such issues include PND, undiagnosed PTSD and, tragically, maternal suicide following childbirth. Women are disclosing their experiences of depression, suicidal thoughts and emotional detachment from their baby. There are also reports of hypervigilance around their baby (extreme vigilance, a state of being highly or abnormally alert to potential danger or threat all the time). In addition, the submission mentions flashbacks and nightmares, withdrawing socially, having difficulty maintaining employment, sexual dysfunction, and marital and family breakdown. Some women fear becoming pregnant again, leading to lack of intimacy, and conflict with partners.[8]

In the report, *Birth injuries: the hidden epidemic*, commissioned by the Australasian Birth Trauma Association (ABTA), Birth Trauma Association (BTA) and Make Birth Better (MBB) in May 2022, 8 key themes arose. When asked, 'Can you tell us a little more about how the physical birth injuries might have affected your life?', the 8 themes arising from the 794 respondents were:

- impact on self-esteem and mental health
- misdiagnosis/delayed diagnosis
- fear and isolation
- ability to be physically active
- impact on relationships and work
- medical gaslighting
- sex life and intimacy
- future births and growing families.[9]

This is distressing and damning reading, but please stay with me and keep breathing.

The HRiC found that it was rare to find a woman who understands what she may experience in hospital, such as strict time limits placed on different stages of labour. Often, these haven't been disclosed to her before she attends the hospital. For instance, the following advice, downloaded from the Department of Health (Victoria) website on 7 June 2019, provides an example of blanket demands for prior acceptance: "If you are in a high-risk group, healthcare professionals have an obligation to put your health and the health of your baby above your preferences. Understand that some decisions might therefore be out of your control."[10]

When hospital protocols are undisclosed, they cannot and should not trump the fundamental human rights of any person. In addition to being a violation of women's human rights, mandating procedures and protocols without disclosing them before the woman engages the services of a health care provider is a breach of the consumer protection provisions under the Australian *Competition and Consumer Act 2000*.[11]

Women reported feeling shocked, unprepared and terrified by sudden intensive changes in approach, often preceded by hours of neglect in labour. Any decision to continue labouring or to have an unscheduled caesarean section is not made by informed choice when undisclosed policy or guidelines are used to influence women. The 'consent' that is finally given is where the women simply gave up after hours of badgering, taunting or abuse. This is coercion rather than consent. Women are suddenly told that they are out of time, not *allowed* to keep labouring, or that their baby will die if they do not submit to interventions. 'Pulling the dead baby card' to frighten women into submission is alive and well in obstetric practice today.[12]

The HRiC also reported that women were kept on their backs to labour for the convenience of the care provider and that mandatory periodic vaginal examinations are used, with strict time limits for stages of labour. In some instances, there has been a 'husband stitch' without consent. This is an extra stitch at the entrance to the vagina to make it nice and tight for the husband, never mind how uncomfortable that will be for the mother.[13]

We also see reports of quick cord-clamping and cutting, removing the newborn to speed up placenta delivery, and denying mother and baby skin-to-skin contact immediately after or in the first few hours after birth. Reports also indicate bans on vaginal birth after caesarean (VBAC), twin vaginal delivery and breech vaginal delivery in some facilities.[14]

I am so saddened to be the bearer of such news. I know it is shocking, gut-wrenching and somehow unbelievable. Yet this is the lived reality for some women. And this is why we are here – to stop this happening to you and future mothers. Please use your practices to sit with the emotions, that you may be feeling. Do what you need to do to nurture yourself. It's understandable if you need to pause awhile – with more tea and chocolate and a heartfelt hug from me. If you can – and only when you feel ready – it's worth having a listen to the interview with human rights lawyer Bashi Kumar-Hazard about 'Obstetric violence, and the rights of women over body autonomy' on *The Midwives' Cauldron*.

- **Dr Amali Lokugamage** 'Obstetric Violence and Human Rights' YouTube.
  https://www.youtube.com/watch?v=Ziy5kSFm7U8

- *The Midwives' Cauldron* S2 #13. 'Obstetric violence, and the rights of women over body autonomy'
  Apple 🎙 Spotify

Birth trauma

Birth trauma isn't always caused by obstetric violence. In *Birthtime*, Professor Hannah Dahlen discusses trauma in birthing: "So, what defines birth trauma? Well, I think women get to define that, not us. For some, it's physical implications. For some, it's psychological and emotional implications. For some, it's cultural and spiritual implications. But what women have said to us is the biggest thing that causes traumatic birth is not being listened to, not having choices, feeling violated, feeling out of control, and then later not having anybody tell them what happened, why it happened, and helping them move on to resolve it."[15] We cannot judge what another person may feel as traumatic.

Professor of midwifery studies, Soo Downe, comments in *Birthtime* that "traumatic birth, which is often treated as just not a nice birth, is much more than that. It's actually a profoundly distressing disconnect from notions of humanity".[16]

Language, respect, acknowledgment, presence and compassion are all so important to the emotional wellbeing of the woman. The work of MBB in the UK defines post-traumatic stress symptoms (PTSS) as different from PTSD, which are both different from PND. Often, symptoms are expressed when women have left maternity services. Symptoms can appear 3 to 6 months after birth, with few supportive services available and a lack of screening or understanding. Mothers, while exhausted, often feel a sense of failure, shame and guilt, all while putting the children first. They fall between the cracks of available care and are often misdiagnosed as having PND.[17]

Birth trauma is a 'silent epidemic' in the words of Emma Svanberg in *Why Birth Trauma Matters*. She uses the analogy of a car accident, proposing that family, colleagues and your GP would be concerned if you and your partner were in an accident. They would ask how you are and would provide physical and emotional support where needed. Apply this to birth. In this same situation, you arrive at hospital and everyone asks about the car, not you and your partner. No matter the physical damage or emotional hurt to you, you should be happy because your car is undamaged. You can't be traumatised, or feel sad or depressed. You just have to get on with it and not complain because your car is okay. A year later, your car accident is celebrated, evoking all those memories and flashbacks, but once again your experiences are pushed aside.[18] What?

In the words of Vanessa Olorenshaw: "A woman's birth experience is something which she keeps with her for the rest of her life. It is no small thing. Yet the treatment of women during labour and immediately afterwards can be shameful and fails to respect the sacred period of birth and the fourth trimester."[19] Failing to recognise the potency of the experiences that birth and early mothering has on mothers for the rest of their lives, shows a shocking lack of regard for women. In *Birthtime*, Debby Gould talks about, "Those feelings, and the feelings that come up time and time again for a negative birth, regardless of what path the birth took – feelings of being powerless, out of control, and their expert insights into their babies and bodies aren't listened to."[20] This has to change.

The BESt study highlights women's responses about obstetric violence and birth trauma. This shocked Dr Hazel Keedle so much it led her to further research in this area. Her work found that one in 10 women experiences obstetric violence. She found that the least birth trauma experienced by mothers is with continuity of midwifery and independent midwifery care.[21] Her findings on this issue are discussed with great compassion with *Great Birth Rebellion*, 'Obstetric Violence and Birth Trauma'.

- **Make Birth Better** 15-minute video. https://www.makebirthbetter.org/free-resources
- *Great Birth Rebellion* #23. 'Obstetric Violence and Birth Trauma' Apple 🎙 Spotify

---

In addition to what we have just discussed, the old saying 'leave your dignity at the door' when you enter the birth room needs to stop. This attitude of demeaning disregard before a woman enters the birth room is distressing and fear inducing. The birth room needs to be regarded as a sacred space where the woman is to be respected at all times, because her dignity and feelings of safety are of paramount importance.

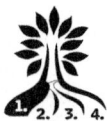

The Physical, Hormonal and Emotional Influences on Assisted Birthing

There is no right way to give birth. None. Your way is unique to you. If all the bells and whistles are needed, then they are needed. It's still yours. Remember, there is no place for judgement here. As Vanessa Olorenshaw writes, "I cannot subscribe to the idea that a woman who gives birth assisted with pain relief, or instruments, or surgery is a lesser mother or a failure. It is anti-feminist and anti-woman. Not my cup of tea."[22] Agreed. Right, nag over, here goes …

Medically assisted labour and birthing, like induction or augmentation, are different from physiological labour. The naturally occurring cascade of hormonal physiology does not occur in the same way in assisted labour and birth. The influences on how a mother experiences labour progress, assessment, and experience in birthing between physiological and medically assisted labour and birth is like comparing apples to pineapples. Here we are going to discuss how to optimise a medically assisted birth so you are part of the process and the experience is yours, rather than 'done to you'.

Birth is a neuro-psycho-social event in all births

Assisted birth needs to be supported in such a way that the neurohormonal, physical, emotional and social aspects of birth are honoured. The evidence for promoting **oxytocin** is powerful. This is achieved through social support that creates a significant effect on neurobiological processes. The brain and body work as one and have evolved to respond to social and emotional support. Yet, "Psychological aspects of labour and birth have received little attention in maternity service planning or clinical practice."[23] Maternity care needs to optimise the environment to support neuroendocrine processes even when birth interventions are used. We know that a decrease in pain, fear and stress, due to having midwifery one-to-one support and other trusted support in labour, benefits the woman. This acknowledges the crucial role that endogenous oxytocin plays in the psychological and neuroendocrinological process of labour.

Clare Goggin's book *Why Caesarean Matters* discusses the findings of a 2013 Cochrane Review that looked into 23 trials with 15,000 women from 16 countries. It found that women with continuous support that enhanced physiological labour felt greater control and competence and a reduced need for obstetric intervention.[24] Our maternity care needs to fully support these processes, especially when birth interventions are needed. Individual emotional support empowers women and increases the chance of a positive birth experience, even if labour is long or requires intervention. Mind and body, emotion and physical sensation are not separate, but one. Attitudes need to change and environments need to support this unique social event.

Hormonal interplay with intervention in birthing

The way the music plays through the body is different in induction and augmentation. If hormones are the musicians, the composer needs to write a different composition to perform the music of assisted birth.

As mentioned before, the baby signals the mother through transference of certain hormones through the placenta to stimulate increased oestrogen and the production of oxytocin receptors in the uterus and breast. They are letting Mum know they are ready for the eustress of labour, to adapt to being born, to breathe and to feed.[14] With induction, it is not possible to know where the baby or mother's body is in this development and communication process.

The preparation, separation and liminal phases are occurring in a hospital environment, often in less time than a physiological process; therefore, the mother's body has less time to adjust and build beta-endorphins, potentially making the experience of pain quite intense.

The baby is also affected by where they are in the phase of signalling their readiness for labour and birth. Their capacity to adapt through the release of cortisol may alter during induction, due to how ready they are for the eustress of labour and birth. They may produce more cortisol during an induced labour, as it may be more stressful to them and affect their transition to breathing and breastfeeding.[25]

It's absolutely possible to support the hormonal cascade that is the experience of physiological labour when caring for a woman who is having a medically managed birth or intervention. It is using everything we have already discussed with Ally and adapting it to assisted birth. Midwives, doulas and partners need to be more physical in supporting the mother. This additional support for optimising oxytocin, prolactin and beta-endorphins (while reducing stress hormone responses) is a vital part of the process in assisted birth.

There is a vast reservoir of knowledge in Dr Sarah Buckley's *Hormonal Physiology of Childbearing* [26] and Dr Kerstin Uvnäs Moberg's books on oxytocin.[27] Dr Buckley's research into the hormones of labour and responses to intervention leads "towards promoting, supporting, and protecting physiologic childbearing, as far as safely possible in each situation".[28] That's what we are going to explore now.

A medically induced or augmented birth is monitored more closely than an undisturbed birth, especially for a serious condition such as pre-eclampsia. This is a condition associated with the placenta, where symptoms include raised blood pressure and protein in the urine. Monitored closely in pregnancy, the decision to induce is made for the safety of mother and baby. Here, obstetric knowledge and care is vital, because it is only resolved once the baby is born.

Getting labour started and vaginal examinations in medically managed birth

Vaginal examinations are a part of medically managed birth, for assessment of how to begin the process and to decide on the method and medication that will be required. Vaginal examinations during medically managed labour shouldn't be a painful, undignified or stress-inducing experience. They are done on a regular basis during managed labour. As we have discussed before, the optimal situation is to keep adrenaline lowered and oxytocin maintained. Having listened to *The Midwives' Cauldron* podcast about vaginal examinations, remember it's all about your comfort, sense of dignity and safety, not ease of access for the practitioners.

More in-depth information about vaginal examination, with consideration of women's previous experience of sexual violence, is explored with compassion in the *Great Birth Rebellion* podcast #10.

- *Great Birth Rebellion* #10. 'Vaginal Examinations' Apple 🎙 Spotify

---

The ripening of the cervix for induction uses the hormone **progesterone**. Prostaglandin gels or pessaries are inserted next to the cervix to encourage softening, thinning and opening of the os (opening in the cervix) until the membranes can be accessed.

A balloon catheter may be needed first, to stimulate opening by irritating the cervix. Balloon catheter insertion is uncomfortable. Furthermore, the lithotomy position is used for access. Dignity and respect, with as much gentleness as possible, are of paramount importance during the insertion of the catheter. A balloon is filled on the inside, beside the membranes and outside of the cervix in the vagina. Cramping and contractions (produced in response to prostaglandins stimulated by pressure of the ballon on the cervix) can be uncomfortable, and each woman's response to induction will vary due to where she is in the oestrogen preparation-for-labour phase. The aim is to open the os until access to the membranes becomes possible.

Artificial rupture of membranes

Rupturing the membranes (ARM) is the second part of induction. The amniotic sac needs to be broken before an infusion of Syntocinon can be given, due to a possible risk of amniotic fluid passing into the woman's circulation.

If ARM is required, practitioners are currently taught to do this with the woman in a supine position. They make a hole in the amniotic sac with what looks like a long crochet hook or a finger glove with a hook on it, so that the liquid surrounding the baby can come out. Occasionally, someone assists by placing pressure on the top of the uterus to press the fetal head firmly down into the pelvis to prevent the umbilical cord flowing in front of the head with the gush of fluid.

The woman should not be asked to bunch her fists and place them under her sacrum for better access by the practitioner, because this is extremely uncomfortable. A pillow should be placed under the sacrum. This procedure can be done with respect, as gently as possible, with low lighting, comfort from the support partner, soft whisperings, music, aromatherapy … all things we have discussed to provide an environment of calm.

Induction and augmentation with Syntocinon

Induction and augmentation with Syntocinon are discussed together here, because the action of the drug on the body is the same. However, protocols for its administration vary between institutions. Synthetic oxytocin does not move from the bloodstream into the brain.[29] With induction, after ARM some institutions allow a grace period of 2 hours before starting the infusion. Nipple stimulation and/ or expressing breastmilk to encourage oxytocin and contractions involves the birthing mother in the induction process. Aromatherapy clary sage is often used to support contractions too, and we can make use of pressure points, rebozo sifting, yoga stretches and more, as mentioned with Ally.

Also discussed with Ally, oxytocin is released in pulses to generate contractions. While this is happening naturally, beta-endorphins rise, providing pain relief. While synthetic oxytocin acts on the oxytocin receptors of the uterus to make it contract, a feedback cycle to the mother's brain could lead to naturally occurring oxytocin release as well. This would support further contractions. The dose of Syntocinon is increased every 30 minutes until 4 to 5 contractions occur within a 10-minute period. This process of inducing contractions rapidly, with lack of time for the woman to adjust and build her own beta-endorphins, can mean that pain becomes intense. Needing pain relief via an epidural is completely understandable.

As we discovered with Ally, plasma oxytocin levels during physiological vaginal birth show a maximum of 3 peaks in 10 minutes, with a giant peak that is the reflex to push. On the other hand, an intravenous infusion of Syntocinon is a sustained level that may become 3 to 4 times higher than in spontaneous labour. It is little wonder the experience is so intense.

Synthetic Syntocinon has several side effects. Uterine hyperstimulation can occur which is when contractions are too close together so the baby doesn't get enough oxygen. Continuous fetal heart and uterine contraction activity monitoring is required.[30] In addition, overexposure to Syntocinon causes desensitisation of oxytocin receptors, contributing to reduced ability for the uterus to contract after birth increasing the risk of postpartum haemorrhage. The use of Syntocinon also contributes to prolonged pushing and instrumental birth. On the other hand, there is a possibility that synthetic oxytocin increases social skills and lowers anxiety after birth.[31]

To assist you in your decisions about induction due to post-dates, and for insight and support into induction for medical reasons, please use the resources on the following page.

The use of ARM, augmentation and induction with Syntocinon bring on contractions more quickly. Maternal guilt and that nasty inner voice can hit women who want or need an epidural when they feel they are not 'achieving' the hopes and wishes they held for birthing. Remember the map? There may be unexpected detours, bogs to cross, cliffs to climb, rivers to navigate. You planned for an altered journey. Feel free to throw that nasty inner voice back into the cesspit where it belongs, along with guilt.

- Wishlist 🎙 *Great Birth Rebellion* #33. 'Induction of Labour' Apple 🎙 Spotify
- Wishlist 🎙 Dr Reed Blog. 'Induction of Labour for prolonged Pregnancy'
  https://www.rachelreed.website/blog/induction-of-labour-for-prolonged-pregnancy
- Dr Rachel Reed Blog. 'Induction: a step by step guide'
  https://www.rachelreed.website/blog/induction-step-by-step
- Dr Sarah Buckley Blog. 'Labour Induction: Making Choices'
  https://sarahbuckley.com/labour-induction-making-choices/

Medically managed induction is in a different realm from physiological labour. They are totally different. Making this an empowered, respected experience for the birthing woman is vital. Here, all the optimising suggestions of environment, touch and support are needed to keep the mother's parasympathetic nervous system present. Maintaining feelings of safety and love assists her to sink into the state of altered consciousness, to release, to find comfort, to rest and snooze between contractions, which supports the release of beta-endorphins. With skilled support in pain-coping strategies, this is all possible.

Epidural analgesia (EDA)

It's important to understand the effects that epidural analgesia (EDA) have on labour and birth. EDA affects the physiology of hormones in labour, and blocks nerve fibres from the uterus and vagina that are associated with pain. EDA may also block the nerve fibres that produce the oxytocin high to trigger the Ferguson reflex to push. EDA reduces the endogenous release of oxytocin and circulating oxytocin, lessening contractions and leading to an increase in augmentation. The side effects of this have already been discussed.

Mothers who have EDA express less satisfaction with their birth experience and their wellbeing. This is due to reduced levels of endogenous oxytocin production, which interferes with the amnesic effect of oxytocin. Amnesia in this experience is forgetting the pain of birthing.[32]

Another effect of EDA is that the mother's chest doesn't display the flushing and increase in warmth that it does in a vaginal birth without EDA. The response is that newborns show less interaction during skin-to-skin contact.[33]

The Australian Society of Anaesthetists website has a page called 'Epidural Anaesthesia for Childbirth'. It provides comprehensive information about epidurals. It is important to know the possible complications of epidural pain relief before going into labour. Anaesthetists are required to gain a woman's consent before providing an epidural and they have to talk about possible side effects before she signs the consent form. This inevitably happens when the woman is in pain, has decided to have an epidural and wants the anaesthetist to get on with it. The opportunity to discuss side effects is only in the minutes between contractions, so, is this really informed consent? These are the side effects they will tell you about.

- For one in 8 women, an epidural does not fully work.

- For one in 20 women, if a caesarean section is needed, the epidural is not sufficient and spinal anaesthesia or a general anaesthetic is required.
- For one in 50 women, there is a significant drop in blood pressure which affects the fetal heart as insufficient blood is being passed through the placenta. This is why an IV is put in beforehand.
- For one in 100 women, there will be a severe headache.
- For one in 1000 women there will be some nerve damage (a numb patch on a leg or foot, or having a weak leg), which is temporary and rare.
- For one in 13,000 women, some nerve damage lasting for more than 6 months can occur. It is rare but can be permanent.
- For one in 50,000 women, there will be an epidural abscess (infection) / meningitis. This is very rare.
- For one in 100,000 women, there is an epidural blood clot or unexpected anaesthetic spread. Very rare.
- For one in 250,000 women, there is severe injury including paralysis. This is very rare.

In addition, a study by Dr Daniela Menichini and associates clearly highlights other side effects of epidural analgesia. In the study, 250 women had epidural analgesia (EDA) and 250 did not. The rate of occipito posterior positions (OP) was 4 times more frequent in the women with EDA. This is due to the side effect of lowered tone in the pelvic floor muscles after epidural insertion, reducing the ability for the fetal head to rotate. Firm muscles of the pelvic floor provide a surface for the fetal head to rotate against in advanced labour. The need for augmentation with oxytocin and the rate of caesarean sections were significantly higher for women with EDA, with longer labours and longer second stage of labour (the emergence phase). Early breastfeeding was significantly lower in the mothers who had EDA.[34]

A trial called BUMPES explored the outcome of upright positions versus lying down position in the second stage of labour in first time mothers with a low dose epidural. It found that lying down in the second stage of labour, waiting for the fetal head to descend, corresponded with more spontaneous vaginal births.[35]

Please don't panic! At least we are now aware of the effects of EDA. We can lessen these effects by changing positions for progress in labour, supportive actions like side-lying release and in the emergence phase to wait for the head to descend deeply into the pelvis and vagina while resting in a left side-lying position. Also nipple stimulation, hand expressing, massage and all that positive love stuff we have explored in stimulating oxytocin and prolactin to assist with birthing, bonding and breastfeeding. For information on the what, why and how of epidurals in labour, look at the Australian Society of Anaesthetists and Pregnancy Birth and Baby websites.

Remifentanil patient-controlled analgesia

Remifentanil is a strong, fast-acting pain relief used during labour. It is becoming more common than morphine as pain relief in labour in some hospitals.

Remifentanil belongs to a group of medicines called opioids, similar to morphine, but it works faster and wears off quickly. It is given through a drip into a vein in the arm or hand and attached to a pump. The labouring mother controls the dose using a button (patient-controlled analgesia or PCA). The pump is programmed to give small doses whenever the button is pressed, usually at the beginning of a contraction. The effect will wear off between each contraction. 'Gas and air' (entonox) can be used as an additional form of pain relief while using the PCA. Remifentanil is an alternative to an epidural and may be an option for someone who cannot have an epidural due to spinal damage.

The mother's body metabolises (breaks down) Remifentanil rapidly, which is why she needs to press the pump button as each contraction begins. Although it will not provide complete pain relief, the mother can feel 'in control of' and able to cope with the contractions. There is more mobility than with an epidural. Remifentanil may cause drowsiness, dizziness, itching and nausea. It can also slow the mother's breathing rate, so it is recommended that the mother has her oxygen saturation monitored. The full effects of Remifentanil wear off within 10 to 20 minutes after the last dose.

The baby's heart rate will be continuously monitored during PCA. Information from the NICE guidelines suggests there is no difference in respiratory depression (slow to breath after birth) in the neonate (new baby) between Remifentanil and other opioids. Remifentanil is metabolised by some enzymes in the neonate after birth to an inactive compound.[36]

- **Australian Society of Anaesthetists website.** Epidural Anaesthesia for Childbirth.
  https://asa.org.au/epidural-anaesthesia-for-childbirth

- **Pregnancy Birth and Baby website.** Pain relief during labour.
  https://www.pregnancybirthbaby.org.au/pain-relief-during-labour

- **Pregnancy Birth and Baby website.** Epidural pain relief in labour.
  https://www.pregnancybirthbaby.org.au/epidural

Synthetic oxytocin for the emergence phase

Prolonged use of synthetic oxytocin in labour reduces the number of oxytocin receptors as an attempt to prevent overstimulation of contractions. This is called oxytocin desensitisation and it could also compromise labour progress and pushing efficacy.

Oxytocin desensitisation means the woman is at higher risk of bleeding after birth. In this instance there is excessive blood loss because the uterus has not contracted strongly enough where the placenta was attached. Therefore, any medically managed birth needs synthetic oxytocin to 'actively manage' the emergence phase of placental birth and prevent postpartum haemorrhage.

Usually, an intramuscular injection of Syntocinon is given immediately after the birth of the baby. Waiting to administer the injection is perfectly safe and allows the placenta to continue passing the baby's own blood, as explained when we discussed delayed cord-clamping. When it is administered, there is no transfer to the baby.[37]

Postpartum haemorrhage is a serious complication of childbirth. The *Great Birth Rebellion* podcast provides reassuring yet honest information on placental birth and postpartum haemorrhage.

- *Great Birth Rebellion* #24. 'Placental Birth' Apple Spotify
- *Great Birth Rebellion* #25. 'Postpartum Haemorrhage' Apple Spotify

Checking the perineum after birth

As mentioned with Ally, it is not unusual for some tearing of the perineum to occur. First-degree tears involve the skin only. Second-degree tears involve some of the muscle of the pelvic floor. We will discuss second-degree tears in more detail, and the use of glue instead of suturing to assist repair, more comfort and healing with Alysia in Chapter 6.

Episiotomy is a deliberate cut to the perinium. It is used with instrumental forceps assisted birth and to speed up the birth of the baby if there is concern the baby is in distress. It is rarely used in vacuum assisted birth. Episiotomies are sutured, but there is now research to suggest a medical grade glue will be enough for some episiotomy repairs, which makes healing more comfortable.

Third- and fourth-degree tears of the perineum are more serious tears. They extend from the perineum to the anus (anal sphincter) or rectum (inside passage that holds poo). They include some degree of muscle that controls the opening and closing of the anus. Third- and fourth-degree perineal tears need surgical repair, done in theatre under spinal anaesthesia. This means the woman is awake, but totally numb during the surgery. Third- and fourth-degree tears may be associated with short- and long-term complications, and can affect physical, psychological and sexual wellbeing. We will explore this in the social part of Tree Root 3.

While not all third- and fourth-degree perineal tears can be prevented, it is possible to reduce the risk of their occurrence. Upright, forward leaning and left lying positions where the sacrum is free to move all help. Knees in, calves out position and warm compresses on the perineum during the emergence phase can also help. Sitting semi reclined on the bed for prolonged periods of time in labour or during pushing is not advised. The mother should not be coached or directed to push as this is associated with increased significant tearing. This type of tear is experienced by about 3% of all Australian women who have a vaginal birth, and 5% of women having their first vaginal birth. This rate is above the reported average for similar countries.

Most women who experience a third- or fourth-degree perineal tear recover well with appropriate treatment and support, although some will need specialised care to optimise their recovery.[38]

This all sounds very scary, but it is part of what we need to know. The predominant message is that women need more information about pelvic health and specialist pelvic health physiotherapy care for recovery after birth. The following resources are here to inform you fully about prevention, incidence, repair, care and recovery.

- **Wishlist** 🌿 Information on third- and fourth-degree perineal tears video.
  https://www.safetyandquality.gov.au/publications-and-resources/resource-library/third-and-fourth-degree-perineal-tears-clinical-care-standard-2021
- *Great Birth Rebellion* #19. 'Perineal bundle' Apple 🎙️ Spotify

---

Caesarean birthing

There is no oxytocin production in pre-labour caesarean birth, so the mother has not experienced the hormonal cascade of labour and birth.[39] There is less oxytocin production with skin to skin immediately after elective caesarean birth too, with a lower warmth response on the mother's chest.[40] However, the infusion of synthetic oxytocin after caesarean birth to reduce bleeding helps produce the effects that would happen in skin to skin after vaginal birth.[41]

Mother and baby have lower oxytocin levels after a caesarean birth. Separating mothers and healthy newborns following caesarean birth (such as paediatric checks done for convenience in some institutions) may be stressful to the mother. Such separation deprives her of the opportunity to increase oxytocin and reduce stress hormones for herself and her baby that skin-to-skin contact provides. It also impacts postpartum prolactin levels.[42]

Two days after elective caesarean birth, a mother releases one peak of oxytocin rather than the 5 peaks that occur after labour and birth.[43] This pattern is associated with a decrease in prolactin for breastmilk production. Here, some supportive actions to facilitate bonding and breastfeeding are:

- antenatal expressing of breastmilk to have a store of colostrum available
- keeping mum warm in theatre (warm blanket on her chest before the baby is placed there)
- prolonged skin-to-skin contact
- skin-to-skin contact for dad
- not separating healthy mum and baby for 'routine baby checks by a paediatrician' during theatre and in recovery
- unrestricted breastfeeding
- providing adequate pain relief for mum.

All that lovely supportive stuff we have been talking about is really important here.

Caesarean birth for 'absolute indications' and 'debated reasons'

For some women, birth by caesarean is the only way to birth their baby. We chatted about this with Ashleigh. This is called an 'absolute indication'. One example is placenta praevia. These account for a much smaller percentage of caesarean births than the 70% for 'debated' reasons, such as breech, failure to progress, previous caesarean birth and fetal distress.[44] (*Fetal distress* is concern about lack of oxygen and nutrients getting to the baby.) The National Institute for Health and Care Excellence (NICE) guidelines do not recommend a routine caesarean for a suspected small-for-gestational-age baby, or continuous heart rate monitoring in labour in a healthy woman.[45]

Caesarean birthing can be magical and empowered. 'Gentle', 'natural', 'woman-centred' are some of the ways we can describe support during the birth. Drapes can be lowered so that the birthing mother and partner witness the gentle birthing of their baby. The baby can be passed to the mother's chest immediately, with time for blood to transfer through the cord. In *Birth-Ed*, consultant obstetrician Florence Wilcock says, "If you lie on the operating table in the maternity theatres of my Trust, you will look up and find butterflies and cherry blossom on the ceiling."

Some women take a more active role. They scrub up like the surgeon and lift their baby from their abdomen to their chest. This is described in Chapter 3 with Ashleigh, and in the *Great Birth Rebellion* #39, 'Maternal assisted caesarean section'. For a mother birthing by caesarean, having a known midwife and/or doula during your pregnancy, birth and postpartum is just as effective in all the ways we have described before. We will be looking in depth into caesarean birthing in Tree Root 2.

Florence Wilcock is a huge advocate for reducing 'debated' reasons for caesarean birth. In *Why Caesarean Birth Matters* by Clare Goggin, Wilcock states: "My job is to master the art of being there only at the critical time, to run in and save the day, keep calm whilst doing so and to never get that judgement wrong. An impossible balance of risk vs choice, art vs science, clinical outcomes vs maternal experience."[46]

- *Birth-Ed* S2 #6. 'Caesarean birth with consultant obstetrician Florence Wilcock' Apple 🎙 Spotify

Vaginal birth after a caesarean section

Birthing vaginally after a caesarean section (VBAC) is profoundly important to women on so many levels. The term VBAC has been replaced with TOLAC, trial of labour after caesarean, which automatically places the woman under the assumption that she is on trial in her efforts to birth vaginally. This puts her on the back foot. It implies that VBAC/TOLAC can be 'successful' (pin that gold star on the woman's notes), or 'unsuccessful' or 'failed' (oops, black mark instead of that gold star). This fails to consider how the woman feels. Language needs to change.

The non-evidence-based ingrained belief of 'once a caesarean always a caesarean' led to a significant increase in caesarean births between 1980 and 1985.[47] Yet efforts to assist VBAC dropped to an all-time low in 2008, at around 6% in the USA.[48]

The UK 'Green Top' guideline no. 45 currently states:

- It is possible for a woman to have a "successful VBAC" at a rate of 3 out of 4 women, or 72–75%, if they have had one previous caesarean delivery and no previous vaginal birth.

- It is possible for a woman to have a "successful VBAC" at a rate of almost 9 out of 10 women, or up to 85–90%, if they have had one previous caesarean delivery and at least one previous vaginal birth.

- An "unsuccessful VBAC" is more likely with induced labour, no previous vaginal delivery, a body mass index (BMI) greater than 30 and previous caesarean for labour dystocia.[49]

With those kinds of statistics, and with self-belief and strong support, VBAC is not only possible, but safe for most women.

There is so much fearmongering about birthing vaginally after a caesarean. One such fear is that the scar on the uterus might rupture. In 2010, research showed that for Australian women attempting vaginal birth after one prior caesarean section, 0.01% had uterine rupture without labour and 0.15% had uterine rupture with spontaneous labour. This is very low. However, "risks were increased three- to five-fold for any induction, six-fold for prostaglandin combined with oxytocin and 14-fold for augmentation."[50] The research concludes that "careful consideration should be given to the use of oxytocin for augmentation of labour or induction by any method for women with a previous caesarean in view of increased risks of uterine rupture."[51] Allowing labour to happen in its own time is ideal.

Many women beginning the journey of VBAC are traumatised from their previous birth, so finding a care provider who is enthusiastic about supporting VBAC makes a world of difference. Continuity of care with a midwife increases the likelihood of vaginal birth. It is also important to point out that, even if a caesarean birth occurs again, the opportunity to have laboured benefits the woman for the cascade of hormones. The fulfilling feeling of having tried everything is healing, because the woman has been in control.

- **Pregnancy, Birth and Baby website.** 'VBAC'
  https://www.pregnancybirthbaby.org.au/vaginal-birth-after-caesarean-vbac

- **Patient information pamphlet on VBAC. website.** RANZCOG
  https://ranzcog.edu.au/wp-content/uploads/Vaginal-Birth-After-Caesarean.pdf

- **Wishlist** *The Midwives' Cauldron* S3 #13. 'An Interview with Dr Hazel Keedle – talking all things VBAC' Apple Spotify

Practice offering: Mountain meditation for challenging times

Practising yoga is extremely important if there are complications during pregnancy and assisted birthing. The effect of yoga for high-risk mothers on hospital bedrest demonstrates that as few as 2 sessions a week reduces both anxiety and depression. Having a complication such as raised blood pressure doesn't stop women from practising yoga. The effects are beneficial. Gentle yoga practice is also possible with placenta praevia and discomfort like symphysis pubic pain if you use adapted positions. The breathwork, visualisations and meditations are invaluable, particularly for women with a complication, anxiety or depression in pregnancy.[52]

All the breathwork you have practised so far is useful to help you find calm in situations of anxiety and fear of the unknown. Have a think about what breath practice resonated most with you and felt the most comforting. Harness this practice at these times to promote the vagal response of calming the nervous system to reduce the adrenaline and cortisol flooding through the body.

This offering may be helpful as a meditation during challenging times. You could use it as a foundation for developing your own.

- Return to your breath. Notice the rise and fall of your chest and begin your chosen practice.

- No matter where you are, scan through your body from head to toe, and soften.

- Feel into your body and notice where pain, tightness and emotion are held.

- Wiggle a little to release tightness and tension. Whisper to your body, asking the tightness and tension to release.

- Breathe into that space and feeling, holding it with respect because it's part of you and needs acknowledging.

- Breathe. Find your rhythm.

- Take yourself to a mountain, standing almost at the top. You feel cold, tired, lonely, frightened, with painful feet. The top is too far, too hard, too challenging to reach.

- Find your breath again. With that breath, breathe in the universe. See its vast, unending energy. Breathtakingly beautiful.

- Bind this energy into your body; let it flood through you, reaching into the depths of your being. Feel your body begin to warm.

- With each breath in, draw this infinite energy into yourself and know you are not alone; find your strength, determination.

- With each breath out, breathe back into the universe, sending gratitude and warmth in return.

- Breathe it all in. No matter how tired, fearful, emotional or in pain, take that first step to keep climbing.

- Breathe in the universe, or whatever has come to you that gives you the powerful feeling of overcoming what is holding you back.

- Each breath in, another step forward. Each breath out, release it all back to the universe, knowing you are held.

- As you reach the summit, look at that magnificent view and know what you have achieved.

- You are the mountain. You are the beautiful view. You are the strength. Look at you. You are amazing.

Practice offering: Yoga postures for assisted birth

This flow is offered with yoga postures altered for comfort in assisted labour and birth. Movement is possible and should be supported when you are attached to an infusion and/or fetal heart monitor. Most of these postures can still be used while being supported with a mobile epidural. The value of everything you have learned and practised is harnessed here so you feel a part of, and empowered in, your labour and birth.

Privacy, movement, fluids, snacks, touch, massage, sound, smell, soft lighting and your trusted birth support all enhance your experience in assisted birth. In particular, use nipple stimulation to encourage your own endogenous oxytocin to flow through your body. Rebozo is effective to support assisted labour. A video on how your birth support can do rebozo is provided in a goody box on page 104.

You still have the power of choice. Your labour, your birth, your body, your baby. You are part of the assisted birth process and the warm-up for labour flow is very useful here.

Again, there is no one-size-fits-all flow or schedule. Use what works for you in any order.

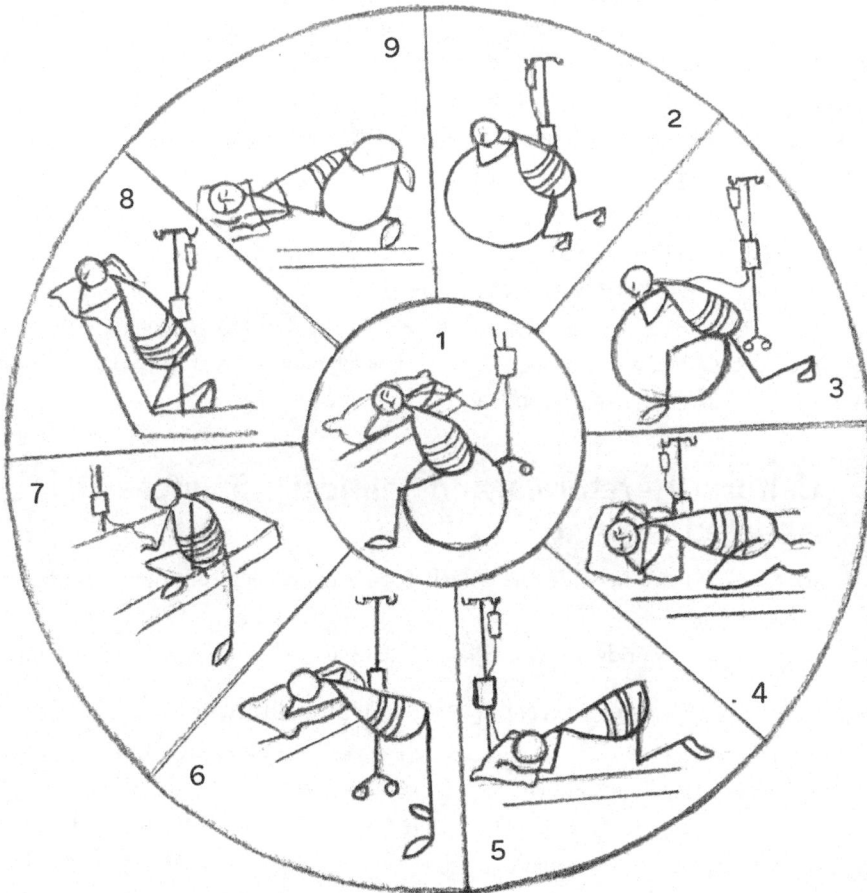

1.   Sit on a birthing ball with your feet facing outwards. Picture the pelvic floor open as you exhale and soften into the position. Rock from side to side and make circular movements. For support, lean forwards on the bed, arms crossed, head resting on a pillow. Your birth support provides pelvic pressure, if wanted.

Sound out "ooooooo", "aaaahhhh", "mmmmmmmmm" as you wish. Long exhalations of golden thread breath. Rest between each surging contraction. Do nipple stimulation to encourage your oxytocin. Listen to your body and move as you need to.

Use the ocean, tree, lotus, meadow or your own meditation. Harness the senses of the body to take you where you want to be during surging contractions.

2. Lean over a birthing ball, be on all fours, lean against a wall, or arms wrapped around your birth support. Do the Cow to Cat sequence as many times as you like. Soften the pelvic floor. Make circles or figure of 8 to the right, then left, when in all fours. Pelvic pressure.

3. Forward lunge, hands on the floor. Front foot turned outwards at 45 degrees. Soften the pelvic floor. Rock forwards, backwards and in small circular motions. Repeat on the other side. Pelvic pressure if wanted.

4. Supported wide-legged Child's pose. Rest here as much as you like. Soften the pelvic floor. Long exhalations of golden thread breath. Rest between each surging contraction. Pelvic pressure.

5. Supported Puppy pose.

6. Standing forward lean with your upper body supported by the raised bed, or arms over your partner's shoulders. One foot at a time out at 45 degrees, then facing inwards. Rock side to side, circles, figure of 8. Repeat on the other side.

7. Sit sideways on the bed with your right leg bent at the knee and your left leg dangling off the edge. Place the hands on the sofa or bed, left foot firmly on the floor. Lean your body forwards and feel the stretch to the outside of the right hip. Repeat on the other side.

8. Upright kneeling, supported by your partner, or beside the bed with a pillow under your knees, or on the bed with a pillow for your arms and head over the top of the mattress. Feet outwards in the first phase of labour and inwards near you when your baby is to be born. KICO.

9. Supported side-lying posture for rest or birth on the bed as you need. Place cushions or a peanut ball between your knees. Choose a meditation that feels right for you in this moment. Hold your mind, body and soul with love, wonder and appreciation. You are extraordinary.

Cultural, Herstorical and Political Influences on Assisted Birthing

It's time for more herstory and a look at current research, practice and future trends. "Argghh! Not more!" I hear you cry. Well, this is the most important bit of herstory and the cultural effects on birthing practices worldwide. Please hang in there, as it is powerful knowledge to hold.

Another technology added – external fetal heart monitoring

Cardiotocography (CTG), another term for external fetal heart monitoring (EFM), was introduced into birthing in the 1960s without any evidence to support its use.

At Yale in the US in the 1950s, Edward Hon and colleagues came up with a theory that fetal heart rate monitoring would prevent birth asphyxia (lack of oxygen to the baby in labour). The use of CTG was presumed to reduce the incidence of cerebral palsy by half, and reduce other neurological damage and fetal death. No randomised controlled trial was ever done, and the inventors' claims were based on guesses and clinical tales. Yet EFM technology and theories were embraced by the medical profession.

Hon and his co-investigators were undisclosed stockholders, directors, investors and patent holders in Corometric, an EFM machine manufacturing and sales company founded by Hon. In addition, much of their later research work was secretly financed by Corometric.[53] Nothing like a bit of one-sided prejudiced research and non-disclosure of personal interests to fill the pockets with cash!

Despite 5 decades of research and evidence that EFM does not prevent or predict cerebral palsy or that it is caused by birth asphyxia, EFM is still used. It does not predict stillbirth, acidemia (too much acid in the blood that can affect how organs work), or neonatal encephalitis (brain swelling in a newborn baby). It is also costly to mothers and babies who are injured by unnecessary caesarean sections.[54] Although EFM is proclaimed to be a safety device, Sartwelle et al claim it is used without mothers' consent, which contravenes foundational bioethical principles. The Obstetric Societies of Australia, New Zealand, the US and Canada all agree that EFM does not provide any long-term benefits for children. The United States Preventative Task Force rates EFM as a 'D' for prevention of cerebral palsy, which is the lowest grade of reliable evidence.[55]

So, why is EFM still used so much? EFM manufacturers make billions. As do trial lawyers. Billions of dollars are spent on cerebral palsy litigation in industrialised nations. This continues to be a 21st century epidemic.[56]

As Dr Sara Wickham states in a Facebook post, "It's important to remain aware of the economic issues that relate to knowledge, research and evidence, as there is an inbuilt bias towards researching the use of tests and interventions which can be developed for profit."[57] Where does the Hippocratic Oath of 'do no harm' come in to question the motivation for continuing the use of EFM? The bioethical principle of acting in the best interests of the woman is not being fulfilled.

In Ashleigh's chapter, I shared the **wishlist** 🌿 YouTube video with Dr Kirsten Small about EFM. Now is a great time to revisit that. A 2019 literature review found " ... no difference in the rates of still-birth, neonatal mortality or perinatal mortality between the use of intrapartum auscultation (listening in with a handheld Doppler) or CTG monitoring during labour in populations that include or consist of women considered to be at increased risk for poor perinatal outcome. Intrapartum fetal surveillance guidelines which recommend CTG monitoring for women considered to be at risk are not consistent with the evidence base. Clinicians and professional bodies have an obligation to provide maternity consumers with recommendations that are underpinned by sound evidence."[58]

In an article titled 'Most women who give birth in Australia are monitored with CTG. But it might not be the best approach', the authors looked into intermittent auscultation and continuous fetal heart monitoring in 'low- and high-risk' labouring women. The results are eye-opening. It showed that women want to be "involved in making decisions about their labour". In assisting the woman to make decisions about how she wants her baby listened to in labour, their research suggests: "Intermittent auscultation is generally the recommended monitoring technique when there are no risk factors. But all major international fetal monitoring guidelines advise CTG monitoring should be used for women considered to be at high risk, despite the evidence. As a consequence, clinicians don't always explain fetal monitoring choices to women with risk factors in a way that helps them make up their own mind about how they want their baby to be monitored during labour." [59]

For low-risk women, they wrote: "Given caesarean section is associated with a higher rate of complications for the mother such as heavy bleeding or infection, and increased rates of miscarriage and stillbirth in subsequent pregnancies, intermittent auscultation is the safer monitoring option for low-risk women." For high-risk women, they conclude: "Poor outcomes such as cerebral palsy and perinatal death occur more often in high-risk women but remain relatively uncommon. Research shows the use of CTG rather than intermittent auscultation doesn't reduce the likelihood of these outcomes but does increase the risk to women by making it more likely they will give birth by caesarean section."[60]

The article 'Midwives must, Obstetricians may' highlights how midwifery autonomy is compromised because it is governed by policy. Midwifery approaches to support fetal wellbeing in EFM is restricted, while the obstetrician's autonomy under the same policies is retained.[61] Women are coming up against guidelines and clinician preference that are not founded on sound evidence.

There are other things to consider with having EFM/CTG. Remember that your consent is required before any monitoring commences. With EFM your movement is confined to the length of the cables that attach the machine to your abdomen. Therefore, women are often steered to a bed because it is easier to keep track of the fetal heartbeat if the woman is still and sitting semi-reclined. But this does not allow the sacrum to move outwards and becomes more uncomfortable. The fetus has become primary over the woman's physiological needs of labour.

We do have methods for continuous fetal monitoring that allow movement. Called *telemetry*, a cable-free device is strapped or stuck to the woman's abdomen and the results are available on a central console at the midwives and doctors station. However, whenever EFM is used, a trained professional should be present with the woman at all times. EFM is not a babysitter or substitute for midwifery observational care. Machines do not always differentiate between the woman's and the baby's heartbeats. Only continual in-person assessment can do that.

Having read all this, it is clear to see how midwives are working in situations of restrictive practice and under observation. With this knowledge, I hope you have gained the confidence to negotiate intermittent fetal heart monitoring suitable for your unique circumstances. Please don't allow yourself to be placed in a position for the convenience of EFM and care provider access. There is no need to be sat on a bed, immobile, in order to be monitored. It's not about a machine; it's all about you.

You can ask for the mobile EFM and do all the moving you want. You can position your body however you feel you need. Sit on a birthing ball, take time out to shower. It's your body, your baby. Intermittent listening can be done then. Even with an epidural and synthetic oxytocin, when EFM is strongly recommended, be on your side, have a belly and back massage, and all the snacks, love and support that works for you.

Environment is important. Ask the midwife to turn off the volume of the monitor and turn away the digital display, so you don't concentrate on it. That's for the midwife to be observing, not for you and your support team to be anxious about or focused on. If you want, ask your midwife to explain exactly what the graph is indicating for curiosity's sake, then let it go and concentrate on yourself.

- Wishlist 🎙 Reminder: 'Electronic fetal heart monitoring' Dr Kirsten Small YouTube.
  https://www.youtube.com/watch?v=aGdknPVOhiw
- Wishlist 🎙 *The Midwives' Cauldron* S4 #4. 'Listening to babies during labour' Apple 🎙 Spotify
- Dr Rachel Reed Blog. 'Listening to baby during labour'
  https://www.rachelreed.website/blog/listening-to-baby-during-labour

Caesarean birth has quite a history

The first recorded 'successful' caesarean section on a living woman was in Germany in 1610. The mother died 25 days later, but her child lived.[62]

Successful caesarean birth was hindered by 4 important factors. The first, opium and whiskey were inadequate anaesthesia. Secondly, hygiene and bacteria were unheard of, so death from infection was extremely high. Thirdly, the church believed that to interfere by surgical means was to interfere with the will of God, because for women "in sorrow thou shall bring forth children".[63] Medical advocates of pain relief and anaesthesia had a battle with the church to practise this medicine. Fourthly, knowledge was scarce. How did one go about abdominal surgery to get a baby out?

In 1876 in Italy, practitioners needed permission from the Bishop of Padua before doing a caesarean section on a woman with rickets. (Because of poor diet and lack of vitamin D, in rickets the pelvis does not grow normally and vaginal birth is impossible.) Both mother and baby survived.[64] Incidentally, the first pre-planned caesarean in Australia was in 1885 for a woman with a vaginal tumour. It was performed by Dr John Cooke in Melbourne.[65]

From 1880–1920 there was a big leap in progress towards safer caesarean surgical practice – the procedure we now call the 'bikini line cut', 2 cm above the symphysis pubis, into the lower section of the womb.[66] In Chapter 1 with Leisja, we met Professor Ian Donald, the founder of ultrasound in pregnancy. He was prophetic when he stated in 1959 that "caesarean section is now performed with increasing impunity, thanks largely to antibiotics, improved anaesthesia and the availability of blood transfusion [...] but it would be a great mistake to regard it a means of finding a happy outcome to all our obstetric afflictions".[67]

The rise of caesareans between 1970 and 1988 in the USA was attributed to reduced fertility (fewer births), due mainly to the use of the oral contraceptive. There was a large increase in caesarean births, from a rate of 5% in 1970 to 24.7% by 1988, which far exceeded the population growth of 2% at that time. During the same period, external medico-legal pressures became associated with labour and birth. Medical malpractice premiums increased. At the same time, interventions in labour and birth increased as 'defensive practice' due to the fear of malpractice suits. This became culturally embedded and influenced the growth in caesarean rates.[68]

Between 1996 and 2011, there was another rapid rise in caesarean births in the USA without any clear evidence that it reduced maternal and perinatal mortality or morbidity, clearly indicating its overuse.[69]

Let's refer back to how anthropologist Holly Dunsworth debunked the myth of the obstetric dilemma that humans' pelvises evolved to be insufficient for birthing. In addition, in the *Birthtime* documentary, Dr Melissa Cheney states: "No evolutionary biologist can possibly digest the possibility that 33% of women need a caesarean section in order to get a live baby. It simply cannot be true."[70]

The human fetal head and the maternal pelvis have co-evolved over 500,000 years or 2,500 generations to accommodate each other. The birthing process and natural selection, along with survival of the fittest, has obviously occurred because we are here today. In relation to this non-existent dilemma, Margaret Jowitt states: "The obstetric solution is to bypass the pelvis and deliver by caesarean section."[71]

In a study on trends and projections of caesarean section rates globally published in 2021, data was collected from 154 countries between 2010 and 2018 (which counted for 94.5% of the world population). It saw caesarean rates between 5% in sub-Saharan Africa and 42.8% in Latin America and the Caribbean. Australia and New Zealand were at 33.5% (higher than the USA and Europe). Projected trends will see caesareans increase to 45% in Australia and New Zealand by 2030. This means that 38 million women worldwide are expected to be birthing by caesarean each year.[72] According to the WHO's 2015 'statement on caesarean section rates': "Since 1985, the international healthcare community has considered the ideal rate for caesarean sections to be between 10–15%."[73]

Placing all this into the Australian context, the latest data from the Western Australian Department of Health shows that caesarean section rates are steadily rising. Currently, 41.4% of WA births are by caesarean section.[74] However, this is an average of all hospital data and sadly does not reflect what is actually happening in the private and public sectors. Obtaining individual hospital data is extremely challenging. The latest available (displayed graphically on Birth Savvy's blog) was the 2017 WA hospital caesarean rates.[75] It has been hard to get transparent private hospital data into the public domain since then. The highest rate of caesarean birth was in a private hospital at 57% and the lowest in a public hospital at 24%.

The average between the private (57%) and public (24%) would reflect WA caesarean rates at 40.5%, which belies the truth of what is actually going on. Private hospitals are responsible for high caesarean section rates and this negates the work of public hospitals to keep the rates lower. The currently available national statistics from 2021 show that the average rate across hospitals is 38%. We need transparent rates of caesarean birth from every hospital.

It is important to know that women may choose to birth by caesarean for individual reasons. Whether from significant fear of childbirth (*tocophobia*) or a previous traumatic birth, these are known as *maternal requests*, and account for 3–4% of caesareans in Australia.[76]

The medical journal *The Lancet* has a large resource base of research for professionals towards reducing global caesarean section rates.[77] The Federation of International Gynaecologists and Obstetricians (FIGO) position paper 'How to stop the caesarean section epidemic' requests "the help of governmental bodies, UN partners, professional organisations, women's groups, and other stakeholders to reduce unnecessary caesareans".[78]

We have already discussed some of the things that FIGO suggests, including equal physician fees for surgical and vaginal birth. Hospitals should be obliged to publish annual caesarean rates, and hospital financing should be partly based on those rates. Women should be informed properly of the benefits and risks of caesarean birthing. With the money saved from reducing the number of caesareans, we should be investing in resources, better preparation for labour and birth, better care, adequate pain relief, practical skills training for doctors and midwives, and more.[79] The 2014 USA Obstetric Care Consensus to reduce first-time caesarean births notes that more than half of all first-time caesareans are for labour dystocia (labour slowing down or stopping) and non-reassuring CTG from fetal heart monitoring.[80]

As discussed with Ally in Chapter 4, modern data illustrates that natural physiological labour stages take longer than current timeline limits. The Obstetric Care Consensus offers many advisory strategies for practices, audits and policy change to reduce the number of caesarean sections. If the evidence around fetal heart monitoring is also acted on as discussed above, this would be another vital element towards reducing unnecessary caesarean births.

The UK has similar guidance from NICE for reducing the overuse of caesarean birth. However, and this is a big however, Australia doesn't have any such protective measures in place. "There is no national policy or campaign to address overuse of CS."[81] This needs to be addressed as soon as possible. In its intrapartum guideline of 2014, NICE stated: "low-risk multiparous women (have given birth before) planning to give birth at home or in a midwifery-led unit (freestanding or alongside) is associated with a lower rate of interventions and the outcome for the baby is no different compared with an obstetric unit." And advised: "low-risk nulliparous (first time giving birth) women that plan to give birth in a midwifery-led unit (freestanding or alongside) is associated with a lower rate of interventions and the outcome for the baby is no different compared with an obstetric unit. ... that if women plan birth at home, there is a small increase in the risk of an adverse outcome for the baby."[82] That's a high percentage of low-risk women who should be offered birthing at home or in birthing/freestanding centres. This was suggested in 2014. It's now 2025 ... Delay, delay ...

As previously mentioned, the WHO considers the ideal rate for caesarean sections to be between 10% and 15%. But what happens in countries where safe caesarean birth is not available? Dr Catherine Hamlin is an Australian gynaecologist who worked in Addis Adaba, Ethiopia, in the 1960s, caring for women with obstetric fistulas caused by obstructed labour. Fistulas are a result of little or no available obstetric care and are common in parts of Africa where women are often married very young and become pregnant before they are fully grown. Their pelvises are small, which impedes the progress of labour. Without obstetric care like a caesarean section, the baby often dies and the stillborn baby is delivered days later. The result of prolonged pressure on the pelvic organs causes an opening between the bladder or bowl and vagina. Urine and sometimes poo come through the fistula opening and out of the vagina. These young women are then shunned by their community.[83] So, while I am ranting at the overuse of caesarean birth in our country, there are thousands of women and babies worldwide who would benefit from such care.

Matricentric feminism in the labour room

The 'good' and 'bad' mother narrative that was introduced with Samantha in Chapter 2 spills over into the birthing room too.

In 'Understanding Obstetric Violence as Violence against Mothers through the Lens of Matricentric Feminism', Nicole Hill explains how the narratives and myths of the good mother are used to coerce women in labour and birth, making them vulnerable to obstetric violence. These narratives and myths say that a birthing woman needs to be an obedient patient who follows doctors' advice and adheres to medical protocols. If she speaks up for herself, declines certain obstetric care and interventions, and fights for her basic human rights in childbirth, she is labelled a 'bad' mother. Hill highlights how women "who have had bad experiences in birth may not report these events for a variety of reasons: in an effort to avoid thinking about them, if they suffer from feelings of guilt because they believe their reactions will not be validated or they feel they have no right to the emotions they have, or they think they must be 'making a fuss about nothing'... silenced because their emotions are perceived as trivial".[84]

This is further illustrated in the HRiC submission to the Australian Rights Commission. It highlights how the identity of good and bad mother can be used to coerce women who disagree with care providers to "perform obediently as against undisclosed care provider interests and mandated facility-based policies; and meet social expectations of feminised behaviour and adhere to harmful stereotypes of what constitutes a good mother".[85]

Social, Economic and Media Influences on Assisted Birthing

Birth injury. Without scaring you, what is it?

How well a woman is prepared for birth, and whether she is able to birth in the position she chooses without restriction, affects the outcome of birth injury. Being informed, even if these injuries are not common, is important.

The range of significant trauma to the perinium can be third- or fourth-degree tears, which include the anal sphincter, and tearing or damage to the bladder or urethra, which may cause difficulty urinating, leakage or pain. Pelvic floor muscle or nerve damage, and weakening of the muscles that support the bladder, uterus and rectum lead to issues like incontinence or prolapse.

The risk of these injuries is increased with instrumental birthing and also occur as physical complications of caesarean birth. If not recognised and treated correctly with intense pelvic health physio follow-up, birth injury can be seriously debilitating.

Social impact of severe birth injuries

A perineum can't show itself off with a plaster cast and pair of crutches. It's hidden. Silent suffering occurs because of our poor knowledge about the possibility of birth injury and lack of language or knowledge of our own anatomy. Without understanding or language, we utter whispers of "down there isn't the same as before birth". Little knowledge and shame around birth injuries prevents women from asking for help and sharing with fellow sufferers in solidarity.

Trying to negotiate a complicated system of professionals and out-of-pocket costs is hard, especially while sleep deprived, possibly anaemic, breastfeeding and looking after other children. These women are often also struggling with significant psychological trauma and physical symptoms from their birth experience. When made to feel that they should be happy because they have a live, healthy baby, these mothers suffer in silence. Feeling isolated, a failure, and unable to speak up, they go under the radar.

Dr Kara Thompson, an obstetrician and gynaecologist, states: "We need to lift the shroud of shame and stigma and reveal the hidden burden of women's birth injuries that have been ignored for too long … We must move from a system that ignores and dismisses birth injuries to one that treats them with as much respect, care and urgency as an injury sustained in other aspects of life." [86]

You have already seen the 8 key themes in the *Birth injuries: the hidden epidemic* report that arose in response to the free question: Can you tell us a little more about how the physical birth injuries might have affected your life?

Three in 4 respondents (73%) said they received treatment for their condition, yet 6 out of 10 (60%) mentioned treatment has only partially been effective, and one in 4 (24%) said they still have a problem. Only 16% said treatment had been completely effective, and so 84% are living with the problem without a solution. [87]

Complications such as an infected perineal wound, faecal incontinence, a vaginal prolapse or a *fistula passage* (an opening between organs) can be debilitating. They can cause interference with bonding, and can affect a woman's sex life, mental health, and her social and work life. They may also contribute to relationship breakdown. And yet they remain invisible to the outside world. "If a patient with a leg injury is unable to mobilise, they will be seen by a physio. If a woman has a torn anal sphincter, she will go home and wait." [88]

Society needs to talk about these injuries so mothers know they are not alone. "Women are suffering birth injuries and are left feeling unprepared, unheard, disbelieved and dismissed. This needs to change," Dr Thompson adds. "Devaluing birth injuries also sends a clear message to women; your injuries do not matter. … No use complaining about it. Suffering is, after all, a woman's lot." [89] Women have heard this message loud and clear and internalised it. Don't make a fuss? Well, no more. Treatment needs to be matricentric, and it must understand the needs of these mothers.

The framework of care put forward by Dr Thompson begins with awareness and preparation of the woman before birth. We want to ensure that the question, 'Why didn't anybody tell me?' is not uttered by a shellshocked new mother. Women need to know that, with current practices, about 5% of mothers will sustain an anal sphincter injury in a first vaginal birth. This increases to about 8% of women having their first vaginal birth after a caesarean section. Forewarned is important. Women are not children to be coddled, but must have their intelligence respected. Withholding information is failing to provide women with unbiased holistic care.[90]

Diagnosis is vital. Dr Thompson's writing exudes frustration and anger at a system that has little compassion for women's care, treatment, support or the research into such a significant issue. It is an issue that currently often creates months or years of suffering – with multiple professional visits that are even less accessible for women with financial constraints.

Overstretched staffing ratios in an overstretched system affect the simple consideration of pain relief for the mother in hospital. Many women do not have access to a physio before discharge home. Many have little to no knowledge of what to look out for, how to help themselves or where to go for help. "Diagnosis and care must start immediately after an injury. This should include access to inpatient physiotherapy for all women after birth, improved postpartum education, safer midwifery staffing levels, and delayed discharge until all injuries have been properly assessed and managed."[91] The lack of adequate numbers of women's health physios is a systemic failing.

The use of ultrasound to diagnose pelvic floor and anal sphincter injuries in the postpartum period requires upskilling for staff to recognise, diagnose and treat. This would be a vital element on the road to treatment and recovery, and would reduce waiting times for specialised urogynaecology and colorectal care. Such care should be trauma-informed, given with utmost respect, be culturally safe and provided within the public system, by a team of dedicated professionals in a birth injury clinic. It should include sexual health, social work and mental health support.[92] Recommendation 6 of the NSW inquiry proposes to "fund postpartum services, including physiotherapy and supported exercise programs, to support those who acquire a pelvic floor injury as a result of birth".[93] This needs to happen nationwide as soon as possible. This is when the village-in-waiting is desperately needed. Boundaries on visitors ought to be respected, because the mother needs to rest, recover, heal. Be nurtured. Getting her pain or discomfort under control is the priority. She may also need more time to establish breast-feeding. Mum will be extra tired with the physiological recovery she has to do. The village needs to step in, cook up a storm, care for other children, advocate for the mother, and help her get to appointments and treatment. It's about supporting her in all the ways we have already described, with compassion, tenderness, empathy and understanding. No judgement. No expectations. Just love and support.

The emotional cost of birthing

We have been looking into the economic costs of childbirth, but what about the emotional and psychological costs? What about the ongoing costs of physical complications, social implications and the silent suffering of the mother? As we have discovered, a fifth of women experience PND. This is only the reported figure; many women suffer in silence and shame. What about the costs of one in 3 women being traumatised by their birthing experience and one in 10 of those women developing PTSD? What about undiagnosed significant birth injuries and the lack of facilities to properly care for women?

Then there are the emotional costs of the experience of coercion and obstetric violence in labour and birth. There is the fear of reliving the experiences and having them dismissed and trivialised when a complaint is made. There is the fear of becoming pregnant again and fear of childbirth due to previous trauma. Women are making the decision to freebirth because they are scared of being retraumatised and do not feel supported to avoid birth trauma, because there is a lack of services to provide the care they need.

The cost of psychological and physical impacts on women due to our current system of care is immeasurable and is breaking many mothers.

The 2023 NSW inquiry into birth trauma received over 4,000 stories of birth trauma.[94] In the inquiry, Professor Hannah Dahlen presented findings from a survey of more than 8,000 Australian women about their birth experiences in 2019, which found that one in 10 reported obstetric violence. She stated: "No means no [in consent] except apparently in childbirth, and it's time to change that.... This is the 'me too' of childbirth."[95] The inquiry describes how women are not being informed about the complications that can happen in our current culture of childbirth, which limits their ability to give informed consent.

Amy Dawes, president of ABTA, stated in the inquiry: "RANZCOG said we can't inform women about all the dangers associated with birth, [but] we need to stop infantilising women … Why aren't we talking about this before women are in the birth suite?"[96] Women are highly invested in their pregnancy and possibilities about birth, especially when they have been exposed to so much negativity. 'Protecting' them from information takes away their autonomy, right of informed choice and consent. Who has the right to deny women information? Nobody.

Unlike the UK and the USA, Australia does not have a Patient Bill of Rights. If all states had one and it included this suggested statement, maybe all practitioners would consider consent before any investigation or procedure: "You are entitled to informed consent at all times when in touch with a healthcare facility/provider." The ICM's Bill of Rights for Women and Midwives states: "Every woman has a right to participate actively in decisions about her healthcare and to offer informed consent."[97]

The current majority system of institutionalised, fragmented care is set up to do exactly what it means to do. This time-controlled, one-size-fits-all, provider-convenient conveyor belt delivery of maternity care fails women. When informed consent for confident choice isn't given the time it needs for proper consideration, and women's voices are ignored, our current maternity system of care fails women.

Here, with Katie, we are finding ways to change this, in order to reduce the emotional and physical cost of birth trauma, injury, PTSD and PND. *Birthtime*'s original question is: "What would it take for all women to emerge from their births physically well and emotionally safe?"[98] Dr Andrew Bisit stated: "A profound sense of safety needs to be established through all aspects of continuity of care, including being listened to and being loved. Then a woman who's had a complication can feel physically safer after it, because all those things were attended to."[99] How simple, yet beautiful is his statement? Yet how can we achieve this profound sense of safety and love? We already have that answer …

"It's a known midwife, somebody that they know right from the beginning. This is the person they've told their story to, not only about their emotional background, their partner, what's going on in their life, etc. They're telling that person everything. They don't want to go to a clinic where they're seeing all these different midwives and having to explain those things over and over and over again to all these different people," states Valyrie Painter in *Birthtime*.[100] Again from Birthtime, Dr Kirsten Small says: "We know the evidence supports continuity of care. We've got big randomised controlled data, more than 17,000 women in trials, not just low-risk women, but women who have all kinds of mixed complexities in their pregnancy. These women do better in this model where you have lower rates of intervention. We have less babies dying in that model. That's really important."[101]

Midwifery COC is supported by Professor Caroline Homer AO, a leading midwifery researcher, who states: "Despite the need for more research into ways to effectively implement this model of care in practice, is it ethical to withhold access to midwifery COC from the majority of women in Australia, given the strength of evidence, the supporting policy documents and the demand from women?"[102]

The WHO's 2018 'Recommendation: for intrapartum care for positive childbirth experience' states: " … respectful maternity care – which refers to care organised for and provided to all women in a manner that maintains their dignity, privacy and confidentiality, ensures freedom from harm and mistreatment, and enables informed choice and continuous support during labour and childbirth – is recommended."[103] There it is in black and white. It is patently unethical to ignore the overwhelming evidence that continuity of known midwifery care meets the needs of women so that they emerge from their births physically well and emotionally safe. There is also an obvious need to give women known COC for a minimum of 6 weeks after birthing, with at least a 3- and 6-month physical and mental health review, so that women emerge physically well and emotionally safe postpartum.

The effect of birth stories in the media

There are 2 main media sources for women exploring pregnancy and birthing information. The first is where women upload their lived reality of birth for others to learn from. The other is vastly different: a form of 'reality television', where women's unique experiences are 'deconstructed' and rewritten as entertainment.[104]

Pregnancy message boards such as BabyCenter provide a platform for mother–authors to share their pregnancy, birthing and mothering stories to be read, felt and understood by hundreds if not thousands of other women. Here on pregnancy and birthing platforms, mother–authors are held in the spirit of personal sharing and remembrance. Quite often these platforms are structured, beginning with early to late pregnancy loss, premature birthing and loss. Then come the birthing stories, organised into type and location. They may be written with humour, sarcasm or anger. Each woman's experience is unique in her social and cultural situation and personal influences. So often, the main theme of the stories is how these women were treated in birth – were they involved in shared decision-making and "perhaps most crucially, whether [their] rights as a labouring woman were fully respected".[105] In contrast, the genre of childbirth reality television is destructive towards women's lived experiences. Being "offered up to the public in the guise of educational entertainment", criticisms include that "these programs co-opt women's stories, editing them to conform to a rigid storyline in which labouring women and their babies must be rescued by technology".[106] Furthermore, "researchers are discovering [that] merely viewing these programs has been shown to increase women's fear".[107] Learning about birth through the medium of reality television can be seriously misleading and may damage women's perceptions about birth.

Witnessing this stereotype is toxic: the hysterical woman in labour, who suffers if she doesn't have pain relief and is 'out of control', who is treated like a child, is misinformed and denied informed consent. On such shows, mothers' voices and wishes are smothered initially by medical establishment that appears to "find their requests to control the conditions under which they labour bothersome".[108] Then mothers' voices are manipulated again by "producers who insert their own commentary, often scrutinizing and judging each mother as they co-opt her personal story".[109] Mothers' voices and needs are not what matters in this medium of entertainment. Tragically, birthing women are even "sometimes blamed for problems they may have experienced in pregnancy and birth, suggesting a punitive surveillance approach to care". [110] Where and how a woman learns about pregnancy, birthing and early mothering matters. Here, I am returning to the theme of finding sources that nourish you and align with your philosophy and values. I decline to infuse your brain with the negative imagery of reality television and associated media. There is a movement on social media similar to the #metoo phenomenon, with tags such as #metoointhebirthroom, #mybirthtoo, #birthtrauma, #birthisafeministissue, #birthjustice, #obstetricviolence, #enough. Awareness is growing as change needs to happen.

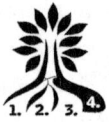

Self-identity, Beliefs and Values, and Spiritual Influences on Assisted Birthing

This section offers information for building self-trust and self-advocacy, and using your strengths, values and resilience for finding healing and post-traumatic growth, if needed. We are reclaiming and reframing identity towards healing the spiritual self, if that feels meaningful to you. This may help you reconcile previous pregnancy loss, pregnancy difficulties and birthing trauma.

Remember, not every mother is traumatised by her birth or develops postnatal depression. This book is full of information to prevent and support birth trauma and PND. However, until changes to our current birthing system occur, trauma in birth will continue.

The 4Ss: silencing, self-blame, shame and stigma

Some themes have evolved during the writing of this book. These are the 4 S's, where the inner voice runs rampant: silencing, self-blame, shame and stigma. I wish to explore these as a way of recognising what might be happening for you and helping you move towards a resolution.

Silencing

The theme of silencing has threaded through each chapter. Silencing women's experiences is intricately linked to self-blame, leading to shame and fear of stigma. These emotions keep the continuous cycle of silence going. The HRiC observed that, when women who have been mistreated attempt to complain, "their attempt to explain their pain and injuries and the impact of abuse and mistreatment is viewed either as a waste of time or treated suspiciously as someone's attempt at extracting compensation".[111]

Remember women wishing to avoid the 'bad mother' label? That is fully present here because she does not want people to know she can't cope, is not taken seriously, or is treated with suspicion.

Self-blame

Vanessa Olorenshaw writes: "Where antenatal classes seek to prepare women for birth, there is no escaping the fact that the phrase 'nobody told me…' is often spilt from new mothers' lips. Nothing prepares you; and, paradoxically, we have just lived through an extremely physical process, which may or may not have been traumatic, painful, or complicated. I commented to a midwife that becoming a mother was like learning to drive the day after being run over by a bus. That said, at heart, it is less the external appearance or our births which matter, but the feelings we have about our births."[112]

Women ask themselves, *Why didn't I know this beforehand? Where did I go wrong?* They blame themselves for:

- not being endlessly positive about pregnancy when feeling ghastly
- being anxious and fearful in pregnancy and about birthing
- not being prepared enough for birth because 'it didn't go as planned'
- failing to live up to the myth of a 'perfect birth'
- feeling broken by the labels 'failure to progress' and 'poor maternal effort'
- being shellshocked by birth and early mothering.

Shame … Shame … Shame …

Shame is the painful feeling of humiliation and distress for:

- failing to live up to the 'perfect mother myth'
- not being 'grateful' for a live, healthy baby, no matter the birth experience
- finding it all overwhelming and needing help and support
- struggling with isolation, boredom and bone-deep exhaustion
- resentment towards their partner who sleeps through the baby crying and can walk out the door as if their life has hardly been touched
- resentment when nobody recognises that a caesarean section is major abdominal surgery and would usually mean 6 weeks off work with rest
- resentment over becoming invisible, the baby becoming first for everyone and in everything.

Stigma

Stigma is when someone sees or treats you in a negative way because of a behaviour or a characteristic. This could be for:

- mental health issues or being labelled with PTSD, PND
- feeling a disgrace as the mother who 'isn't coping', keeping emotional and physical suffering hidden
- being a mother who doesn't like being a mother
- having flashbacks and nightmares
- feeling disconnected from her baby
- disclosing all these psychological and physical struggles to a health professional.

On top of this, a mother may fear that her child will be removed because she isn't coping.

Reaching out and finding support

Dear mother becoming, if any of this rings true for you, it is not you who has failed, but a system and culture that has failed you. It's going to take work to change the narrative in your head, but please believe in yourself. You have more strength and resilience than you give yourself credit for.

Well … this chapter has been tough reading. Here, I would like to guide you to the resource podcasts. They will help you realise that self-care and support are of paramount importance. They offer ways to acknowledge and begin to heal birth trauma and understand mothering challenges. Your spirit matters, dear mother.

- **Wishlist** *Birth-Ed* S1 E9. 'Healing and Preventing Birth Trauma with Dr Rebecca Moore'. The founder of MBB in the UK, she is dedicated to reducing birth trauma and healing women who have experienced it. Apple Spotify

- *Healing Birth with Carla* #45. 'Midwifery, Matrescence and Birth Trauma Healing' Apple Spotify

---

Where can you find help and support?

Birth trauma goes hand in hand with PND, but not always. Remember, one in 5 women experiences PND.

- **The Gidget Foundation website.** Provides a free 'Start Talking' telehealth service and is full of useful supportive information for partners and families too. https://www.gidgetfoundation.org.au/support/start-talking-telehealth. Phone: 1300 851 758; Email:self-referral: contact@gidgethouse.org.au

- Wishlist 🌿 MBB UK PDF guide 'Am I Traumatised?' Please read through this and note the symptoms and emotions that pop out for you. It may be a place to start to identify what is happening to you, to begin to understand why, and to find a way forward. Having this acknowledgment is a good starting point when going to your GP. ' See the free downloads on https://www.makebirthbetter.org/pdf-downloads-parents and click on 'Am I Traumatised'.

- **Australian Birth Trauma Association (ABTA) Birth Trauma Care Guide PDF.** A source of information about the kinds of care that are available for physical and/or psychological trauma. https://birthtrauma.org.au/wp-content/uploads/2020/05/ABTA-Birth-Trauma-Care-Guide-May-2020.pdf

- **ABTA Peer2peer support program, website.** Facebook and online support groups. https://birthtrauma.org.au/wp-content/uploads/2020/05/ABTA-Birth-Trauma-Care-Guide-May-2020.pdf

- **The MHM 'Mental health toolbox' website.** Mentioned with Samantha in Chapter 2. https://maternalhealthmatters.org.au/

- **The COPE website.** 'Recovering from traumatic birth'. Your postcode can be put in at the bottom of the page to find birth trauma counselling support near you. https://www.cope.org.au/preparing-for-birth/things-dont-go-plan/recovering-from-a-traumatic-birth/

- **PANDA has a helpline that is a safe place for you to go to talk.** Especially when you can't think straight and are too exhausted to read much. Its national helpline 1300 726 306 is available Monday to Saturday. They can help you begin to make a plan for yourself, and they understand that it is important to be heard when feeling big emotions of powerlessness, hurt, sadness, dismissal and not being taken seriously. https://www.panda.org.au/articles/what-happens-when-i-call-the-panda-helpline

- **PANDA website** 'Healing after birth, ways to look after yourself' https://www.panda.org.au/articles/childbirth-trauma-and-recovery

Be brave, dear mother. There are people who see you, don't judge you, won't think less of you or doubt your ability to mother. We acknowledge how much you have been through and are still experiencing. You are not alone. You are important. You matter. So, do reach out.

Taking back control, reclaiming and reframing your identity, speaking up, reaching out for help and support, obtaining your medical notes, and debriefing with a counsellor or birthing trauma specialist may help you. Most hospitals provide a debriefing service, yet this may not be an appropriate place to go as you explore your trauma experience. Returning to the place of trauma with the same individuals can be re-traumatising. Please consider doing debriefing with somebody who understands the paperwork and can guide you through your experiences.

Post-traumatic growth as part of healing means recognising the psychological change people experience after a traumatic event. It doesn't suppress the distress caused, but rather acknowledges it. This process of recovery allows you to reflect and grow from understanding the experience. The experience never leaves us, because this is a part of our life, always remembered. However, the effect of the emotional response can be reduced and managed.

Recommendation 41 of the NSW birth trauma inquiry recommends establishing formal debriefing clinics that are attached to all public hospitals with maternity services to provide "an evidence-based framework for effective debriefing, the ability for clinics to establish a feedback loop to the hospital for improvements to services, including options to provide feedback online and an option to debrief with a health practitioner who is independent from the service who provided the care if requested".[113] Recommendation 30 is to establish debriefing and psychological services for maternity clinicians as well, and is equally important. Bring them on!

Making a complaint

If you have a complaint to make, please consider how this may affect your mental health, and think about whether it is the right time for you to do so. I mention this because of some HRiC findings: women who pursue making a complaint about human rights violations mostly did so for altruistic reasons – because they didn't want other women to experience the same thing. Yet after approaching their care provider first, not being satisfied and then making a formal complaint, these are some of the experiences women had:

VM said: "[I] was belittled, laughed at, ignored and told I had 'issues' by delivery staff, the hospitals' risk manager, the hospitals' CEO, and ... the Board that is supposed to regulate hospitals. These people did nothing."[114]

AW said: "I've tried to write my story to [redacted]. Every time I try though, I hear [redacted]'s voice jeering at me, telling me I'm just a baby, crying for not getting her way. If writing my story helps just one woman avoid the abuse I've experienced, it was worth the pain of remembering."[115]

Again, it's distressing reading, because the current system for making a complaint isn't working in the woman's favour. The HRiC also notes that if a human rights lawyer is to be present with the woman, hospitals in Australia decline requests for a meeting.[116]

Recommendations 40, 42, and 43 of the NSW inquiry into birth trauma talk about supporting the Health Care Complaints Commission to resolve complaints more quickly, and with more accessible trauma-informed support to complainants throughout the process. It recommends pregnant women be provided with information that outlines pathways to ask questions, raise concerns and make complaints. It also recommends considering the public reporting of complaints data relating to maternity care and birth trauma, and its referral processes, including complaints that may have allegations of assault.[117] The last needs to be done, not considered.

If enough copies of complaints sent to hospitals are also sent to members of parliament, ABTA, MCN and the MCA, how might this speed up change? Harnessing the power of women's voices by making their experiences seen, heard and acknowledged. Women advocating for themselves through speaking up and making a complaint. Who knows where that explosion of voices may take us towards changing the culture of birthing?

As Dr Rachel Reed states in *Birthtime*: "Women need to step up and say, 'No, we need better than this. We are worth better than this.'"[118] Also in *Birthtime*, Deborah Pascali-Bonaro, an internationally renowned pregnancy, birth and postpartum doula trainer, states: "It's really going to take knowledge and it's going to take a huge movement of people speaking up. Then it's going to take politicians to be brave enough to say, 'We have to mandate that we can't allow the abuse of women and mothers and babies anymore.'"[119] *Birthtime*'s Jessie Johnson Cash said, "I think if men were the ones that were giving birth then we would have a completely different system than we do now."[120] Too right.

- The ABTA website. Guidance and support about making a complaint. https://birthtrauma.org.au/raising-a-concern/

- MCA website. Guidance on making a complaint. https://www.maternitychoices.org/complaints-template

- The MCN website. Representation services to take what happened further. https://www.maternityconsumernetwork.org.au/services-3

  It is possible to email both MCN and ABTA, if you don't know where to start, can't find what you are looking for, or are so emotionally fogged that you just need to find clarity of the process.

- The MCN website. Information about obstetric violence. A pamphlet, provides definitions of exactly what this is, how it can be reported to the police as a medical crime and how they can assist you with it. https://www.maternityconsumernetwork.org.au/_files/ugd/76e9eb_9d2874906d854b8c9b6f8ad40295350e.pdf

- Other assistance available to you is the Women's Legal Services Australia website. https://www.wlsa.org.au/members/

- Add the ICM Bill of Rights for Women and Midwives to your email of complaint to reinforce the importance of human rights in childbirth. https://internationalmidwives.org/resources/bill-of-rights-for-women-and-midwives/

Practice offering meditations. Loving kindness and on *Bhāva*

This has been a challenging chapter to read, full of deeply felt emotions. It may have provoked incredulity, frustration, uncertainty, anxiety and sometimes anger. I hope it has also harnessed knowledge so you can work within the current birthing culture to optimise all the powerfully important supportive actions to make your birth your own. Not 'done to you', but an embodied part of the experience, no matter how you birth.

The following meditation is offered as a way of returning to yourself. Come back to your values, your strengths, inner knowing, feminine intuition and self-trust. Calm the raging storm of emotions, thoughts and feelings. Take back control and learn a method to move forward with purpose, passion and intent.

This practice supports the perspective of knowing in the depths of your soul that you did not fail, that you are not broken. It is particularly potent when looking into healing the experiences of disempowered and traumatic birthing. It uses your inner strength to transition through your experiences and find some sense of resolution, peace, acceptance and healing.

To begin, we will build on the loving kindness meditation offered with Liesja in Chapter 1, doing the same with the attitude of holding compassion:

May I be compassionate to myself.

May I receive compassion from others.

May I extend compassion to others.

The next part of the practice offering is a meditation on *bhāva*. Bhāva is to meditate on an intent.[121] An intention that is filled with love and affection for yourself. To meditate with bhāva moves you towards cherishing yourself through transitioning into mother. As you listen to your heart, mind and soul, find an intention to express love and affection for yourself as you evolve in your unique journey of mother becoming. Your intention could be:

I am enough.

I will speak to myself with kindness.

I will notice joy in the little things.

Messy home, who cares?

I will be patient with myself.

Rest is precious.

I respect and love myself.

Within your bhāva, hold the values, strengths and self-trust you have found as these pages have unfolded. Be aware of your part in the ever-evolving mystery of our world and universe.

- Return to your breath … Notice the rise and fall of your chest and begin your chosen breathing practice for this bhāva meditation.

- Feel into your body, heart, mind and soul, noticing where tightness or emotions arise.

- Breathe into those places and feelings while holding them with respect.

- Whisper with love and kindness to wherever you hold or feel these sensations, acknowledging, owning, softening.

- Breathe … Find your rhythm and hold your bhāva, intent, within your heart. See the words. Whisper them in your mind or aloud. Attach a visualisation to them.

- Breathe in your intention, infusing it with love and affection. See the words, embody the feelings, harness your strength. See it manifest.

- With each breath out, allow the intention to dissipate, visualising it as light softly emanating from your body, with the sense of surrender into the universe.

- Each breath in, your bhāva settles a little more into heart, mind and body.

- Each breath out, release into the universe, knowing you are held by your own strength and courage and the love of others.

Mother Becoming Inspired Actions for Assisted Birthing

We pause on our journey once more. Boots and backpack off. Plenty of snacks and tea as you find the words to express what has come up for you from reading Katie's chapter. Your feelings need acknowledging with a way to move through them. Here, we are going to cultivate an attitude of grace rather than anger.

In this context, grace is filled with dignity and respect towards ourselves and other mothers. It is awake and powerful in informed autonomy, placing potent awareness in your hands. Practise grace with wise and non-judgemental inquiry as you work through all you have read and the feelings that arose for you. Hold yourself with quiet courage and an open heart, drawing from the power of your inner strength as all you learned sinks in.

Giving voice to grace is to give voice to women, because we can harness our power and qualities in a non-threatening way as a foundation for cultivating infinite change.

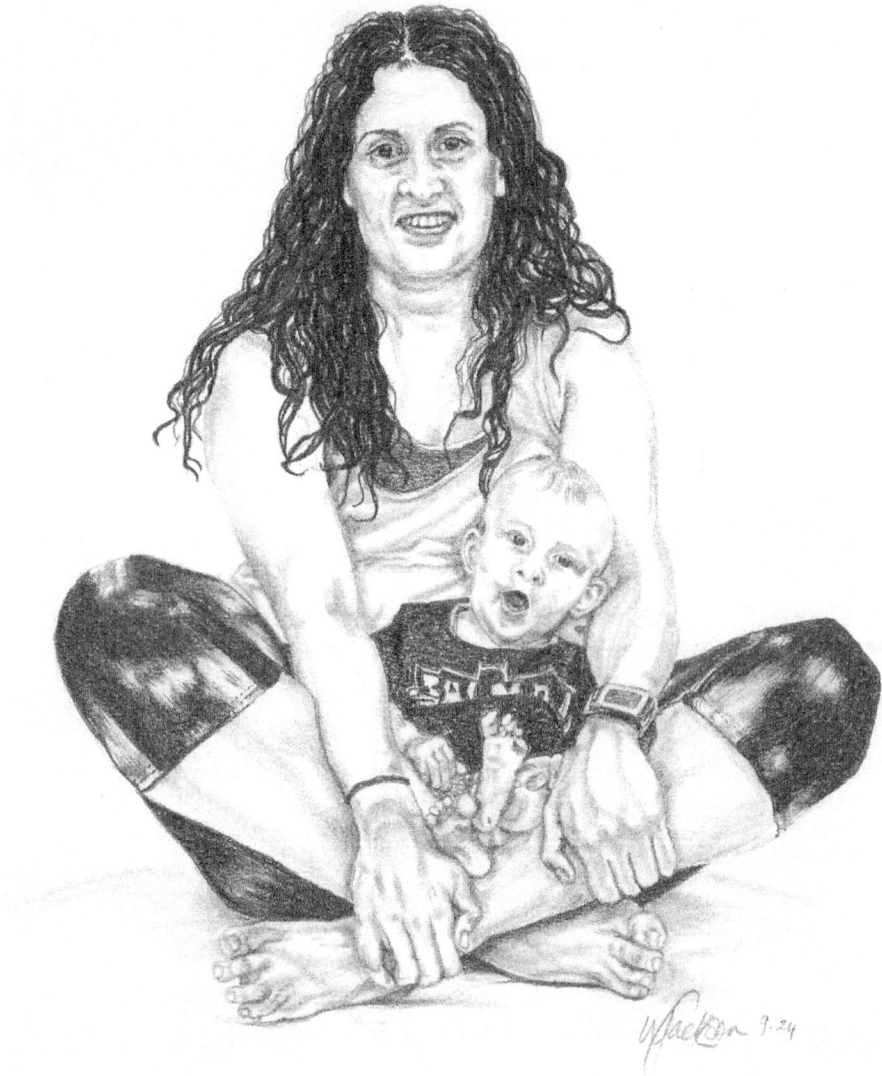

Katie and Mason in my postpartum yoga class. Look at those gorgeous faces. Katie's smile, evidence of her incredible strength and courage in her journey of recovery while experiencing postpartum depression. Her arms hold Mason safely while he chants his own song during class.

How might it be for you ...

- If human rights in childbirth were respected above institutional convenience, were written into policy, and practised with utmost respect for the woman's choices?

- If all states had a Patient Bill of Rights and it included the suggested statement: "You are entitled to informed consent at all times when in touch with a healthcare facility/provider", in line with the ICM Bill of Rights for Women and Midwives?

- If the Australian Health Practitioner Regulation Agency (AHPRA) and other registration bodies took women's human rights into consideration first when elevating practice standards?

- If we used the ICM Bill of Rights for Women and Midwives as a resource?

- If all practitioners reflected on consent before any procedure?

- If birth-planning or mapping were a foundation for strong, respectful conversation?

- If obstetricians approached the care of women by looking at women's deep underlying needs and also reflected on their own?

- If a two-way process of negotiation and reciprocal respect were formed?

- If bias in information-giving and coercion through fear tactics were stopped?

- If we respected a woman's intelligence and intuition to make choices for herself?

- If all care providers in maternity care had mandatory training in trauma-informed care for birth?

- If we were given time for labour to happen in a supported environment without pressure to intervene?

- If we listened to women?

- If RANZCOG started similar guidance for reducing induction and primary prevention of caesarean birth in line with ACOG in the USA and RCOG in the UK?

- If evidence of best practice (such as the issue of EFM) were put into clinical practice in a timely fashion?

- If women felt reassured that their care would be based on evidence of best practice, standards and guidelines, with consumer and other advocacy involvement?

- If federal and state governments demanded transparency and accountability for the rising intervention, induction and caesarean rates?

- If all hospitals were required to publish their statistics?

- If COC, home birthing, birth centres and freestanding birth homes increased, reducing the emotional and physical costs for women, as well as making financial savings?

- If women's health were no longer subject to silence, taboo and shame?

- If women's pelvic health were valued as highly as sports injuries?

- If birth injury were better diagnosed and treated in a coordinated, easily accessible, holistic manner to meet women's needs?

- If we had long-term support and specialist women's health physios?

- If the costs of childbirth weren't just a monetary matter?

- If maternal emotional wellbeing, satisfaction in her experience, and decreasing birthing trauma and PND were higher on the agenda?

- If, when a previous traumatic experience (including traumatic birth) were disclosed, women were given trauma-informed care?

- If we had the opportunity to receive mental health support and discuss how the obstetric team could avoid potential triggers?

- If Recommendation 41 of the NSW birth trauma inquiry for establishing formal debriefing clinics happened?

- If the mother were supported by an independent person in birth debriefing?

- If recommendations 40, 42, and 43 of the NSW inquiry into birth trauma to resolve complaints more quickly, and with more accessible trauma-informed support to complainants throughout the process, were adopted?

- If women who needed to complain received support, acknowledgment and apologies, and knew that changes would be made?

- If all mothers who experienced disrespect, abuse, coercion and birth trauma made a complaint to their birthing place and copied it to the MCA, ABTA and their member of parliament?

Assisted Birthing References and Wishlist

1   R Shiller, *Why Human Rights in Childbirth Matter*, Pinter and Martin, 2016, p134. ISBN 9781870665801

2   A Lokugamage, Presentation on Obstetric Violence and Human Rights. YouTube https://www.youtube.com/watch?v=Ziy5kSFm7U8

3   *Birthtime The Documentary* and *Birthtime The Handbook*, Clark and Mackay. 2021. p33. https://www.birthtime.world/

4   *Birthtime The Handbook*, p71.

5   V Olorenshaw, Liberating Motherhood: birthing the Purple Stocking Movement. Womancraft Publishing, 2016, p76. ISBN 978-910559-192

6   Application of the Human Rights Act of Queens land to the provision of public maternity services in Queensland. 2020. p4. https://www.maternitychoices.org/_files/ugd/369522_f10169bc2f114782bf-cfddfb77b5ccb4.PDF

7   Human Rights in Childbirth Website https://www.humanrightsinchildbirth.org/rights.html

8   Human Rights in Childbirth submission to the Australian Human Rights Commission to the Free & Equal: An Australian Conversation on Human Rights, 2019, p8. https://humanrights.gov.au/sites/default/files/2020-09/sub_149_-_human_rights_in_childbirth.PDF

9   A Dawes, G Beard, C Pistone, S Callaghan (Australasian Birth Trauma Association) K Thomas, K Myers (Birth Trauma Association) E Docherty, N Wilson, S Ballard (Make Birth Better Birth Injuries: A Hidden Epidemic international survey 'Birth Injuries: Improving Diagnosis and Treatment'. Australasian Birth Trauma Association (ABTA), Birth Trauma Association (BTA), and Make Birth Better (MBB) May 2022. https://static1.squarespace.com/static/5ed8a1b746cc235b44a50be1/t/62d8447c-29f06e731352577a/1658340476879/Birth+injuries_+the+hidden+epidemic_SUMMARY+%281%29.PDF.

10   Human Rights in Childbirth submission to the Australian Human Rights Commission, p13.

11   Human Rights in Childbirth submission to the Australian Human Rights Commission, p13.

12   Human Rights in Childbirth submission to the Australian Human Rights Commission, p17.

13   Human Rights in Childbirth submission to the Australian Human Rights Commission, p13.

14   Human Rights in Childbirth submission to the Australian Human Rights Commission, p13.

15   *Birthtime The Handbook*, p34.

16   *Birthtime The Handbook*, p34.

17   Make Birth Better, Register for free 15-minute video https://www.makebirthbetter.org/free-resources

18   E Svanberg, *Why Birth trauma Matters*. Pinter and Martin, 2021.,p23-4. ISBN 9781780666105

19   V Olorenshaw, *Liberating Motherhood: birthing the Purple Stocking Movement*. Woman Craft Publishing; 2016; p64. ISBN 978-910559-192

20   *Birthtime The Handbook*, p31.

21   H Keedle, R Lockwood, W Keedle, D Susic, H Dahlen, 'What women want if they were to have another baby: the Australian Birth Experience Study (BESt) cross-sectional national survey'. BMJ Open 2023;13:e071582. doi:10.1136/ bmjopen-2023-071582 https://bmjopen.bmj.com/content/13/9/e071582

22   Olorenshaw, *Liberating Motherhood*, p70.

23   I Olza, K Uvnäs-Moberg, A Ekstro¨m-Bergström, P Leahy-Warren, S I Karlsdottir, M Nieuwenhuijze, S Villarmea, 'Birth as a neuro-psycho-social event: An integrative model of maternal experiences and their relation to neurohormonal events during childbirth'. 2020. p1 DOI:10.1371/journal.pone.0230992

24   C Goggin, *Why Caesarean Birth Matters*. Pinter and Martin, 2018, p62. I BN 9781780665405

25   R Reed, *Reclaiming Childbirth as a Rite of Passage: Weaving ancient wisdom with modern knowledge*, Word Witch. 2021, p114-5. ISBN 978-0-6450025-1-5

26   SJ Buckley, 'Hormonal physiology of childbearing: evidence and implications for women, babies, and maternity care, Childbirth Connection Programs, National Partnership for Women & Families'. p i,v-xx. 2015 https://nationalpartnership.org/wp-content/uploads/2023/02/hormonal-physiology-of-childbearing.PDF

27   K Uvnäs Moberg. *Oxytocin. The Biological Guide to Motherhood*. Praeclarus Press, 2014. ISBN 9781939807809

28   Buckley, Hormonal physiology of childbearing, p i.

29   Buckley, Hormonal physiology of childbearing, p xiii.

30   K Uvnäs Moberg, *Why Oxytocin Matters*. Pinter and Martin, 2019, p127-8. ISBN 9781780666051

31   Uvnäs Moberg, *Why Oxytocin Matters*, p125, 126.

32   Uvnäs Moberg, *Why Oxytocin Matters*, p113-115.

33   Uvnäs Moberg, *Why Oxytocin Matters*, p117-118.

34   Daniela Menichini, Nicole Mazzaro, Simona Minniti, Alba Ricchi, Maria Teresa Molinazzi, Fabio Facchinetti, Isabella Neri. 'Fetal head malposition and epidural analgesia in labor: a case-control study'. The Journal of Maternal-Fetal & Neonatal Medicine. 2022 Dec;35(25):5691-5696. https://doi.org/10.1080/14767058.2021.1890018

35   The Epidural and Position Trial Collaborative Group. 'Upright versus lying down position in second stage of labour in nulliparous women with low dose epidural: BUMPES randomised controlled trial'. https://www.bmj.com/content/bmj/359/bmj.j4471.full.pdf

36   NICE guideline NG235, Intrapartum care [D] Evidence reviews for remifentanil patientcontrolled analgesia, September 2023. p15 https://www.nice.org.uk/guidance/ng235/evidence/d-remifentanil-patientcontrolled-analgesia-pdf-13186672961

37   SJ Buckley, K Uvnäs Moberg, Z Pajalic, K Luegmair, A Ekström-Bergström, A Dencker, C Massarotti, A Kotlowska, L Callaway, S Morano, I Olza, C Meier Magistretti, 'Maternal and newborn plasma oxytocin levels in response to maternal synthetic oxytocin administration during labour, birth and postpartum – a systematic review with implications for the function of the oxytocinergic system'. BMC Pregnancy Childbirth 23, 137 2023. https://doi.org/10.1186/s12884-022-05221-w

38   ❦ Wishlist The Australian commission on Safety and Quality in Health. 'Information for wom-
      en-Third- and Fourth-Degree Perineal Tears Clinical Care Standard. https://www.safetyandquality.gov.
      au/standards/clinical-care-standards/third-and-fourth-degree-perineal-tears-clinical-care-standard/infor-
      mation-women-third-and-fourth-degree-perineal-tears-clinical-care-standard

39   Uvnäs Moberg, Why Oxytocin Matters, p110.

40   Uvnäs Moberg, Why Oxytocin Matters, p116.

41   Uvnäs Moberg, Why Oxytocin Matters, p12-16.

42   Uvnäs Moberg, Why Oxytocin Matters, p110-112.

43   Uvnäs Moberg, Why Oxytocin Matters, p111.

44   Goggin, Why Caesarean Birth Matters, p37.

45   Goggin, Why Caesarean Birth Matters, p40.

46   Goggin, Why Caesarean Birth Matters, p16.

47   National Library of Medicine. Caesarean Part 4. https://www.nlm.nih.gov/exhibition/cesarean/part4.html

48   Obstetric Care Consensus: 'Safe Prevention of the Primary Cesarean Delivery'. The American College
      of Obstetricians and Gynaecologists. Society of Maternal-Fetal Medicine. 2014; p2. https://www.acog.
      org/-/media/project/acog/acogorg/clinical/files/obstetric-care-consensus/articles/2014/03/safe-preven-
      tion-of-the-primary-cesarean-delivery.PDF

49   Best-Practice Guideline. Birth after Previous Caesarean Birth RCOG 'Green Top' Guideline No
      45: https://www.rcog.org.uk/media/kpkjwd5h/gtg_45.PDF

50   GA Dekker, A Chan, CG Luke, K Priest, M Riley, J Halliday, JF King, V Gee, M O'Neill, M Snell, V
      Cull, S Cornes. 'Risk of uterine rupture in Australian women attempting vaginal birth after one prior
      caesarean section: a retrospective population-based cohort study'. BJOG. 2010. Dec;117(13):1672. p1358
      doi: 10.1111/j.1471-0528.2010.02688.x. https://pubmed.ncbi.nlm.nih.gov/20716251/

51   GA Dekker, et al, Risk of uterine rupture, p358.

52   A Gallagher, D Kring, T Whitley, 'Complimentary Effect of yoga on anxiety and depression for
      high-risk mothers on hospital bedrest'. Therapies in Clinical Practice. 2020; 38: 101079 doi: 10.1016/j.
      ctcp.2019.101079. https://pubmed.ncbi.nlm.nih.gov/32056815/

53   TP Sartwelle. JC Johnston. B Arda. M Zebenigus. 'Cerebral palsy, caesarean sections, and elec-
      tronic fetal monitoring: All the light we cannot see'. Clinical Ethics 2019. 0(0) p1–8. p 3.
      5. DOI:10.1177/1477750919851055

54   Sartwelle et al., 'Cerebral palsy, caesarean sections, and electronic fetal monitoring. p4.

55   Sartwelle et al., 'Cerebral palsy, caesarean sections, and electronic fetal monitoring. p4.

56   Sartwelle et al., 'Cerebral palsy, caesarean sections, and electronic fetal monitoring. p5.

57   Wickham, Facebook. https://www.facebook.com/photo/?fbid=980243990128621&set
      =a.227369068749454

58   KA Small, M Sidebotham, J Fenwick, J Gamble, 'Intrapartum cardiotocograph monitoring and perinatal
      outcomes for women at risk: Literature review'. Women and Birth. Elsevier Ltd. 2019. p7 https://doi.
      org/10.1016/j.wombi.2019.10.002

59   S McCutcheon, The Conversation. 'Most women who give birth in Australia are monitored with a CTG
      but it might not be the best approach'. https://theconversation.com/most-women-who-give-birth-in-aus-
      tralia-are-monitored-with-ctg-but-it-might-not-be-the-best-approach-147262

60   McCutcheon, The Conversation.

61   KA Small, M Sidebotham, J Fenwick, J Gamble, 'Midwives must, obstetricians may: An ethnographic exploration of how policy documents organise intrapartum fetal monitoring practice'. Women and Birth. Volume 35, Issue 2, March 2022, Pages e188-e197 https://doi.org/10.1016/j.wombi.2021.05.001

62   C de Costa, *Hail Caesar. Why one in three Australian babies is born by caesarean section*. Boolarong Press, 2008, p28. ISBN 978192105280

63   de Costa, *Hail Caesar*, p31.

64   de Costa, *Hail Caesar*, p35.

65   de Costa, *Hail Caesar*, p39.

66   de Costa, *Hail Caesar*, p41.

67   de Costa, *Hail Caesar*, p5.

68   National Library of Medicine. Caesarean Part 3. https://www.nlm.nih.gov/exhibition/cesarean/part3.html

69   National Library of Medicine. Caesarean Part 3.

70   *Birthtime The Handbook*, p43.

71   M Jowitt. *Dynamic Positions in Birth. A fresh look at how women's bodies work in labour*. Second Edition. Pinter and Martin, 2020, p13. ISBN 9781780666907

72   A Pilar Betran, J Ye, AB Moller, J Paulo Souza, Jun Zhang, 'Trends and projections of caesarean section rates: global and regional estimates'. BMJ Global Health 2021;6:e005671.p 1-8. doi:10.1136/ bmjgh-2021-005671 https://gh.bmj.com/content/bmjgh/6/6/e005671.full.PDF

73   World Health Organization, Statement on a caesarean section rates. 2015. https://www.who.int/publications/i/item/WHO-RHR-15.02

74   Western Australian Mothers and Babies Report. Australian Institute of Health and Welfare. 2023. https://www.health.wa.gov.au/Reports-and-publications/Western-Australias-Mothers-and-Babies-summary-information/data?report=mns_cs_y

75   Birth Savvy Blog, https://birthsavvy.com.au/c-section-rates-perth-and-regional-wa/

76   Australian Mothers and Babies. Australian Institute of Health and Welfare. 2021. https://www.aihw.gov.au/reports/mothers-babies/australias-mothers-babies/contents/labour-and-birth/method-of-birth

77   The Lancet Series. 'Optimising Caesarean Section Use'. 2018. https://www.thelancet.com/series/caesarean-section

78   GHA Visser, D Ayres-de-Campos, ER Barnea, L de Bernis, Gian Carlo Di Renzo, MF Escobar Vidarte, FIGO position paper. 'How to Stop the Caesarean Section Epidemic'. p1358. https://www.thelancet.com/PDFs/journals/lancet/PIIS0140-6736(18)32113-5.PDF. 11/ajo.13529

79   GHA Visser, et al, FIGO position paper. 'How to Stop the Caesarean Section Epidemic'. p1358

80   Obstetric Care Consensus: 'Safe Prevention of the Primary Cesarean Delivery. The American College of Obstetricians and Gynaecologists'. Society of Maternal-Fetal Medicine. 2014. https://www.acog.org/-/media/project/acog/acogorg/clinical/files/obstetric-care-consensus/articles/2014/03/safe-prevention-of-the-primary-cesarean-delivery.PDF

81   Jyai Allen. Jocelyn Toohill. Debra K Creedy. Emily J Callander. Development of a co-designed, evidence-based, multi-pronged strategy to support normal birth. ANZJOG Obstetrics and Gynaecology; 2022. 1-5. P 2 DOI:10.1111/ajo.13529

82   World Health Organization, Statement on a caesarean section rates. 2015. https://www.who.int/publications/i/item/WHO-RHR-15.02

83   C de Costa, *the women's doc*. Allen and Unwin, 2021, p165. ISBN9781760529147

84   N Hill, (2019). Understanding Obstetric Violence as Violence against Mothers through the Lens of Matricentric Feminism. Journal of the Motherhood Initiative for Research and Community Involvement, 10(1/2). Retrieved from https://jarm.journals.yorku.ca/index.php/jarm/article/view/40566. https://jarm.journals.yorku.ca/index.php/jarm/article/view/40566/36737

85   Human Rights in Childbirth submission to the Australian Human Rights Commission, p17.

86   K Thompson, 'Birth injuries are a feminist issue. An obstetrician explains why'. Conversation Article. https://womensagenda.com.au/latest/birth-injuries-are-a-feminist-issue-an-obstetrician-explains-why/#:~:text=An%20obstetrician%20explains%20why,-by%20Kara%20Thompson&text=%22We%20need%20to%20lift%20the,been%20ignored%20for%20too%20long.%22

87   A Dawes et al, Birth Injuries: Improving Diagnosis and Treatment, 3.1, Diagnosis and Treatment.

88   Thompson, Birth injuries are a feminist issue.

89   Thompson, Birth injuries are a feminist issue.

90   Thompson, Birth injuries are a feminist issue.

91   Thompson, Birth injuries are a feminist issue.

92   Thompson, Birth injuries are a feminist issue.

93   New South Wales Parliament Legislative Council Select Committee on Birth Trauma, Report. 2024. p xv, xv. ISBN: 978-1-922960-38-2x. https://www.parliament.nsw.gov.au/lcdocs/inquiries/2965/FINAL%20Birth%20Trauma%20Report%20-%2029%20April%202024.PDF

94   ABC. 'NSW birth trauma inquiry described as 'me too' moment for mothers receives record 4,000 submissions'. https://www.abc.net.au/news/2023-09-05/nsw-birth-trauma-inquiry-day-one-me-too-moment-for-mothers/102812906

95   ABC. NSW birth trauma inquiry described as 'me too' moment for mothers.

96   ABC. NSW birth trauma inquiry described as 'me too' moment for mothers.

97   International Confederation of Midwives. Bill of Rights for Women and Midwives.2024. https://internationalmidwives.org/resources/bill-of-rights-for-women-and-midwives/

98   *Birthtime The Handbook*, p17.

99   *Birthtime The Handbook*, p102.

100   *Birthtime The Handbook*, p103.

101   *Birthtime The Handbook*, p103.

102   CSE Homer. 'Models of maternity care: evidence for midwifery continuity of care'. Med J Aust. 2016 Oct 17; 205(8):370-374. p373. doi: 10.5694/mja16.00844. https://www.mja.com.au/system/files/issues/205_08/10.5694mja16.00844.PDF

103   WHO 'Recommendation: for intrapartum care for positive childbirth experience'. 2018. https://www.who.int/publications/i/item/9789241550215

104   H Palladino, (2015). Motherhood's Opening Chapter: Birth Stories as Performance and Counter Performance Across Dueling Media Platforms. *Journal of the Motherhood Initiative for Research and Community Involvement*, 6(1). Retrieved from https://jarm.journals.yorku.ca/index.php/jarm/article/view/40245 https://jarm.journals.yorku.ca/index.php/jarm/article/view/40245/36426

105   H Palladino, Birth Stories as Performance and Counter, p108.

106   H Palladino, Birth Stories as Performance and Counter, p114.

107   H Palladino, Birth Stories as Performance and Counter, p113.

108   H Palladino, Birth Stories as Performance and Counter, p113.

109   H Palladino, Birth Stories as Performance and Counter, p113.

110   H Palladino, Birth Stories as Performance and Counter, p113.

111   Human Rights in Childbirth submission to the Australian Human Rights Commission, p26.

112   Olorenshaw, *Liberating Motherhood*, p65.

113   New South Wales Parliament Legislative Council Select Committee on Birth Trauma, p xviii, xx.

114   Human Rights in Childbirth submission to the Australian Human Rights Commission, p26.

115   Human Rights in Childbirth submission to the Australian Human Rights Commission, p27.

116   Human Rights in Childbirth submission to the Australian Human Rights Commission, p.26.

117   New South Wales Parliament Legislative Council Select Committee on Birth Trauma, p xx.

118   *Birthtime The Handbook*, p91.

119   *Birthtime The Handbook*, p145.

120   *Birthtime The Handbook*, p87.

121   L Roche *The Radiance Sutras*, Sutra 74 of Yuki Practice Transmission, Sounds True, 2014, p289. ISBN 978-1-60407-659-2

Wishlist

1. *Great Birth Rebellion* #33. Induction of Labour Apple Spotify

2. Dr Rachel Reed Blog 'Induction of Labour for Prolonged Pregnancy' https://www.rachelreed.website/blog/induction-of-labour-for-prolonged-pregnancy

3. The Australian commission on Safety and Quality in Health. 'Information for women-Third- and Fourth-Degree Perineal Tears Clinical Care Standard. https://www.safetyandquality.gov.au/standards/clinical-care-standards/third-and-fourth-degree-perineal-tears-clinical-care-standard/information-women-third-and-fourth-degree-perineal-tears-clinical-care-standard

4. *The Midwives' Cauldron*, S3 #13 VBAC, vaginal birth after caesarean, an interview with Dr Hazel Keedle. Apple Spotify

5. *The Midwives' Cauldron* S4 #4 'Listening to babies during labour' Apple Spotify

6. *Birth-Ed* S1 E9. 'Healing and Preventing Birth Trauma with Dr Rebecca Moore'. Apple Spotify

7. Make Birth Better. 'Am I Traumatised?' See the free downloads on https://www.makebirthbetter.org/pdf-downloads-parents and click on 'Am I Traumatised'.

Chapter 6

First Few Hours and Days with Alysia

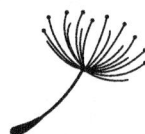

Meeting Alysia

Alysia and I met on the birth day and passing of her beautiful stillborn son, Thomas. I was their midwife. This book is in memory of Thomas.

To journey with Alysia and her loved ones through the experience of knowing their expectations and dreams had come to an end is hard to describe. To try to care in such a way that you ease some of their suffering, grief and pain, while acknowledging it is an honour to be there for them, is impossible to put into words.

Later, Alysia told me that she thought I was the cruellest person on the planet when I told her I was going to lift her son to her chest after she birthed Thomas. Yet holding him immediately after birth and for many hours are her most precious memories, she then said.

Being there for the pregnancy and birthing of her rainbow baby, Nicholas, – the life birthed after a previous baby was lost – we all experienced a sense of completion, filled with gratitude, love, wonder and grief. These emotions held us connected in the precious hours after his birth.

The impact that meeting Alysia has had on my life is almost impossible to articulate. She is a gift. It isn't my place to tell her story, but I can say that to be part of her journey and life is a privilege. It fills my heart with love.

Mum of Thomas and Nicholas, here is Alysia's letter to you.

"I always felt my son was cheering me on as I studied."

Dear Reader,

What an honour for me to be able to share my experiences with you in the hope of offering some insight or support for your journey ahead. Firstly, perhaps a trigger warning. I will be talking about stillbirth, grief, PTSD and PND.

Please know that it is not my intention to cause anxiety or worry, but that I share in the hope of shaking off some of the 'mystery' or 'taboo' surrounding stillbirth. I wish for this to help others feel not quite so alone or improve their understanding of how to care for and support those who have lost their child.

Well, hello! My name is Alysia and I am a midwife. I wasn't always a midwife though, and that's a long story, so best you make that cup of tea and settle in.

I was 30 years old when I was pregnant with my first baby. A low-risk pregnancy, very unremarkable. I did all the classes and appointments, gave myself crippling anxiety as most first-time mothers do, as we navigate and avoid all the things we can and can't eat, drink, smell or even make eye contact with. I was lovely and naive and did everything right.

One night, when I was 39 weeks pregnant, we'd gone for dinner for my husband's birthday. We ate cake and I mentioned that baby was usually very active after cake but wasn't tonight. (I didn't know the importance of fetal movements and patterns back then.)

The following morning, I hadn't felt baby move at all either, so I went to my hospital. They couldn't find his heartbeat. Sadly, he had passed. We were in absolute shock, completely unaware this could happen.

It's not something that is talked about or brought up. I asked for a caesarean section, but they explained a vaginal delivery was safer. Our family was called, and after many investigations, we were sent home to process the events. We would go in for an induction. At that point, I couldn't have cared less about my future, but in hindsight I'm so incredibly grateful for the opportunity to birth vaginally, as it would shape the woman and mother I am today.

I was admitted to hospital for induction, grief-stricken, shellshocked and numb. A warm and gentle midwife introduced herself to me and my family. She spoke softly, nurturing yet powerful, strong and knowledgeable. She explained what to expect, the care plan and my options. Her name was Wendy Jackson. Sound familiar? Well, you might even know her ... She wrote this book!

As I laboured, Wendy sat with us. Quiet, knowing, caring. Marvelling at me, showing me and proving to me what my body was actually capable of and the strength it had in a time when I felt it had betrayed me.

My baby boy was born and, as she told me she would, Wendy delivered him onto my chest. I specifically remember thinking how cruel it was when she told me she was going to do this. Yet once he was on me, I felt a calmness. A possessiveness. A stillness.

He was my baby. I was his mother. And this time with him would be all I had. He stayed with us overnight until we were ready to leave, held by his dad and family. We cried for him. Gosh, how we cried. We marvelled at how perfect and beautiful he was. We had photos taken by an organisation dedicated to this. Heartfelt. When it was time to be discharged from hospital, we left with empty arms and an empty car seat. At home, we closed the door to his nursery, grateful that our family had packed away most of it to save us the heartbreak.

Family stayed for a week or two, nurturing us, feeding, cleaning, arranging difficult events and services. A few weeks on, our family needed to return to work and my 'village' had to disperse. Life continued and I had to get on board, ready or not. But I wasn't ready. My body wasn't ready. Still carrying all the hormones, breast changes, producing breastmilk, stretch marks, weight gain, repairing and recovery from delivery. It wanted to nurture a little baby, but there wasn't one.

When I was at the shops, I couldn't even look at a baby. I had to answer awkward questions from friends and colleagues about when they could visit me and my baby.

In the background of all my grief, trauma and heartache, I valued my body and its abilities. My body's incredible ability to have created and carried him all the way to term. My ability to value the time and memories I had been able to make with him in pregnancy and birth.

My midwife had reminded me of that. My power. My strength. My motherhood. Wendy had not only helped me birth my baby, but she also helped me rebirth myself into a powerful woman. To see the glory, strength and beauty in our bodies, even in a time of deep grief and trauma. She changed the path of my grief. She inspired me. What Wendy had shown me, I wanted to show others. Their beauty, strength and power. Six months on, I was accepted into university where I began my studies to become a midwife.

I wanted to show women how *amazing* they are, not just during labour and birth, but in pregnancy, after birth, being a mother, everything. So much focus and pressure is on one single event, on how this baby arrives! What about the 9 months of *growing* a complete tiny person, the discomforts, the responsibility, physical changes, anxiety and fatigue? All irrelevant until the baby is born! And then it's the mum guilt, about the birth, caesarean section, breastfeeding, breastmilk supplementation, bed-sharing, dummies, returning to work. The judgement. Good grief, what are we doing to each other?! All mummas need is information. Not judgement. They can make their own decisions with the right information.

Wendy and I stayed in contact throughout my university studies, even working alongside each other at the hospital where I'd birthed. My midwifery graduation day coincidentally fell on my son's fourth birthday/anniversary day. There's no better way to know I was on the right path.

I always felt my son was cheering me on as I studied. There were times my grief was overwhelming, where I couldn't stop myself crying, my chosen career far too confronting given my trauma and grief. Somehow I kept going. Somehow things kept falling into place. I trained at the hospital where my son had been born. What a powerful way to stay connected to him and a reminder of my motivation.

I worked as a midwife for several years before trying for another baby. It was another boy. I couldn't have been happier or more anxious! I was about 14 weeks when my mum passed away from cancer. How grateful I was that she had been able to celebrate my pregnancy before she went. The anxiety I experienced was intense. Grief and trauma resurfaced. I reached out to Wendy, who identified a disconnection between me and my baby. We meditated, yoga-ed and spent hours working on bonding and recreating a strong mentality and being present.

It would have been easy to remain cautious and disconnected with my rainbow baby until he was born to safeguard me from further stress and grief. Yet to my mind, it is only in hindsight you find value in those moments. If something were to happen with this baby too, I would want to have these memories of him to hold and keep.

Wendy was there for my second baby's birth, as was midwife Sue, who had taken over from Wendy after Thomas's birth. What a celebration that was, birthed in the same hospital as his big brother all those years before. I finally got to hold my baby and plan for our future together. I was excited to start breastfeeding and doing all those mothering jobs I would educate new mums on every day at work.

I was elated being a mum. I felt ready, knowledgeable and confident. After all, I educate mums every day in this. I am literally *qualified* to be a mum! I've got this! My first breastfeed was beautiful. I gazed down at his perfect little face and hands, drinking in how soft and adorable he was ... Marvelling at his deliciousness ... Not noticing increasing nipple pain ... Wait! *Ouch!*

By the second breastfeed, my nipples were in trouble. His latch looked fine though. Fortunately, the postnatal midwife was also a lactation consultant. He wasn't able to latch without nipple trauma, so I started expressing, resting my nipples and finger feeding. I had expressed breastmilk antenatally, which helped to feed him.

That's when my 'mumma bubble' popped and the reality of a baby set in. He cried, I expressed, he fed. He napped 30 to 60 minutes at a time, then I cried. We fed, we napped, he cried, I cried etc. … What a mess. My little baby boy was my world. I held him every second I could. I couldn't get enough of him. I spent hours gazing at him as he slept on me, and as I fed him, or pumped, or tried to breastfeed. Although it was lovely, it was so tiring. Slowly, my baby bubble engulfed me. Silly me for thinking, just because I could settle anyone's baby, I could settle my own! Or that I would be prepared for motherhood! Ah, such innocence!

And so, determined in my journey to breastfeed, I continued to express and feed for a few weeks until my boy could latch without causing trauma to my nipples. It was going well; I was getting on track. Then a worldwide pandemic hit. COVID.

Suddenly, my village was gone again. Not just *my* village, but everyone's village. My husband, struggling with his PTSD and fear of attachment with this baby, was suddenly my only support. And life continued. Food shopping, bills, cleaning, appointments …

I became too tired to eat or drink. I would get anxious if my baby cried. Even though he was so difficult to settle, I was worried about leaving him too long, so I woke him. I didn't care to go anywhere, see anyone. It was scary to go outside because of this pandemic too. I was in a constant state of wired anxiety. I stayed with him on my lounge all the time. I lost weight, wasn't sleeping, wasn't eating well. I was short-tempered, irritable and easily overwhelmed. It was perplexing that I could find joy in my little boy, be so enamoured with him, but find no joy in anything else.

Hello Postnatal Depression. There are not enough pages in this book for my experience, but I know this is discussed in these next 2 chapters. I see you. You are stronger than you think.

You've got this. Now go build your village.

Love Alysia x

Dear Mother Becoming,

Wipe your tears, make a cuppa, breathe and sit with the emotions that reading Alysia's letter has evoked. What an extraordinary woman she is. After her devastating experience with Thomas, what an incredible legacy to him Alysia has achieved in becoming a midwife. Here with Alysia, we are honouring all the families who have experienced loss, grief and the utter devastation of a stillborn child. This chapter is written to honour the memory of Thomas, big brother to Nicholas, and son of Alysia and Steven. This is written for all parents who have a stillborn child, because the first few hours and days is all the precious time they have to be together.

As this chapter unfolds, we talk about and discover the myriad of miracle happenings in the first hours and days, with a sense of awe and reverence for the extraordinary physiology that occurs. Discover the immense capacity of being a new mother in the phase of integration, enchantment and bonding, and the sensations this phase evokes. A new beginning, a new life, a new journey, all the while remembering

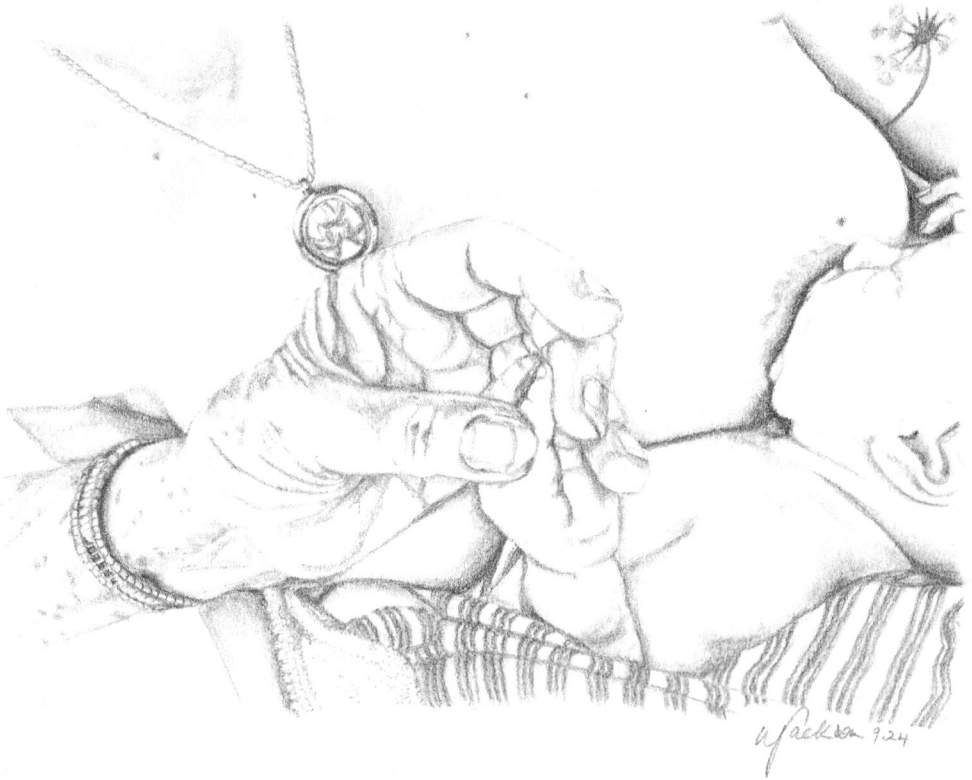

Alysia's mother passed in her early pregnancy and she wore some of her mother's ashes in a necklace while in labour and birthing Nicholas. The tattoo on her left arm of the dandelion clock is in memory of her son Thomas. While Nicholas breastfeeds, his Great Nana holds his hand. The 3 generations of women are together, connected in deep sorrow and joy.

and acknowledging the baby who never drew breath or got to grow into an older sibling. Here, I hold and value the depth of emotion felt by these families, and recognise that the birth of a rainbow baby holds so many raw and powerful mixed emotions.

Transitioning with utmost respect to continue our conversation, welcome to the world of being a mother. Look at what you have achieved and created! A little human bean! You are utterly awesome, no matter your birthing journey. Please know that deep in your bones. However exhausted, elated, bamboozled, overwhelmed and anxious you are for this new little life, you are also utterly awesome, even if the enormity of the responsibility has just hit you.

Postpartum begins as soon as the placenta is birthed. This generates enormous changes in a mother's body over the first few hours and days. The intertwining between mother and newborn in the first few hours is magical. The effects of oxytocin, prolactin, adrenaline and beta-endorphin are heard loudly within the mother and baby, and assist the process of childbirth as a rite of passage. The phase of integration is expressed in bonding, through the emotional and physical actions of the newborn, specifically the breast crawl, being skin to skin, finding nurture and nourishment in the first breastfeed. There are the embodied sensations like the enchantment of eye-gazing, maternal touch and smell in exploration of her newborn, and feeling the emotions in the first few hours of becoming a mother, a father, a family.

The umbilical cord as a physical connection may have been cut or left to dry and released via lotus birth, but the invisible connection of a psychological and emotional umbilical cord is forever with the mother. As part of honouring this, we'll be talking about creating a ceremony to welcome your child into the world and new rituals to recognise such an occasion. You can play and sing a song that means so much to you. You can say a phrase, a quote, a prayer, your own words, whatever resonates with you while the cord is cut.

On becoming a mother, the concept of thinking for yourself alone no longer exists. Each and every thought now encompasses your child. Your maternal brain evolves a new way of thinking, responding and behaving as the self-identity of 'mother' and all that that entails changes you to your core.

It's so important to still see her. That a woman becomes a mother does not define all she is. "Ah, so-and-so's mother." You are so much more – evolving and growing, bringing everything you were to a profound otherness. Maintaining a matricentric focus is vital to support the woman's transition into this otherness, because mothers become invisible in our society once they have given birth, when all the attention becomes focused on the baby. If the mother is well, the baby will be well. It's as simple as that. See her.

Postnatal care in western society is the "poor relation of the birth world".[1] This is why it is often called the Cinderella service. With the current attitude of shifting the focus to the baby and most of the gifts to the new parents being soft toys, baby clothes and flowers – well, mum and dad or parent-partner can't eat those. Although well-meaning, this doesn't recognise or acknowledge the true needs of a new family. This shift happens in the current healthcare model, where the mother's physical and emotional recovery, as well as support with breastfeeding and transition to motherhood, are secondary.

This phase, the fourth trimester, is the area that needs the most investment in care and resources.

- **Wishlist** 🎙 Reminder: *The Midwives' Cauldron* S2 #1. 'Why Postnatal Recovery Matters with Sophie Messager'. Gentle nag: if it wasn't the right time to listen then, please listen and share with your support now. Smiley face. ^Apple 🎙 Spotify

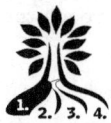

🌱 The Physical, Hormonal and Emotional Influences on the First Few Hours and Days of Mothering

[1.][2.][3.][4.] A new score of music begins to play. The musician of pregnancy, **hCG,** rapidly reduces after the birth of the placenta, alongside **oestrogen** and **progesterone.** All quietening in approximately one week. The soft background sound of oestrogen allows breast swelling and diuresis (peeing a lot) as you carried more fluid from pregnancy. Progesterone, having been produced by the placenta, has been inhibiting the sound of **prolactin.** Prolactin, now free to be heard, makes its presence on breastmilk production loud and clear.

There is an orchestra playing in the newborn too in the precious first few hours after birth, with musicians **adrenaline, oxytocin** and **beta-endorphin** at high levels. This helps the newborn baby with alertness, bonding and feeling calm.[2]

Medically, the terminology of the first 24 hours is known as the *acute phase*,[3] yet relating to the rite of passage terminology, we call it the *integration phase*.[4] This name allows for the recognition of the importance of emotional, social and psychological factors in the transition to becoming a mother, and from intra-uterine to extrauterine life for the baby.

Postpartum hormonal rave rather than symphony

The hormonal musicians prolactin and oxytocin are intricately linked in the physiology of the post-partum experience. The rise in oxytocin at birth increases the temperature over the mother's chest and breast tissue, and contracts the smooth muscle in the *alveoli* (milk sacs) and small milk ducts, allowing for 'milk ejection' as the baby suckles.[5] This high level and early suckling assists the oxytocin receptors in the uterus to keep it well contracted to prevent heavy bleeding from where the placenta was. Oxytocin helps the uterus to return to its almost pre-pregnancy size, a process called *involution*, which is usually completed by 6 weeks.[6] So, feeding in the early days coincides with continued uterine contractions or *afterpains*, which can be intense.

Oxytocin release is in rhythmical peaks in breastfeeding, as it is in labour, and is stimulated by the suckling of the newborn. Released within minutes of the start of suckling, oxytocin allows the *letdown reflex* to occur, by contracting the smooth muscles around the alveoli, so that colostrum is ejected towards the nipple. The letdown reflex is also activated by tactile stimulation, and by visual and auditory cues in the mother as she responds to her newborn. The baby kneading the breast with their little hands, and hand expressing evoke this response too. When there are a high number of oxytocin pulses in the first 10 minutes of feeding, more breastmilk is given and oxytocin levels remain elevated for a further 20–30 minutes.[7] Oxytocin also increases the mother's sense of smell and the formation of memories. It plays a major role in bonding.

Prolactin levels peak at birth and early postpartum; they are produced and released in direct response to the newborn's suckling for 10–20 minutes, with raised levels lasting for about an hour.[8] This isn't to suggest that feeds are to be limited to 10–20 minutes. Far from it. This information is to let you know what your hormones are doing. The longer the suckling, the longer prolactin is stimulated. Oxytocin also affects prolactin production. Although oxytocin is produced in the posterior pituitary gland, it also releases into the anterior pituitary gland, where prolactin is produced in response to suckling.

This makes sense of the timings of release and stimulation of each hormone, and explains how intricately interwoven they are. It highlights how important oxytocin is in lactation. Prolactin has a circadian rhythm, with higher levels produced at nighttime than in daytime suckling.[9] It is associated with beta-endorphin production too, which enhances the feel-good factor of calm that suffuses through the mother when feeding her baby.[10]

As we have discussed, stress hinders oxytocin production, which reduces contractions in labour. It affects the rhythm of lactation and milk ejection too, and is associated with a reduction in prolactin release. Oxytocin production in itself reduces stress in the mother, as does prolactin. Babies born by elective caesarean do not have the same levels of oxytocin in their body because they have not been through the physiological adaptations during labour and birth. So, the closeness of skin-to-skin, touch, stroking, kissing, warmth and the mother's voice, with uninterrupted access to the breast and feeding, all assist with newborns' sense of safety, love and bonding. This, in turn, stimulates oxytocin and prolactin.

Both musicians play a key role in neuroplastic changes in a mother's brain, in her psycho-emotional adaptations to mothering and her interactions with her child. With the closeness between mother and baby, boundaries are removed. It is like a continuation of pregnancy, but the umbilical cord is substituted by the close skin-to-skin contact.

Recommendation 24 of the NSW birth trauma inquiry is to "review hospital practices to ensure that, wherever possible, parents and baby are able to remain together after birth and have skin-to-skin contact".[11]

· **Healthy Births, Happy Babies #94.** 'Your hormones and the miracles in the first hour' Apple 🎙 Spotify
A dive into Dr Sarah Buckley's research on how 4 main hormones affect a mother in biological bonding in the first hours, as well as sensitive advice when intervention occurs.

Baby breast crawl and baby-led attachment

The extraordinary abilities of a newborn are witnessed in the breast crawl. This is where a healthy, vigorous baby is placed onto the mother's abdomen and chest immediately after birth. Time seems to be suspended as the baby opens their eyes, cries and begins to move with a stepping reflex, reaching towards the breast, grasping, licking, in search of the nipple through smell, sight, taste, hearing and touch. Glands on the areola secrete odours that guide the newborn.

Newborns are attuned to gazing at the shape of faces and seeing the darkness of the areola. The taste of colostrum and breastmilk are familiar, as they are similar to the tastes of amniotic fluid. Alongside this, they hear the familiarity of their mother and father's voices, which is comforting. Touch, being held, skin to skin, and feeling safe and secure all regulate the newborn's heartbeat, breathing and temperature.

· **Newborn doing the breast crawl.** YouTube. https://www.youtube.com/watch?v=a9SH55UzCSo
· **Wishlist** 🌿 Baby-led attachment visual guide and video. **The ABA website.** https://www.breastfeeding.asn.au/resources/baby-led-attachment

---

Skin to skin, the golden hour (or 2)

Skin-to-skin time in the first few hours is the precious integration part of a woman's rite of passage and should be honoured, no matter how she births. "Skin-to-skin and nipple contact may maximally stimulate hormonal systems for mother and newborn at this time, with long-term benefits to maternal adaptations and maternal-infant attachment (via 'biologic bonding'), and breastfeeding."[12]

Smell is of great importance to the newborn and mother, so feel free to decline the baby being bathed for the first day at least. Also consider not wearing perfume, aftershave or strongly scented deodorants, because this is overpowering to the newborn's senses. Ask your care provider to wash perfume off and request that visitors refrain from wearing anything strongly scented, including strong essential oils.

If the sudden wave of intense love doesn't happen, is something wrong? No. This feeling and connection doesn't always happen immediately, or in the first few days or weeks. Sometimes, the coming down from an intense, exhausting, maybe dramatic or traumatic experience of birthing may not allow space for such feeling. The mother needs time to reconnect with herself, as cortisol from stress hormones settles and the intensity of the experience begins to sink in.

Occasionally, some mothers feel disconnection and ambivalence towards the baby. It's okay. There is nothing wrong with the mother; she is not broken and hasn't failed. Sometimes, it just takes time.

Being able to talk to somebody about those feelings, having them acknowledged without judgement and finding ways to negotiate them is enough. You can discover why you may feel this way and find a way forward – whether that is resolution, understanding or acceptance – moment by moment, day by day. Bonding is an ongoing experience and can be fulfilled even with delay.

- *The Midwives' Cauldron* #8. 'The things they don't tell you about skin-to-skin contact!' ^{Apple} Spotify
  Information about separation if baby needs to be in NICU; the importance of skin-to-skin kangaroo care with mum, dad or another human; caring for baby while in NICU; advice and support about lactation in these circumstances.

- Reminder: *Birth-Ed* S1#15. 'The first 24 hours with Marie Louise' ^{Apple} Spotify
  Myriads of magical happenings highlighting the incredible euphoria, strength, fierceness and protection a mother often feels towards her newborn.

Your body in the first 24 hours

Talking about the other physical aspects of the first few hours and days means acknowledging the discomfort of afterpains and possible perineal injury, stinging when passing urine due to grazes on the vulva, and that all-important first postpartum poo. You'll also learn how to soothe the perineum and vulva.

On the first day, the temperature of the mother is higher at birth, warming her baby. The pulse is higher too, with a mixture of fatigue and elation. The uterus weighs about 1 kg at this time; after one week, it will have already reduced to 500 g, with very heavy blood loss to begin with, which gradually eases as the uterus shrinks.[13] The bladder wall may be a bit swollen, not so toned, because it has been overstretched and the urethra compressed during birth. All this leads to a reduced urge to wee, with a possibility of retention of urine.

Oh, and the good old discomfort of wind, then constipation, due to the remnants of hormones relaxin and progesterone! There may be haemorrhoids too. All these are extremely important things to consider for the mother's comfort in the first days.

Mothers are quite often surprised how lax the abdomen feels, a bit like a jelly wobble. With a strange feeling of laxity of the pelvic floor and a tender perineum, the overall sensations are a lot to adjust to – particularly when considering the fatigue from labour, birth and then the demands of a new little being who needs warmth, love, feeding and a clean bum. All this doesn't bring about a good night's rest. A marathon runner or elite athlete gets to rest, recover and restore. A new mother doesn't. Often we don't recognise that a woman who births by caesarean is recovering from major abdominal surgery alongside her transition into mothering. Also, the hormonal swing from dropping hCG, progesterone and oestrogen, and the increase in prolactin and surges of oxytocin, make interesting ingredients for an emotional cocktail!

The expectations that mothers have of themselves at this time need to be grounded on the basic elements of love, touch, rest, nutrition, warmth and comfort. This is why considered, respectful, kind, gentle, nourishing and supportive care is so incredibly important for new mothers. It isn't about the baby. It's all about the mother. The intensity of so many adjustments in a new mother's body in the first hours, days and weeks is extraordinary. There isn't nearly enough noise made about how incredible and utterly amazing these dynamic processes are. Although their bodies are awesome, women need to know how strange their body might feel during this time and how bloody uncomfortable it can all be! Make a fuss of the mother, not the baby! "Wow, Mum, you are out of this world! How can I support you and make you comfortable? By the way, your baby is adorable, but you are just brilliant!"

Fabulous postpartum mum brains in action

Here we return to learning more about fabulous mum brains and the extraordinary neuroplastic changes of mother becoming. Remember we discussed the maternal pregnant brain shrinking and changing before birthing? Well, afterwards, it grows again and rewires in new ways. The research, 'From baby brain to mommy brain: Widespread grey matter gain after giving birth', found a significant increase in grey matter after birth within 4 to 6 weeks, indicative of the massive adaptations and reorganisation in the maternal brain after birth. These neuroplastic changes show the mother's capacity to learn, respond to her newborn and behave in new ways.[14] Mums' brains are just wow!

- **Wishlist** 🌿 **Happy Mama Movement #231**. 'The real truth about how your brain changes with parenthood' Apple 🎙Spotify

  Discusses implications for both maternity and paternity leave and how these brain changes are equipping you for the first days, weeks, months and the rest of your life.

Breastfeeding matters

Charlotte Young, a breastfeeding counsellor and lactation consultant, in her book *Why Breastfeeding Matters* provides insight into the world of breastfeeding. In late pregnancy, a species of good bacteria, *Bifidobacterium*, lives around the nipples, thriving deep inside the milk ducts. When exposed to air, these bacteria release antibiotic chemicals and potent acids that protect against harmful bacteria.[15] Amazing. If you look inside a breast, the tissue appears similar to the shape of a grape vine in full fruit – the trunk and branches are the ducts towards the nipple and the alveoli the bunches of grapes. Skin-to-skin contact during these early hours and days – with baby-led demand feeding – promotes lacto-genesis, which is the change in the colostrum to the transitional milk produced in the first 2 to 5 days.

Colostrum is liquid gold. Yellow to orange in colour, it is thick, nutritious, rich in protein, vitamins and immunoglobulins, and provides immunological protection with white blood cells to destroy harmful bacteria, and an antibiotic defence in the newborn as the gut is colonised. In the first day of life, the newborn's stomach can only expand to the size of a cherry. That means 2–10 ml or 1–2 teaspoons in each feed.[16]

Maddie McMahon, in *Why Mothering Matters*, describes colostrum as more of a medicine than a food in its ability to coat the walls of the gut, preventing harmful substances from entering the baby's bloodstream. Colostrum also acts as a laxative to help baby poo the sticky, dark, greenish-black, tar-like consistency of *meconium* (baby's first poo).[17]

Human babies evolved to lie on their mothers like other primates, as we are a carrying species. Although human babies are the slowest growing and have the longest childhoods, the human brain is the fastest to grow, at a rate of 1% a day to around 65% bigger than the newborn size by 3 months. Fuelled by breastmilk, with its high levels of lactose sugars, omega-3 and omega-6 fatty acids, it is astounding. The area of the brain that directs movement, called the *cerebellum*, doubles in size by 3 months as well.[18]

Pheromones are part of the mix too. They have been crossing the placenta between mother and baby, and they now help the mother recognise her own child. Baby also finds the breast from the delicious lure of pheromones at the nipple and is able to recognise their mother within hours of being born.[19]

Avoiding the use of teats and pacifiers while lactation becomes established means all that suckling on the nipple is telling the mum's brain that, yep, prolactin is needed to produce yummy milk. I would like to mention here that some mothers choose to artificially feed their baby for all sorts of individual reasons. Some physical, some psychological. There is no room for judgement about choice and method of feeding in these pages.

A note for consideration about those supporting you to breastfeed: nobody should touch your breast without permission, as this is an intimate act. Unconsented, hands-on breastfeeding support by health professionals and well-meaning individuals is so routine. Most of the time, talking you through latching your baby is enough. If assistance is needed, then respectful consideration, privacy and consent should be expected. In addition, pressure and pushing on the baby's head causes them to jerk back and can be uncomfortable for them as they may be tender after birth.

Microbiome considerations

Breastfeeding and skin-to-skin (including the partner's rich source) combined with the good bacteria transferred in the womb and vaginal birth build a strong immune system. Exposure to microbes (bacteria, viruses and fungi) colonises the baby externally and internally. This colonisation is the *human microbiome*, which plays a crucial role in your baby's health. These microbes help your baby's body fight off infections, digest food and regulate their immune system. Non-digestible human milk oligosaccharides feed the microbes in your baby's gut.[20] Your baby's microbiome is as unique as a finger print. Continuing to evolve as they start eating solid foods and exploring their environment, their microbiome will adapt and grow more complex, stabilising between one and 3 years of age.

This is important to consider in caesarean birth. When born without passing through the mother's vagina, a baby misses out on exposure to the vaginal and gut microbial soup. Lots of skin-to-skin time with mum and dad is beyond valuable to colonise the baby in caesarean birth. Research is ongoing into *vaginal seeding*, a way to mimic the natural process of vaginal birth. A swab is placed into the mother's vagina and then passed over the baby's skin and mouth.[21]

Supporters suggest that vaginal seeding could reduce the risk of certain conditions associated with an unexposed microbiome, such as allergies, asthma and obesity, though more research is needed to fully understand the long-term effects. Read and listen to the resources provided and discuss the potential risks and benefits with your healthcare provider. Ultimately, it is your choice if you wish to do this for caesarean birth.[22]

- **Wishlist** 🌿 *The Midwives' Cauldron* S2 #7. 'Breastfeeding: the early days' Apple 🎙 Spotify
- **ABA #2.** 'Early days: what do you need to know' Apple 🎙 Spotify Mothers volunteer for this podcast and chat about a range of topics through storytelling; a good resource to add to the list of 'helpful advice' in preparation for your fourth trimester.
- *The Midwives' Cauldron* S2 #4. 'The baby's microbiome during pregnancy, birth and breastfeeding – An interview with Toni Harman' Apple 🎙 Spotify
- **Dr Sara Wickham website.** 'Microbiome seeding – what's the evidence? https://www.sarawickham.com/research-updates/microbiome-seeding/
- *Great Birth Rebellion* #38. Part 2 'Positive Caesarean (seeding the baby)' Apple 🎙 Spotify

The vulva, vagina and perineum in the early days

The first few hours also herald checking the vulva, vagina and perineum for any grazes or tears. This needn't be rushed. Unless there is suspicion of significant blood loss that is not from the uterus, you can decline any interruption to the magical time of skin-to-skin and the first feed. The 'check of the perineum' can wait. Even then, during this examination, the baby can remain on the mother's chest, as well as during any repair that may be needed.

First-degree tears do not need suturing and there is strong evidence for the use of surgical glue for repairing second-degree tears and some episiotomies. This can provide greater comfort to the mother afterwards. In their research, 'Use of surgical glue versus suture to repair perineal tears: a randomised controlled trial', Adriana Caroci-Becker and fellow researchers conclude that "surgical glue (GLUBRAN-2°) has proved to be effective because it has similar or better results in pain intensity and healing process compared to continuous suture with polyglycolic thread (Vicryl rapide°) in the repair of first- and second-degree perineal tears in vaginal births".[23] So, bring on the glue!

Again, when having any repair, it should be approached with sensitivity, privacy and respect for the mother and her comfort at all times.

Emma Brockwell, a physiotherapist, wrote the book *Why Did No One Tell Me? How to Protect, Heal and Nurture Your Body Through Motherhood*. She describes her own naivety of the toll pregnancy and birth would have on her body, and how she underestimated her journey of recovery. She discusses how underprepared she was, even with her expertise, and set out to prevent the same unpreparedness in other mothers.[24] Women and mothers need to know the truth of what to expect after birthing. Practical measures include: taking regular pain relief; placing lightly covered ice packs to reduce swelling on the perineum; pouring warm water down the vulva while passing urine to ease stinging of any vulval grazes (or in the shower or bath as it is sterile after all!); taking a sodium bicarbonate preparation to reduce the acidity in urine and therefore the stinging; and practising cleanliness.

The pelvic floor and perineum can feel really weird in these first days. When attempting to do gentle pelvic floor lifts and releases, the brain-to-body connection might feel a bit detached. Worry not. Even the association of thought to slight connection and action is helpful. And the sooner pelvic floor exercises begin, the better for recovery. Do wait until a catheter is removed though, if one is in place. There is a gentle pelvic floor breathing exercise in the practice offering coming up.

The all-important first poo

Then there's that first poo. Avoid constipation by consuming fibre such as prunes, flax seeds and chocolate. (Yes! Chocolate. The darker the better!) Hydrate and consider taking a stool softener, as straining is associated with developing haemorrhoids and prolapse of pelvic organs.

Take a squatting position on the loo, where knees are higher than hips, by placing the feet on a stool (like the kiddie ones). This removes the kink in the lower spine making it easier for a poo to move through the bowel. Push gently with long breaths in and out. Give yourself time and place a pad on the perineum for support and comfort. With a caesarean scar, place a rolled-up towel over the wound with gentle pressure for support.[25]

The first few hours and days after caesarean birth

Caesarean birth may have been planned and everything went as you hoped. Perhaps both you and your baby are well, able to be skin to skin and breastfeeding with plenty of support on a quiet ward. Alternatively, caesarean may have come after a long, hard labour, complications throughout pregnancy or at surgery, with your baby needing support in NICU. Maybe you arrived on the ward at night, when partners are unable to stay to lift your baby from the cot, and you're waiting for a midwife to come because they are short-staffed. Optimally, you will keep your baby skin to skin and give the first feed, while the midwife and recovery staff check your wound, blood loss, observations and pain relief, until you are ready to move to the postnatal ward. You will have an intravenous drip (IV) and a urinary catheter.

If a general anaesthetic (GA) was needed and your baby is well, they will hopefully be skin to skin with your partner to stay warm and toasty, while you are waking in recovery. This usually takes 30 to 60 minutes. After surgery with a GA, epidural or spinal anaesthesia, you will usually be in bed for 12 to 18 hours before being assisted to have a shower.[26] This depends on what time of day or night your birth was. You get to wear super sexy compression stockings. An injection of Clexane goes with the stockings, usually given just under the skin of the abdomen. This is to thin the blood to prevent any clots forming in the lower legs while mobility is restricted.[27]

Thank goodness you can eat and drink a few hours after the birth, because usually mums are pretty hungry and thirsty. The cannula that had the intravenous fluid going through will be bunged or removed once you are drinking freely. You will still be attached to your new type of handbag, the urine collection bag, for 12 to 24 hours. Different hospitals have differing guidelines for when they are removed.

It is difficult to lift your baby from the cot for breastfeeding during this time. With an IV to navigate, and reduced bodily mobility, you'll need extra support from your midwife or partner to care for your baby. (Oh, how I wish we had clip-on cots, or a cot where the side comes down to form a secure slide between mum's bed and the cot for ease of access.)

Your wound dressing is usually removed after 24 hours. It's okay to shower daily, gently patting it dry and keeping it that way in big, comfy cotton or disposable paper pants that don't rub the wound with a seam. Lovely baggy, comfy clothing is your go-to for a while. Please always check in with yourself on how you are feeling. Know that you are infinitely important and have an increased need for support in caring for your baby and your own mobility needs in the first few days. Your comfort in these early days is extremely important. Taking pain relief regularly optimises early mobility and recovery, which is far better than suffering and struggling.[28] Breastfeeding initiates oxytocin, which in turn contracts the uterus. With a fresh wound on your uterus, afterpains would be significant without good pain relief.

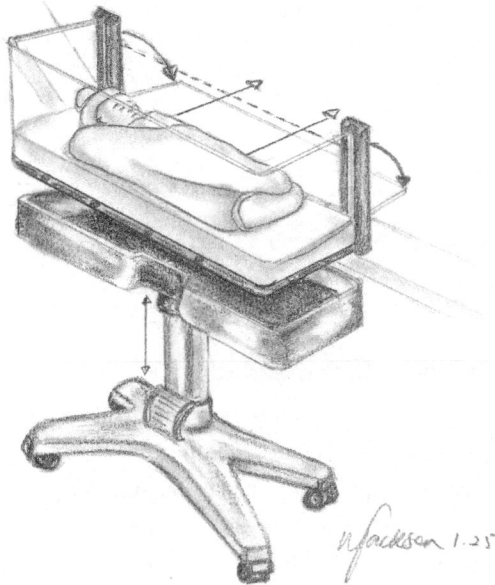

Close cuddle, breastfeeding and bonding cot design by
Wendy Jackson

Belly-binding

As **relaxin** reduces, pelvic bones close. The abdominal wall draws together again after diastasis recti (separation of the abdominal wall muscles) in pregnancy. To support this process and bring comfort, the practice of *belly-binding* using belly bands, rebozo scarves or a traditional bengkung can be used. A bengkung is a long piece of cloth used to bind the mother's pelvis and abdomen as part of ritual postpartum care in many cultures. This is part of recognising the needs of the mother in transition from pregnant to non-pregnant state. Research found that most women experienced improvement in perineal and pelvic discomfort with a belly-bind and would recommend it to other women.[29]

Belly-binding assists the internal organs and maternal posture, for comfort and support. Yet it isn't a substitute for pelvic floor and abdominal exercise, which is discussed more in Chapter 7 with Clémentine.

- *Great Birth Rebellion* #91. 'Belly Binding' Apple 🎙 Spotify
- YouTube 'How to easily wrap a bengkung' https://www.youtube.com/watch?v=XQoMYAPXWl8

Vitamin K for your newborn

Vitamin K is offered for the newborn baby, orally or intramuscularly by injection into the baby's thigh. Consent should be obtained first. Although rare, some babies have what is called *vitamin K deficiency.*

This is the inability for blood to clot and thicken, and such a deficiency may lead to internal bleeding. Therefore, vitamin K is offered to prevent this for those few who are at risk. I'm not going to write in detail about it here, as I am focusing on you, the mother. It is well described and explained in the following resources.

- *Great Birth Rebellion* #35. 'Vitamin K for newborns' Apple 🎙Spotify
- **Dr Sara Wickham's website.** 'Vitamin K Resources' https://www.sarawickham.com/topic-resources/a-decade-of-vitamin-k-articles/

Practice offering: Dandelion clock meditation

Can you be strong enough to be vulnerable to this transition of becoming a mother? Is it time to reflect on the way you usually meet obstacles, anxieties and feelings? Is it with harshness? Perhaps judgement. Maybe both. Becoming a mother is a physical and identity shift, with new demands and ways of living. So, you might explore being soft, if immediate negative reactions and inner voice criticisms arise.

Allow for openness and compassion with your emotions, acknowledging any fear, love, grief, sadness, ambivalence, frustration, disappointment, bewilderment, confusion or anger. Let these emotions be felt instead of buried. Cry or don't. Sit with these emotions. They are as real as you are. Be in the moment. Breath by breath, be aware of the cresting waves of these feelings, not necessarily labelling them as good or bad, strong or weak. Allow them to dissipate with time, trusting in your depth of strength to be present and non-judgemental of yourself. Breathe.

These first few hours and days, like a dandelion clock, are so fleeting, fragile, beautiful. The dandelion seeds are at the mercy of the breeze as it lifts each seed to float away on a breath of wind. Time hovers. You are suspended in ethereal moments. This precious time is so short in the grand scheme of things.

- Scan through your body and soften while holding, smelling, feeding or gazing at your child. Release through the body with awareness of tiredness, with tenderness and reverence at your immense achievement.

- Inhale deeply, expand the lungs fully down to the belly, side ribs and upper chest, re-familiarise yourself with the space your lungs have again.

- Imagine the power of the breath, drawing the dandelion clock close to the face, hovering. Held, floating, fine, soft, fragile and wispy as the soft down of your baby's hair.

- In the space between the in-breath and out-breath, notice the now. Take a picture with the mind's eye to hold always, using all the senses of sight, touch, smell, taste, sound. All that is felt is captured as a treasure. Fleeting yet precious. Present.

- Release the breath and allow the belly to soften, and gently compress the lungs to release all the air. Blow the dandelion clock out into the atmosphere. Free.

- With each breath in and out, a dandelion clock is drawn towards you and then released. Captured in suspension for just a moment. The inhalation of the delicious smell of your child. The softest silken caress of their skin. Crescent eyelashes resting peacefully over kissable cheeks.

- Allow the swell of emotion to break free. Tears of immeasurable elation, love, exhaustion, confusion, transition, grief, pain … all of it, free to fall.

- Moments of time are more valuable than physical wealth. Embodied memories saturated deep into the bones. Breathe them in. Breathe them out. Just be.

Practice offering: Gentle connection to the pelvic floor

- Make yourself comfortable lying on your side. Have a cold pack in place over the perineum before you begin and do this practice when any pain relief has kicked in.

- Soften, while noticing and releasing through the body, noting tiredness and tenderness, yet celebrating yourself.

- Breathe in deeply, expanding fully, down to the belly, side ribs and upper chest, allowing the diaphragm (the layer of muscle between lungs and stomach) to begin to expand as it did before late pregnancy.

- Allow the pelvic floor to soften, remembering that release is just as important as tone for these tissues.

- Breathe out with a long exhalation. As you gently squeeze the air from your lungs, tighten the anus (back passage) as though stopping passing wind. It will feel weird. That's okay. Imagine the anus picking up a blueberry.

- With the next inhalation, soften more deeply through the pelvic muscles. Let it all hang out. (Let the blueberry drop!)

- On the long out-breath, imagine drawing the pubic bone and tailbone together towards the vagina, as though a cord between the 2 tightens a little and allows the vagina to lift. (You could picture a tightrope walker, the vagina being the person walking the rope.)

- As you breathe in, let it all go and completely soften. These slight contractions and releasing of the tissues are promoting blood circulation and healing.

- With the next long exhalation, imagine drawing up through the urethra, as though stopping yourself from passing urine. Breathe in and release fully.

- Now repeat in the opposite direction on each breath cycle, as though you are stopping yourself from passing urine. Then the line drawn between public bone and tailbone lifting the vagina. Then the anus lifting and tightening. Fully release.

In these first few days, a few cycles of this would be great to tune back into your pelvic floor and in preparation for deeper recovery. Practise this while sitting on the loo too, knees above hips, especially for fully releasing when passing urine to completely empty the bladder.

Cultural, Herstorical and Political Influences on the First Few Hours and Days of Mothering

The herstory of breastfeeding and infant sleep

Culture and the herstory of breastfeeding, infant sleep, bed-sharing, co-sleeping and baby-wearing are intertwined with each other because each deeply affects the other. There are 4 resources on the **wishlist** that will debunk myths and reassure you about breastfeeding and both infant and adult sleep. The research-based information will provide reassurance for anxiety or fear around bed-sharing, co-sleeping and sudden infant death syndrome (SIDS). They will also help you establish and maintain breastfeeding more easily, and reduce sleep deprivation.

In *Why Your Baby's Sleep Matters*, Sarah Ockwell-Smith, a specialist in the psychology and science of parenting, poses this question: "When did we, as humans, sever the ties with all our mammalian relatives and decide that we would only listen to our intuition during daylight hours? That our parenting would be relegated to only 12 out of 24 hours? When you think of it like this, the fact that we ignore the cries of our young at night is ridiculous!"[30] Well, as usual, there is history to it.

Ever wondered where the notion of 4-hourly feeding came from? In the Industrial Revolution of the 1800s, women would pay for a wet nurse because they had to work. The wet nurse often had 4 or more babies to feed and care for. Babies were fed on a schedule of taking turns and the woman didn't always have enough breastmilk to feed them all. Often undernourished herself, the babies were given thin gruel. For hundreds of years in the UK, babies were also given opium to keep them calm and quiet. Many died because their breathing was suppressed by the opium. Opium was easily available, sold at the door or in local shops. Although known to cause harm and death, it wasn't until the early 1900s that legislation prevented its availability and use.[31]

If you are interested in the herstory of breastfeeding, listen to *The Midwives' Cauldron*. It's an eye-opening tale, which provides some background to the attitudes and perceptions around breast-feeding now.

> • *The Midwives' Cauldron* S1 #7. 'The herstory of breastfeeding – a fascinating, hilarious, and sometimes gruesome, tour of breastfeeding over the past few hundred years' Apple 🎙 Spotify

Sarah Ockwell-Smith provides a historical snapshot of the effect of baby 'sleep experts' on the expectations, fears and anxieties within the culture of parenting today. Enter Luther Emmett Holt. Born in 1855 in New York, Holt's rigid belief in a parent-led schedule was introduced. The baby was never to feed for more than 20 minutes and no more than every 3 hours, with no night feeds to be given by 5 months of age. He advocated for ignoring the 'attention-seeking' of crying babies. His parenting handbook, *The Care and Feeding of Children*, had a massive impact. Indeed, it is still deeply ingrained in the westernised psyche.[32]

Modern parents – often isolated with minimal support, and exhausted and vulnerable – are open to exploitation from an unregulated industry. So-called 'sleep experts' may use pseudo-science to 'fix' parents' problems and train their baby to sleep, often blaming breastfeeding as the root cause.

Remember how prolactin has a circadian rhythm with higher levels produced at night? Babies feed when hungry, have different requirements for sleep, are unique in their needs and vary in so many ways. Again, one size does not fit all. The baby is able to communicate via behaviour, expression and crying cues to the mother. By recognising those cues, the mother is able to respond to her baby's needs before the red zone of screaming is reached. Feeding, care and the sleep needs of both mother and baby are melded together more calmly when responding to the baby's cues.

Please have a listen to 'Infant sleep! An interview with Lyndsey Hookway'. The sensible, realistic information and advice will dispel so many myths, fears and prejudices. The interview provides a firm foundation of trustworthy knowledge to begin from, and will help you to recognise the cues in infant behaviour. It also talks about how doing the same things in a familiar order is comforting and familiar to the newborn, and they can be done at any time, not just on a rigid schedule.

The short animated video 'Why you might want to put the baby books down' clearly and beautifully describes how our society expects a baby to be 'good'. This definition of good is only if they sleep a lot, feed on a schedule, are not held much, and are calm and quiet when awake etc. The video debunks the unhealthy and mythical unicorn creature of 'the good baby'. It explains how baby-led feeding, rather than a schedule, leads to more satisfied mothers. It also shares how schedules lead mothers to think that their baby is difficult, that they are not very good at caring for their baby, have failed in some way or even have PND.

Ockwell-Smith highlights another significant feature of Caucasian culture that affects sleep – earlier bedtimes for the baby than in non-western culture. In the west, we tend to prioritise 'adult alone time' in the evening. In Asian culture, the baby is part of family activity, feeding, winding down in arms, and going to bed when the parents do. Asian mothers report better and longer sleeping. This appears to lead to better sleep for all.[33]

Here, let's talk about the elephant in the room: co-sleeping and bed-sharing. Co-sleeping is being in the same room. Bed-sharing is baby being in the bed. (Sometimes bed-sharing is called co-sleeping, causing some confusion.)

This is a subject of contention. Parents fear fraught nights and myths thrive – such as bed-sharing will kill the baby and wreck the marriage. Not so. Stepping right into the evidence, the quick-reference visual guide 'The Safe Sleep Seven' by La Leche League clearly highlights the considerations and actions parents need to be aware of to bed-share safely.

You are:	Your baby is:	And you both are:
1. a non-smoker	4. healthy and full-term	7. on a safe surface.
2. sober and unimpaired	5. on their back	
3. a breastfeeding mother.	6. lightly dressed.	

The Australian Breastfeeding Association (ABA) website's 'Position Statement on Safe Infant Sleeping' states: "Co-sleeping can benefit babies by supporting breastfeeding and therefore a baby's health … It is unlikely that co-sleeping per se is a risk factor for SUDI (sudden unexpected death of an infant) but rather the particular circumstances in which co-sleeping occurs."[34]

Breastfeeding and bed-sharing is discussed in *The Midwives' Cauldron* interview with Professor Helen Ball, an anthropologist who specialised initially in primates, then moved into studying infant sleep. In the episode she talks about 'SIDS, bed-sharing and an anthropological look at motherhood and infancy'. She explains how the harmful Victorian and early 20th century attitudes to childcare (developed by men) have damaged mother and baby connections. There is ignorance and disregard of the evolutionary need of babies to be held with unrestricted access to feeding.

Professor Ball also talks about the distressing early herstory of pain relief in labour, again in the late 19th and early 20th century, which knocked the mother out, required her to be strapped to the bed for her own safety, and made her unable to care for her baby. Newborns were taken straight to the nursery as the anaesthetic given to mum suppressed the baby's ability to breathe. While the mother recovered, the baby was given formula and cared for by a nurse. As anaesthetics improved, nurseries took on the role of being a safe place for the baby due to fear about infection instead. We talked about that in Samatha's chapter.

This herstory of separation, formula feeding, ignorance of maternal and infant needs – with imposed schedules and behaviour rules – and lack of support with breastfeeding are still influencing young families today. These attitudes need to be wiped out. Professor Ball's research looked at mothers' behaviours and sleep patterns between those who bed-shared, those who had a clip-on side cot to make it easier to reach the baby, and those mothers who were separated with the baby in a clear plastic cot beside the bed. The difference in maternal and infant sleep, establishing breastfeeding and witnessing the natural behaviour of first-time mothers in keeping their infants safe was astonishing. Bed-sharing proved to provide more sleep and improved establishing of breastfeeding.

There has been so much fearmongering about bed-sharing and SIDS that the damage to families in sleep deprivation and breastfeeding difficulties is immeasurable. Professor Ball states in the interview: "It always seemed completely perverse to me that we tell them, give them so much encouragement to breastfeed, yet we make it so difficult for them from the get-go."

In the ABC *Babytalk* podcast on 'Co-sleeping', Professor Ball talks about her infant sleep research findings, which provide a clear explanation and understanding of the practicalities and benefits of bed-sharing while breastfeeding. It has facts and gives reassurance that bed-sharing while breastfeeding is not a cause of SIDS, with information on how to do it safely. Bed-sharing helps establish and maintain breastfeeding, while improving the mother's sleep and responses to the baby's cues.

Professor Ball also explains that parents 'accidentally' bed-share anyway and are reluctant to tell health professionals about it for fear of judgement. This creates a barrier to talking about safe bed-sharing practices, which should have been discussed in pregnancy. Her research illustrates how mothers are programmed through evolution to sleep and care for their baby in a certain way.

Professor Ball's work debunks the myth that bottle-feeding mothers get more sleep than breastfeeding mothers. They don't. Her work recommends that health professionals talk about safe sleeping practices and do not dismiss bed-sharing. This is the recommendation of the UK NICE guidelines. It states: "The committee agreed that on the basis of the evidence presented, which showed no greater risk of harm when parents shared a bed with their baby compared to not bed-sharing, healthcare professionals should not routinely advise parents against sharing a bed with their baby. They agreed about the importance of parental choice in relation to bed-sharing with their baby assuming they follow safe practices for bed-sharing."[35]

Australia needs to bring advice on safe bed-sharing practices up to date as soon as possible. To begin with, a clip-on cot for ease of access would be amazing for all new mothers in hospital, but particularly for mothers who have birthed by caesarean.

Baby Sleep Information Source (BASIS) is a project of the Durham University Sleep Centre (where Professor Ball works and did her research). They have images to illustrate safe bed-sharing, have an infant sleep app and are a fabulous resource to answer any questions you may have, with information for parents of twins too.

Parent-led care schedules (rather than care guided by a baby's instinctive needs) makes returning to pre-baby life and the workforce the modern ideal. The expectation that the infant will become independent by being able to self-soothe as soon as possible and sleep through the night is a fallacy. Guess what. We didn't evolve that way. And babies *certainly* haven't. With everything you have just learned, is it any wonder parents are exhausted, confused and feel they are doing it wrong or failing?

Babies haven't evolved with social and cultural expectations alongside the Industrial Revolution. Nor should they be expected to. Babies don't pop out knowing they are supposed to sleep through the night and be quiet to be accepted as an 'ideal baby'. They are born with all the primitive instincts to feed when hungry and cry to express their needs because they can't talk. We are more separated from our infants now than at any other time in history. Parents are encouraged to put their babies down as much as possible so they are not being 'manipulated' by a demanding child and don't spoil them.

> - **Wishlist** 🎙 *The Midwives' Cauldron* S4 #3. 'Infant sleep! An interview with Lyndsey Hookway' Apple 🎙Spotify
> - **Wishlist** 🎙 **'Why you might want to put the baby books down'** YouTube. https://www.youtube.com/watch?v=DagfgMeMSXl&list=PLoflLgxNjBdyr7i2Zx-ArwTEU2PwXWgf4&index=5
> - **La Leche League website.** Bed-sharing 'The Safe Sleep Seven'
>   https://llli.org/breastfeeding-info/sleep-bedshare/
> - **Wishlist** 🎙 *The Midwives' Cauldron* S4 #7. 'SIDS, bed-sharing and an anthropological look at motherhood and infancy' Apple 🎙Spotify
> - **Wishlist** 🎙 ABC Babytalk podcast. 'Co-sleeping with Professor Ball' ABC Listen 🎙
> - **BASIS website.** https://www.basisonline.org.uk/co-sleeping-bed-sharing-image-archive/

Our modern society and culture separates parent and baby with cots, baby holders, prams and electric rocking chairs. Along with its inaccurate, ingrained expectations of newborn behaviour, this has led to reducing the collective knowledge of recognition of infant cues. Infant cues communicate their needs to the mammalian carrying species they expect their parent to be.[36]

Baby-wearing

This is why baby-wearing matters. As a species, we need to reconnect with our abilities to nurture our young. In these early months, carrying is one of these abilities. Carrying makes the baby feel secure emotionally. Their heart, respiratory rate and temperature are more regulated. They are calmer when held and rocked. Their sleep is deeper and longer when held close. The upright position helps with wind and reflux, and a spread squat position, with legs either side and with knees above hips, helps them poo.[37] For parents, family members and other adult support, carrying to free-up the hands is probably the least of the advantages. Please do not breastfeed hands-free using the sling to support your baby. You need to be able to see your baby feeding.

The emotional and physical health of carrying – with oxytocin release in the adults – assists with breastfeeding and gives confidence in the parents' ability to recognise and respond to infant cues. Noticing the movements, facial expressions and noises helps parents feel more in tune with their child. [38] This way, they respond to needs before the red zone of screaming and distress arises for all involved. In a comfortable sling or baby carrier, parents may carry a baby on the chest (moving to the back as they get older). This carrier is a small economic investment, which saves emotional and physical energy and distress. It's actually an investment in the family dynamic of bonding, feeding, connection, communication, convenience, time and energy. Win, win, win, win, win.

The TICKS Rule for Safe Baby-Wearing for a sling or baby carrier:

- **Tight** enough to hug your baby close and comfortable for both of you.
- **In view at all times**, able to see your baby's face with a downwards glance. In the cradle position, face up, not turned towards the body.

- **Close enough to kiss,** so able to kiss on the head or forehead.
- **Keep chin off the chest,** where the baby isn't so curled up their chin drops to the chest, because this restricts breathing. A finger should be able to rest between their chin and chest.
- **Supported back,** held comfortably close to the body, the baby's back is supported in its natural position. In a pouch or ring sling the bottom is in the deepest part.

- Babyslingsafety website. Visual guide for baby-wearing. https://babyslingsafety.co.uk/

Making money out of promoting 'not' breastfeeding and the fallout to global health

The politics of breastfeeding have a huge influence on parents-to-be. Here, we are exploring just a few factors.

Milk formula companies undermine breastfeeding. Pregnant and new mothers are bombarded with messaging from milk formula companies, subversively advertising breastfeeding as a 'lifestyle choice' for pleasure or fulfillment. Targeting the mother with ideas of 'bodily autonomy' and of 'getting her body back' gives mixed messages to mothers. This is combined with social pressure to keep breastfeeding invisible; mothers are judged and made to feel ashamed when breastfeeding in public. This situation creates hurdles for women to jump over, before they even birth their baby. Breastmilk is undoubtedly the very best source of nourishment and protection for babies. After all, human mammary glands have had millennia to evolve and get it right.

Investment in breastfeeding support to improve population health

Nutritionist Gabrielle Palmer, in her book *Why the Politics of Breastfeeding Matters*, explores the fallout of not providing breastmilk. "Globally, if all babies were breastfed within an hour of birth, 22 percent of newborn deaths would be prevented."[39] Weak, premature and sick babies can be tube or bottle-fed expressed breastmilk. In Australia, an estimated $120 million could be saved across health systems annually if all babies were breastfed up to 6 months of age.[40] Investment in breastfeeding support and breastmilk banks would be the most sensible, humane move forwards. Ultimately it would improve population health.[19] Some women with rare medical conditions cannot breastfeed, or they have AIDS or have had a double mastectomy. In these circumstances breastmilk banks would be wonderful. A breastmilk bank is a place where donated breast milk is collected, screened and processed. These banks help babies who can't get breastmilk from their own mothers, especially premature or sick infants. If the service of breastmilk banks were expanded to support mothers through breastfeeding difficulties or illness, that would be awesome.

Breastfeeding doesn't make money

However, breastfeeding doesn't make money: " ... despite what they say, there is no evidence that health and wellbeing of infants and mothers is at the heart of what the artificial milk companies do ... The artificial milk companies' relentless marketing has reached a level where global sales were valued at US $44.8 billion in 2014." Sales were projected to reach $70.6 billion by 2019.[41]

The '2023 Lancet Series on Breastfeeding' highlights how milk companies make profits by making normal baby behaviours of crying and sleep patterns seem abnormal, casting doubts on breastmilk and undermining parents' confidence. There are also accusations of tax evasion and political lobbying. The cost to mothers' and babies' health worldwide by undermining the physiological protective process of breastfeeding in the pursuit of profit is an absolute disgrace.[42]

- *The Midwives' Cauldron* podcast S4 #12. 'The unbelievable tactics of the formula industry – Do not think you can skip this episode!' Apple 🎙 Spotify
- **The Lancet Series on Breastfeeding.** YouTube.
  https://www.thelancet.com/series/Breastfeeding-2023

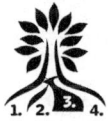

Social, Economic and Media Influences on the First Few Hours and Days of Mothering

The effects of becoming a parent on men and partners

Here with Alysia, we will explore the effects that becoming a parent has on men and partners. The physical, social, cultural, economic and psychological effects on them are huge too. In this journey of mother becoming, the partner evolves too. It is a life-changing experience for them. We have had approximately 200,000 years of evolution in birthing, including the massive upheaval in the past 250 years of industrialisation and globalisation that has formed isolated families. This has affected men's community, connection and support too.

Men have only become part of the birthing room in the past 50 years. Witnessing the birth of a child is momentous. When it involves watching the physiological mammalian labour and birth behaviours in the woman they love, it can be awe inspiring and confronting. Witnessing the emergence of their baby into life elicits emotions and feelings that rock them. The very real awe, reverence, respect, love and fear accompany an overwhelming urge to protect. Surely, this should be respected as a rite of passage for him too.

Believing in the power of the birthing woman they love is of infinite support to her. By providing that sense of safety and strength through holding, massage and words, a partner's presence is far more powerful than words can describe and should not be undermined in any way.

It is really important to say here that being at the labour and birth isn't for every partner. This intensity can be too much and this is by no means a failing. It is a strength to acknowledge this, to ensure that the labouring and birthing woman has the support she needs. This could be her mother, a friend or a doula.

In the early stages of research with male partners, it turns out dads' brains change as well. Fatherhood changes men's brains according to before-and-after MRI scans. The findings have shown several significant changes in the brains of fathers from antenatal to postpartum that did not emerge within the childless men Saxbe and Martínez García followed across the same time period.[43] Also, there were greater changes in the fathers who had more paternity leave allowance; regions of the brain that support goal-directed attention were more developed. This suggests that neuroplastic changes depend on how much they are able to interact with their newborn. A finding like this has implications for the social, cultural, economic and psychological effects associated with parental leave for new families. Dads matter too.

In many of the *Why It Matters...* books mentioned throughout this book, partners and dads are included. Their understanding of the dynamic processes in pregnancy, birthing, breastfeeding and early mothering affects how they feel and act in their role of support, provider, protector and parent. In *Why Postnatal Recovery Matters* Sophie Messager, a doula and antenatal teacher, writes about a dad who was asked by their doula how he was doing. He burst into tears and said, "Not even my own mother asked me that."[44]

Early parenting is tough. Partners are often sidelined in pregnancy, birth and the early months. They are expected to suppress their feelings and anxieties, which all go unacknowledged. Men may bury those emotions deep for fear of judgement, because they are socialised to stay strong, and not feel sad or anxious. Society says "men don't cry" and that it's not cool to talk about or express the emotional stuff.

Although research into the mental health of fathers is relatively new, Mia Scotland, a clinical psychologist and birth doula, explores this in her book *Why Postnatal Depression Matters*. She writes: "The number of men diagnosed with perinatal depression (perinatal being the entire period of pregnancy and postpartum) seems to be on the increase. If you are a man who is going to become a father or has just become a father and you are struggling emotionally, then you are not alone. Estimates range from 1 in 10 to 1 in 4 new fathers experiencing perinatal depression. That is as high for some of the estimates of new mothers."[45]

In our current social culture of the isolated nuclear family, the man may get 2 weeks' parental leave, then needs to return to work full-time to support the family. His life has been turned upside-down too. Yet he is expected to function as he did before on a broken night's sleep, while being the emotional and practical support for the mother of his baby. He is the provider, protector, co-parent and witness to the change and evolution of the woman he loves in her matrescence. The physical and emotional exhaustion is real. Some partners are traumatised by witnessing a traumatic birth, seeing the effects on their partner, feeling angry and helpless. Scotland adds: "In conclusion, perinatal depression matters to father too. Many of the issues are the same for mums as they are for dads, including lack of support, previous history of depression, lack of sleep, loss of previous life, adjustment to change and so on."[46]

A great source of information and support for dads is the *How Other Dads Dad?!* podcast with Hamish Blake. This provides support and plenty of wisdom for fathers from the first episode. It's a welcome change from the stiff upper lip, 'man up', 'suffer in silence' attitude so ingrained into men. Tackling all subjects from the dad's perspective, the podcast provides a place for men to go to listen, learn and know they are not alone in the sometimes-overwhelming changes involved in becoming a dad. They also find out how to understand and support their partner.

Support for dad

Remember, you've also got the Ready to Cope app and COPE antenatal emails for men suggested with Liesja in Chapter 1. The same goes for the COPE postnatal emails for men too. These are weekly to begin with, then bi-weekly, all the way to when the baby is one year old. Resources and support for men is so important.

- *How Other Dads Dad?!* #1. 'What is How Other Dads Dad?' Apple 🎙 Spotify

- *The Good Enough Dad* S1 #9. 'Co-parenting is a whole new ball game' provides frank insight into the realities of becoming a dad. Apple 🎙 Spotify

- COPE website. Postnatal emails for men.
  https://www.cope.org.au/prior-ready-to-cope-for-men-postnatal-emails/

While this book is all about mother becoming, this becoming directly involves men and parent-partners too. If the experiences of the mother improve through understanding and support made available for the brand-new family, then there's the benefit of an overall more healthy family unit. Further places to go for support for fathers are:

- sms4dads.com/About/Project
- thefatheringproject.org
- mensline.org.au
- https://www.dadsgroup.org/
- https://supportforfathers.com.au/resources/just-about-dads/dadtalk/
- https://www.panda.org.au/get-support/support-dads.

Men supporting their partner in breastfeeding

What about dads' involvement in breastfeeding, baby-wearing, bed-sharing and sleeping? We have already introduced the politics around breastfeeding. This continues here with midwife Mark Harris in *Men, Love and Birth*. When talking to men about breastfeeding in this book, he clearly states: "Breasts are not yours," and "they are not even for you."[47]

Harris summarises breastfeeding for men from the point of view of the risks of not breastfeeding for the baby and mother. For the baby, he mentions increased ear and chest infections, admissions to hospital for diarrhoea and vomiting, constipation and higher likelihood of obesity and related diseases like diabetes. For the mother, he talks about higher likelihood of developing heart disease, and breast and ovarian cancer, periods starting sooner and related iron deficiency anaemia.[48]

We are mammals; we are called this because we have mammary glands (breasts with nipples) to feed infant young. As such, Harris suggests looking up the benefits of breastfeeding and gives tips on how to be supportive of it. Swapping breasts after a fixed amount of time feeding is no longer advised. Instead, he recommends waiting until one breast is empty before latching to the other. As well, topping up with formula is not recommended, because it means the breasts have less stimulation and therefore produce less milk. With the best intentions, men can help the mother get some sleep during the night by giving expressed milk via a bottle. This would be more possible in later weeks when breastfeeding is established. Expressing may be much easier once breastfeeding is established too.

Harris also talks of not waking the baby to 'get into a routine' and not being intimidated by professionals (who should have a hands-free approach). If mum's nipples are sore, he discusses avoiding nipple shields without first checking the baby's latch to the breast.[49]

Harris' advice on the role of the man is to be supportive and encouraging, and to not jump to conclusions. When the mother says she is tired, sore or worried about something, he encourages men not to assume it means she wants to stop breastfeeding, nor assume that stopping would fix the problem. He also talks about well-meaning language used by friends and family that can actually be undermining. "Are you going to *try* to breastfeed?" insinuates it will be challenging. For some mums it is, of course. However, with support, these challenges can be overcome.[50]

Harris encourages men to stay connected, to listen, be supportive, and to ignore grandma's advice about a bottle solving the problem, or the advice of others who don't understand breastfeeding. Partners are her strength, believing in her and the baby as they learn together and find their way. Partners can also ensure they have a lactation consultant's details to hand for help, support or to arrange a visit. Calling the ABA may be great support during your fourth trimester.

Baby-wearing is great for bonding with the dad and giving mum a break. Dad's smell, secure touch and voice are all safety-rich cues for the baby.

Midwife continuity of care costs the tax payer less, yet we face a midwife crisis

We don't have enough midwives. Not nearly enough. An article in *The Age* highlights a profession in crisis; midwife shortages are putting strain on maternity wards. Postnatal wards have become a pressure point; mothers are discharging themselves because they are not receiving care. Midwives are reducing their hours to manage burnout and fatigue. Hospitals are unable to adequately staff wards to a level of safety. Women who need induction or planned caesarean are even being pushed back because there are not enough midwives to care for them safely.[51]

The WHO states: "The world is currently facing a shortage of 900,000 midwives, which represents a third of the required global midwifery workforce ... Millions of lives of women and newborns are lost, and millions more experience ill-health or injury, because the needs of pregnant women and skills of midwives are not recognized or prioritized ... Fully investing in midwives by 2035 would avert roughly two-thirds of maternal, newborn deaths and stillbirths, saving 4.3 million lives per year ... Governments must prioritise funding and support for midwifery and take concrete steps to include midwives in determining health policies."[52]

The UN Population Fund response to the WHO report reads: "Gender inequality is an unacknowledged driver in this massive shortage. The continued under-resourcing of the midwifery workforce is a symptom of health systems not prioritizing the sexual and reproductive health needs of women and girls, and not recognizing the role of midwives – most of whom are women – to meet these needs. Women account for 93 per cent of midwives and 89 per cent of nurses ... For midwives to achieve their lifesaving and life-changing potential, greater investment is needed in their education and training, midwife-led service delivery, and midwifery leadership."[53]

Midwives want to do their job well but can't

Midwives want to work within their professional expertise and philosophy of practice, which is in conflict with our current mainstream systems of maternity care. This causes moral distress, because it compromises midwives' knowledge and wisdom and the beliefs that underpin the care they wish to give. This care would improve women's experiences and outcomes. "Discourses in maternity care are affected by the ideologies and philosophies of the maternity care provider. In Australia, obstetricians are the lead professionals, so their philosophies and ideologies are the ones that dictate how policies and services are provided ... Although some individual obstetricians have woman-centred philosophies, the mainstream philosophy is the medical model."[54]

Many midwives are retiring, and more are leaving the profession than entering it. This compounding loss of experience and wisdom being handed down means junior midwives are entering a profession in crisis. Recommendation 29 of the NSW inquiry into birth trauma says we should "investigate ways and take action to address, the midwifery shortage". This includes ways to increase entry into the profession with incentives, appropriate staff level mix, competitive pay and prioritising recruitment of midwives into COC models.[55] Do it now!

Australia needs to train many more midwives. There are some government initiatives to subsidise or offer free postgraduate training for nurses. The provision for direct entry midwives and subsidising their training should be available and well supported in every state.

Midwifery continuity of care provides better health outcomes for mothers and babies

From all we have explored together so far, we know that continuity of midwifery care centred on the woman improves mothers' and babies' physical and emotional wellbeing. When midwives are able to work within their philosophy and autonomy, their work satisfaction increases. So, happier midwives too. Win, win. Women want and need to feel they have a safe, supported choice. Midwives want to provide this and are more likely to be retained in the workforce in this model of care. When comparing current strategic directions for Australian maternity services to other international maternity plans, Australia falls short, particularly in providing woman-centred care, midwifery continuity of care and birthplace options.

The lack of transparency about women's rights to make decisions about their care is also contradictory in most of the strategies and plans put forward. In countries where midwifery is more present and autonomous, the guidelines have greater midwifery contribution. "Maternity strategy/plans should be based on the best available evidence, with consistent and complementary recommendations. Within this framework, priority should be given to women's preferences and choices, rather than the interests of organisations and individuals."[56]

Private practice midwifery, jumping through hoops and cutting of red tape

Privately practising midwives need to jump through a lot of hoops and navigate reams of red tape before being able to offer their services. "Although there have been some recent advances to support private midwives there have also been some concerns, particularly the perceived need for medical dominance in maternity care. Legislation and policies focus on 'risk' … medical model perceives childbirth as inherently dangerous, with women assessed and categorised according to their perceived risk level … The increasing reliance on technology and medically dominated birth contributes to the belief that midwives who provide care in the community and attend births at home cannot be competent. Therefore, to assess their competence they must be closely monitored and controlled."[57]

Women no longer need a referral from their GP to receive Medicare rebates for engaging a privately practising midwife. The Federal Budget 2024 announced an indemnity package to provide intrapartum insurance for privately practising midwives who provide services for low-risk births, homebirth and Birthing on Country. However, the definitions of 'risk in pregnancy' limited women's choices and access to a private midwife and homebirth. The Australian College of Midwives and Homebirth Australia worked hard, together with consumers, to ensure all women had the right to choose homebirth with a midwife who is insured to provide maternity care, no matter perceived risk, and were successful.[58] Cheer!!

Benefits of a private midwife

A boost to support the excellent outcomes of privately practising midwives is found in a study by Dr Yu Gao and associates, 2024.

- Women had significantly lower induction, instrumental and caesarean birth rates.
- Homebirth was at 12.5%, on par with the Netherlands, and 14.5% birthed in a birth centre.
- There was a much higher VBAC success rate at 75.9%, compared to 11.9%.
- There were significantly lower episiotomy rates of 9.55%, compared to 23.9%.
- There were fewer lower birth weight babies.
- There was more postpartum care up to 6 weeks after birth.
- Higher exclusive breastfeeding rates of 84% at 6 weeks were achieved.
- Intervention rates were lower.
- Multidisciplinary and financial modelling showed reduced costs to hospitals.
- $3,707.90 was received from Medicare per woman and out-of-pocket costs were also influenced if private insurance was available to the mother.[59]

Win, win, win, win, win.

From Recommendation 39 of the NSW birth trauma inquiry, we ought to see "consultation to consider legislative change to protect health practitioners when delivering individualised, responsive maternity care, and ensure that consumers' birthing decisions and preferences can be supported and respected".[60] In addition, Recommendation 27 is to "review the regulatory framework and funding arrangements for privately practising midwives, including ensuring these midwives have authority to practise within hospital settings as well as hospital admitting rights".[61] Bring it on!

Midwifery is an entirely separate profession to nursing, with different philosophies and dynamic methods of practice. Midwifery needs representation to government and all perinatal healthcare providers. A major influence for change would be if Recommendation 31 from the NSW birth trauma inquiry were applied to all states, following Queensland's lead, to all appoint "a standalone Chief Midwifery Officer".[62]

Many organisations are working towards improving maternity services. Yet this top-down approach needs a boost to make the changes happen sooner. The greatest influence for change will come from you. We need a groundswell of women's, mothers' and partners' voices, as well as all who support young families, to make so much noise that government and private practice listen. You are part of this change.

Media influence on new mothers

Media influence and the exploitation of new mothers' vulnerability about their body image is rife. In pregnancy, women change what they eat and drink for the health of their baby, which is totally understandable. As their body changes, management of bodily self-identity and aesthetic (how they look) during pregnancy is influenced by celebrity culture and media. Even though they recognise it as 'not normal' or realistically attainable, women still feel pressured by it.

Then, fuelled by the ideologies of 'yummy mummies' in the media, some new mothers are eager to return to their sense of pre-pregnancy self and body after birth. In the real world of motherhood, the likelihood of attaining 'bounce back' in no time is a fallacy which fuels negative body image and a sense of failure.[63]

The 4th Trimester Bodies Project offers the reality of mothers' postpartum bellies and bodies through imagery and stories, and encourages women to acknowledge their new, changed body. It doesn't snap back into pre-pregnancy jeans. As mothers' brains change, so do their bodies, never to be the same again. That's okay. The social norm of body-shaming mothers is cruel, unnecessarily damaging and ignorant. It shouldn't be given air time. Rant not over …

There is pressure from social media on women to reach unreal expectations and ideals of mothering. So many mothers are feeling this pressure in isolation, along with that good ol' mum guilt. Please revisit the 'Postpartum Identity + Mum Guilt' podcast with Dr Nicole Highet here – link in the goody box below.

Mum guilt. Oh, she's a nasty one. Feeling guilty for taking time for yourself to rest. Having a relaxing bath rather than a quick 'pits and bits' wash. Leaving the baby with dad while going for a walk or catching up with friends instead of doing the laundry. How dare you! Then mothers judge themselves against other mothers and may feel as though they are coming up short, in turn feeling guilty for it. That nasty inner voice is manifesting itself as mum guilt and is having an absolute field day with your heart, thoughts and emotions.

Sarah Napthali captures this perfectly in her words: "Guilt is a confusing emotion because although it clearly undermines our happiness, it's easy to tell ourselves that it's a worthy mind state. We see guilt as a way of controlling ourselves. We even say to ourselves, 'I might be doing something wrong but at least I feel guilty – if I didn't feel guilty then I'd be a really terrible person.' In the same way, we use guilt to ward off disapproval from others as we try to convince them that at least we feel really bad about our failure to be perfect."[64]

Other people's assessment of, and opinions on, your mothering don't matter. If you are nourished, supported, getting rest and filling your cup, your baby and family will feel the positive effects too. More oxytocin. Good! Each situation and baby is so unique. So, when your inner voice tells you otherwise, feel free to tell her to take that running jump. Here, return to what you value, your strengths and self-trust. Come back to realistic expectations and allow yourself what you need. It doesn't make you a bad mother. There is no such thing, remember? How will total self-sacrifice and depletion help you? It won't.

Mothers are the fundamental foundation of our society. You matter. Nag complete.

- Reminder: *Seasons of Matrescence* S1 #5. 'Postpartum Identity + Mum Guilt with Dr Nicole Highet, Founder and Executive Director at COPE' Apple 🎙 Spotify

---

🌿 Self-identity, Beliefs and Values, and Spiritual Influences on the First Few Hours and Days of Mothering

An invisible umbilical cord is forever entwined with every aspect of your life now. It is deeply embedded into your evolving sense of identity. You are no longer an individual, but are forever connected to your child. Every thought, plan and action considers another person. Your sense of yourself is deeply changed, affecting your identity as you evolve, renew and redefine yourself as a mother. The woman you have become is a fiercely protective lioness. This transition in identity is normal. It should be acknowledged, understood, valued, supported and respected.

The reality of the early mothering months is the indescribable yet survivable exhaustion and bone-deep fatigue. Understanding this will reframe your thoughts, perceptions and expectations of transitioning to mothering. With clarity about this, treat yourself with kindness and self-compassion always. At this stage of your journey, sink into 'Matrescence with Zoe Blaskey'.

> • *Birth-Ed* S3 #5. 'Matrescence with Zoe Blaskey' Apple 🎤 Spotify

Supporting spirituality in loss

We again honour Alysia and all families who have experienced the birth of a baby who will never take a breath or grow. Reducing this to a percentage of births seems so callous, because every loss is tragic in the extreme. That being said, it's important to say that 1% of babies born each year are either stillborn or die in the first 28 days of life.[65]

Grief has no boundaries, cannot be contained, and has no words to fully describe it. Grief is unique in its embodied experience and expression for each individual. In *Why Baby Loss Matters*, Kay King, a doula and Grief Recovery Method specialist, explores grief in relatable ways. She explains grief as a response to the experience of loss, rather than a single emotion. Our society has lost the language of death, because we avoid talking about it. Acknowledgment of grief comes before recovery, healing or even support. To compare, fix, dismiss, limit or disallow grief does not help, as it removes the autonomy of realistic suffering of the parent. Comments such as, "You can try again," or "Everything happens for a reason," don't help at all. The experience of grief is unique to everyone, with no rules or right path to follow.

Empathy and compassion is powerfully supportive – really listen, be present, refrain from judgement, preconceived ideas or pressing our own beliefs, and be in companionable silence. In this capacity, without doing anything, just being there is infinitely comforting. It's okay to talk about feelings, and acknowledge and recognise the parents' loss. Indeed, ignoring it or displaying pity compounds their grief.[66] "That the NSW Government improve psychological support for parents managing grief following pregnancy loss" is Recommendation 36 of the NSW birth trauma inquiry.[67] Such psychological support is a desperately needed service to bring the suffering of pregnancy and perinatal loss out from under the carpet countrywide.

Alongside the physical expressions of giving birth, blood loss and breastmilk production, there is nowhere for these mothers to go. Mother and baby groups and other social gatherings are closed to them and there are few groups for postnatal recovery after loss. The fourth trimester transition is still happening for the mother who has lost a child – but all those hormones and instincts to reach for her baby have nowhere to go. Some mothers choose to express milk to supply a neonatal unit. All these mothers experience breasts engorging from days 2 to 5, and produce breastmilk for 2 to 3 weeks. The ABA offers resources about choices, support and care for lactation suppression when a baby passes.

Here, the support of a postnatal doula for both parents would be incredibly comforting. A 'closing the bones' ritual may be deeply beneficial for the mother, because she too experiences these physical changes. Apart from the rite of passage of a funeral, this acknowledgment of the mother having commonality with all other mothers may be soothing. Closing the bones is discussed with Clémentine in Chapter 7.

A reminder about SANDS, Bears of Hope and Pink Elephants, organisations that were mentioned with Liesja. Red Nose has 'Hospital to Home' free counselling and peer support on 1300 308 307 available 24 hours. They recognise the double grief of grandparents and provide for them too, as well as siblings, family, friends and the wider community. With easy access referral forms for anyone to use, this is another source of support for families experiencing loss.

- ABA website. 1800 686 268
  https://www.breastfeeding.asn.au/resources/lactation-after-your-baby-dies
- The Pink Elephants website. contact@pinkelephantssupport.com / https://www.pinkelephants.org.au
- Bears of Hope website. 1300 11 BEAR
  https://www.bearsofhope.org.au
- Stillbirth and Neonatal Death Society (SANDS) website. 1300 308 307. https://www.sands. org.au
- Red Nose 'Hospital to Home' 'Guiding Light Peer Support' 1300 308 307 24/7.
- Red Nose website. Online support via intake@rednose.org.au, and rednosegriefandloss.org.au/live-chat. For stillbirth, neonatal death and SIDS. https://rednosegriefandloss.org.au/

Practice offering: Meditation on the invisible umbilical cord and *Bāndhava*

Bāndhava in the yoga of the Radiance Sutras refers to bonding, especially with a maternal relation.[68] Also, a friend or family member. The practice of bāndhava is to meditate on and think about the nature of the bond between you and each individual person you love.

Throughout this book, I have used the analogy of an invisible umbilical cord, forever connecting the mother and child. Bāndhava, on the invisible umbilical cord, whether it is a fleeting thought or a meditation, seems perfect to practise here.

- Do the comfortable wiggle and stretch, checking through the body for tension, with awareness of tenderness. Take a note of how you are feeling emotionally. Hold your baby, feed, gaze at them or rest separately. Whatever you need.
- Practise your preferred breathing as best calms the heart and lowers the blood pressure, towards finding some inner peace. Allow any negative emotions to dissolve, honouring them as being present, yours.
- Feeling heavy, grounded, supported, put some headphones on, allowing the sounds around you to float away. Nobody and nothing else matters right now.
- Picture the umbilical cord as silvery white light, pulsating, a living entity, shimmering. As feelings and emotions are sent, it vibrates with a musical note ...
- Each breath in, absorb the universe. Allow oceans, mountains, planets, stars, space to flow into your heart and dissolve in shimmering light through your body.
- Each breath out, see the umbilical cord, connected from your heart to your child. Through the soft pulsating, silvery white light, send your thoughts. Thoughts like: *I cherish you. I love you. I hope for you. I'm overwhelmed by you. I'm tired. I'm struggling but I'm doing my best for you. I'm learning to love you. I'm your mum.*
- Breathe in the energy all around you.
- In the pause between breaths, see the light shimmer though your body.
- Breathe out and allow the emotion to swell.
- Send it through the bond, a pulse, like your heartbeat, joy, love, hope ...

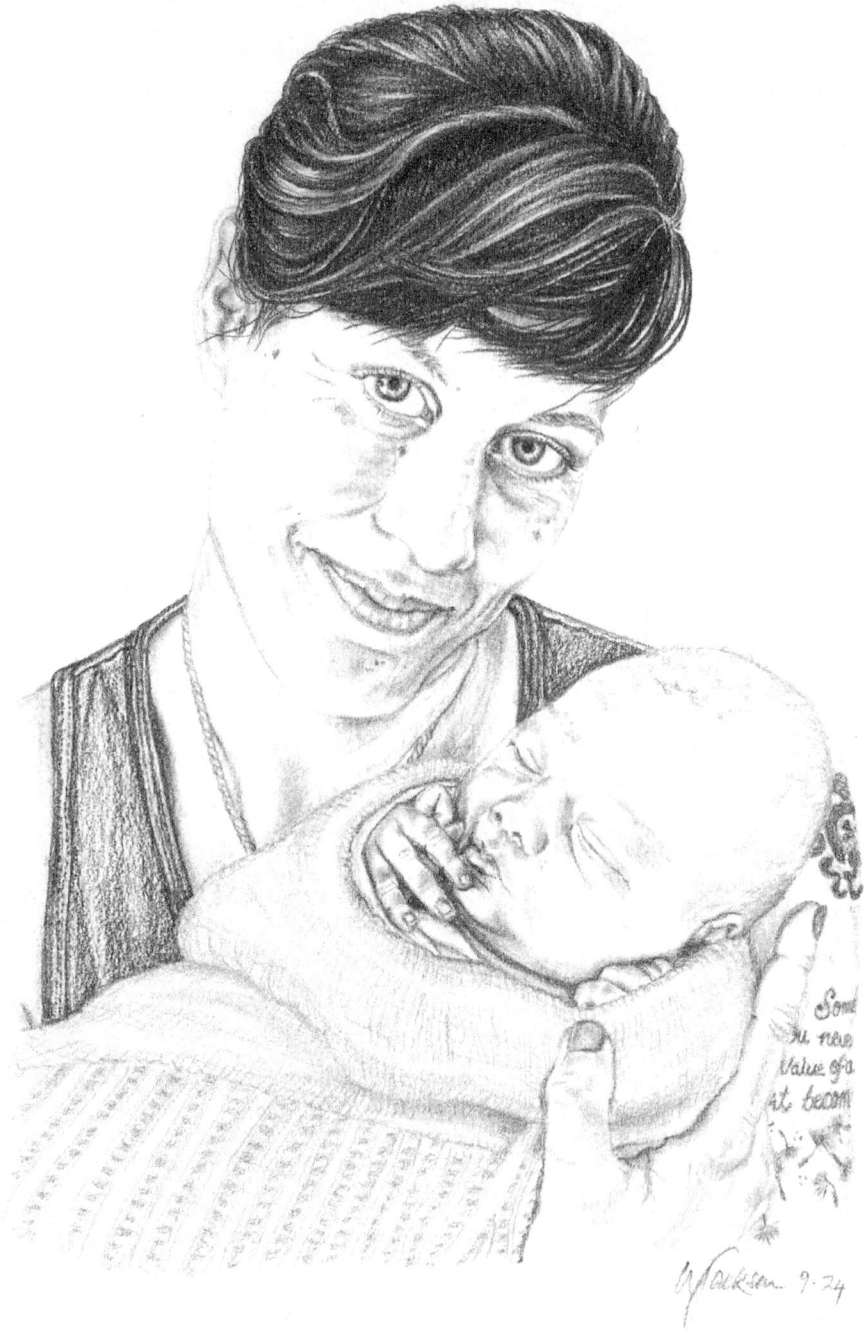

Well, doesn't Alysia's expression say it all? *Look at what I created!* You can see the pride and swelling love flowing out of her as Alysia holds Nicholas up for the camera to capture this precious moment in time.

Mother Becoming Inspired Actions in the First Few Hours and Days of Mothering

Wow! Here you are … a mum! Liesja, Samantha, Ashleigh, Ally, Katie and Alysia have been with you all the way so far. There is more to come. What a journey. These moments, the first few hours and days of becoming a mother – goodness, what a life-altering experience. Let's just take the pack and boots off. Rest a while. Soak it all in.

How might it be for you …

- If skin-to-skin time were supported with deep respect, so your baby can adjust to the transition of life outside the womb and have their first feed?

- If Recommendation 24 of the NSW birth trauma inquiry were implemented to "review hospital practices to ensure that, wherever possible, parents and baby are able to remain together after birth and have skin-to-skin contact"?

- If your baby weren't removed for checks, measurements, weighing, paediatric checks for care provider convenience?

- If your baby could be on dad's chest, if not with mum?

- If you performed ritual, pause, ceremony, acknowledgment, or welcomed your child somehow during cord-cutting?

- If glue were the first choice and common practice for second-degree (and some episiotomy) perineal repair?

- If your comfort came first and all the fuss was about you, celebrating and supporting the mother, rather than focusing exclusively on the baby?

- If practical support like meals, a cleaner, a doula for a day were provided by your village as a way of celebration?

- If clip-cots were attached to the side of mum's bed as standard in hospitals for ease of access to your baby, especially for mums who have had a caesarean birth?

- If safe bed-sharing education were updated with research, recognised as the best way to support breastfeeding, and maternal sleep were supported, rather than shamed?

- If fearmongering about SIDS in this situation were removed?

- If breastfeeding were no longer undermined by the artificial infant milk companies?

- If your belief in your ability to breastfeed were strong?

- If all mothers were championed in breastfeeding, with time for midwives to support them?

- If lactation consultants were subsidised by Medicare?

- If baby-wearing became the norm again, because we evolved that way?

- If Recommendation 29 of NSW inquiry into birth trauma were implemented to "investigate ways and take action to address the midwifery shortage"?

- If we provided more subsidised or free training for midwives to fill the gap in numbers, with direct entry midwifery training available in every state?

- If we supported, valued and provided more COC practices, and supported the autonomy and philosophy of practice to retain midwives?

- If privately practising midwives were better supported and the requirements for private midwifery practice became part of the student midwifery training program?

- If midwives were supported to set up in private practice, with ease of access and admitting rights to hospital if needed?

- If the ongoing Federal Budget conversations came out in favour of supporting privately practising midwives for women who want to access COC?

- If there were a place for you to go other than the emergency department or labour ward when experiencing a stillbirth – like the three-bed unit in Canberra, mentioned with Liesja – as a place of dignity, deep compassion and respect?

- If we implemented Recommendation 35 of the NSW birth trauma inquiry to "ensure dedicated spaces available for parents experiencing miscarriage or stillbirth in all healthcare settings, including private waiting rooms separate from pregnant women, new mothers and babies"?

- If Recommendation 36 of the NSW birth trauma inquiry "That the NSW Government improve psychological support for parents managing grief following pregnancy loss" were acted on?

First Few Hours and Days References and Wishlist

1   S Messager. *Why Postnatal Recovery Matters*. Pinter and Martin, 2020, p8. ISBN 9781780666259.

2   SJ Buckley. 'Hormonal physiology of childbearing: evidence and implications for women, babies, and maternity care, Childbirth Connection Programs, National Partnership for Women & Families'. 2015. p V-XX. p 47. https://nationalpartnership.org/wp-content/uploads/2023/02/hormonal-physiology-of-childbearing.PDF

3   G Chauhan, P Tadi, 'Physiology, Postpartum Changes'. In: StatPearls [Internet]. Treasure Island (FL): StatPearls Publishing; 2024 Jan-. Available from: https://www.ncbi.nlm.nih.gov/books/NBK555904/

4   R Reed. *Reclaiming Childbirth as a Rite of Passage: Weaving ancient wisdom with modern knowledge*. Word Witch, 2021, p218-221. ISBN 978-0-6450025-1-5

5   K Uvnäs Moberg, *Why Oxytocin Matters*. Pinter and Martin, 2019. p57, 88. ISBN 9781780666051

6   G Chauhan, Physiology, Postpartum Changes.

7   Buckley, Hormonal physiology of childbearing, p44.

8   Buckley, Hormonal physiology of childbearing, p145-6.

9   Buckley, Hormonal physiology of childbearing, p142.

10   Buckley, Hormonal physiology of childbearing, p101.

11   New South Wales Parliament Legislative Council Select Committee on Birth Trauma, Report. 2024. P xvii, ISBN: 978-1-922960-38-2. https://www.parliament.nsw.gov.au/lcdocs/inquiries/2965/FINAL%20Birth%20Trauma%20Report%20-%2029%20April%202024.PDF

12   Buckley, Hormonal physiology of childbearing, p47.

13   G Chauhan, Physiology, Postpartum Changes.

14   E Luders, F Kurth, M Gingnell, J Engman, EL Yong, IS Poroma, C Gaser, 'From Baby Brain to Mommy Brain: Widespread Grey Matter Gain After Giving Birth.' Cortex. Volume 126. May 2020, p334-342 https://doi.org/10.1016/j.cortex.2019.12.029

15   C Young. *Why Breastfeeding Matters*. Pinter and Martin, 2016, p21. ISBN 9781780665207

16   Young. Why Breastfeeding Matters, p22.

17   M McMahon. *Why Mothering Matters*. Pinter and Martin, 2018, p46. ISBN 9781780665900

18   McMahon. *Why Mothering Matters*, p47.

19   McMahon. *Why Mothering Matters*, p50.

20   McMahon. *Why Mothering Matters*, p49.

21   T Harman. Human Microbiome. https://microbirth.com/

22   T Harman. Human Microbiome. https://microbirth.com/

23   A Caroci-Becker, W Sousa Brunelli, M de Oliveira Pimentel Lima, A Megumi Ochiai, S Guimarães, O Luiza Riesco, M Luiza Riesco, 'Use of surgical glue versus suture to repair perineal tears: a randomised controlled trial'. 2023. p10. BMC Pregnancy and Childbirth. (2023)23:246 https://doi.org/110.1186/s12884-023-05568-x. https://link.springer.com/content/PDF/10.1186/s12884-023-05565-x.PDF

24   E Brockwell. Why Did No One Tell Me? How to Protect. Heal and Nurture your body through Motherhood. Vermillion, Penguin Rando House, 2021, p2-5. ISBN 9781785043369.

25   Brockwell. Why Did No One Tell Me? p103.

26   C Goggin, *Why Caesarean Matters*. Pinter and Martin, 2018, p25. ISBN 9781780665405

27   Goggin, *Why Caesarean Matters*, p123.

28   Goggin, *Why Caesarean Matters*, p102-3.

29   S Messager, *Why Postnatal Recovery Matters*, p93.

30   S Ockwell-Smith. *Why Your Baby's Sleep Matters*. Pinter and Martin, 2019, p10. ISBN 9781780665450

31   M Obladen. 'Pap, gruel and panada; early approaches to artificial infant feeding'. Neonatology. 2014;105(4):267-74 https://pubmed.ncbi.nlm.nih.gov/24577423/

32   Ockwell-Smith. Why Your Baby's Sleep Matters, p65-6.

33   Ockwell-Smith. Why Your Baby's Sleep Matters, p77.

34   Australian Breastfeeding Association. 'Position Statement on Infant Sleeping'. https://www.breastfeeding.asn.au/position-statement-safe-infant-sleeping

35   NICE Guideline NG 194. 'Benefits and Risks of Bed-sharing'. 2021. p17. https://www.nice.org.uk/guidance/ng194/evidence/m-benefits-and-harms-of-bed-sharing-PDF-326764485977

36   R Knowles, *Why Baby-Wearing Matters*. Pinter and Martin, 2016, p32. ISBN 9781780665351

37   Knowles, *Why Baby-Wearing Matters*, 29-34.

38   Knowles, *Why Baby-Wearing Matters*,54-64.

39   G Palmer. *Why the Politics of Breastfeeding Matter*. Pinter and Martin, 2019, p14. ISBN 9781780665252

40   McMahon. *Why Mothering Matters*, p97.

41   Palmer. *Why the Politics of Breastfeeding Matter*. p15.

42   The Lancet Series on Breastfeeding. 2023. https://www.thelancet.com/series/Breastfeeding-2023

43   D Saxbe, M Martínes García, 'Fatherhood changes men's brains, according to before and after MRI scans'. November 2020 https://dornsife.usc.edu/news/stories/fatherhood-changes-mens-brains/

44   Messager, *Why Postnatal Recovery Matters*. p35.

45   M Scotland. *Why Postnatal Depression Matters*. Pinter and Martin, 2015, p 99. 2015 ISBN 978178066503.

46   Scotland. *Why Postnatal Depression Matters*, p106.

47   Harris, *Men, Love and Birth*. Pinter and Martin, 2017, p138. ISBN 9781870662251

48   Harris, *Men, Love and Birth*, p140.

49   Harris, *Men, Love and Birth*, p142-8.

50   Harris, *Men, Love and Birth*, p139.

51   T Jack.'It's like hospital ramping: Midwife shortage puts strain on maternity wards'. 2022. https://www. theage.com.au/national/victoria/it-s-like-hospital-ramping-midwife-shortage-puts-strain-on-maternity- wards-20220525-p5aobg.htm

52   WHO 'Global Shortage of Midwives'. https://www.who.int/news/item/05-05-2021-new-report-sounds- the-alarm-on-global-shortage-of-900-000-midwives

53   UN Population Fund https://www.unfpa.org/press/new-report-sounds-alarm-global-shortage-900000- midwives

54   C Davison, Looking Back and Moving Forward: A History and discussion of Privately Practising Midwives in Western Australia. 2019. p223, https://espace.curtin.edu.au/handle/20.500.11937/77506

55   New South Wales Parliament Legislative Council Select Committee on Birth Trauma. p xviii.

56   H Dahlen, S Ormsby, A Staines, M Kirk, L Johnson, K Small, B Hazard. V Schmeid.'A comparison of the woman-centred care: strategic directions for Australian maternity services, 2019 comment on the national strategy with other international maternity plans'. Women and Birth. Volume 36, Issue 1. February 2023 Pages 17-29. p 17. https://doi.org/10.1016/j.wombi.2022.04.003

57   Davison, Looking Back and Moving Forward, p223.

58   The Australian College of Midwives.'Consultation on expanding eligibility under the Midwife Professional Indemnity Scheme for low-risk homebirths ACM Submission'. Issued 14 August 2024. https://www. midwives.org.au/common/Uploaded%20files/ACM%20response%20DoHAC%20MPIS%20for%20 low-risk%20homebirths%2014%20August%20Final.PDF

59   Y Gao, L Wilkes, A Tafe, L Ruthenburg, M Warriner, S Kildea.'Women Clinical outcomes and financial estimates for women attending the largest private midwifery service in Australia compared to national data: a retrospective cohort study'. Woman and Birth. Vol 37. Iss 3. May 2024 https://doi.org/10.1016/j. wombi.2024.101591.

60   New South Wales Parliament Legislative Council Select Committee on Birth Trauma. p xviii.

61   New South Wales Parliament Legislative Council Select Committee on Birth Trauma. p xix.

62   New South Wales Parliament Legislative Council Select Committee on Birth Trauma. p xviii.

63   M Patterson, LO'Malley (2013)'Bouncing Back: Reclaiming the Body from Pregnancy', in S O'Donohoe, M. Hogg, P. MacLaran, L. Martens and L. Stevens (eds.) Motherhoods, Markets and Consumption, Routledge, Taylor & Francis Group; 2014. 131-144. ISBN 97804415516495. https://www.academia. edu/23426260/10_Bouncing_back

64   S Napthali. *Buddhism for Mothers. A calm approach to caring for yourself and your children.* Allen and Unwin, 2003, p42. ISBN 978174237701830.

65   Australian Institute of Health and Welfare. https://www.aihw.gov.au/reports/mothers-babies/still- births-and-neonatal-deaths

66   K King, *Why Baby Loss Matters.* Pinter and Martin, 2020 .ISBN 9781780666358

67   New South Wales Parliament Legislative Council Select Committee on Birth Trauma. p xix.

68   L Roche, *The Radiance Sutras*, Verse 48, Yuki Practice Sounds True, 2014, p255. ISBN 978-1-60407-659-2

🌱 Wishlist

1. *Birth-Ed* S1 #15. The first 24 hours with Marie Louise ^{Apple} 🎙 ^{Spotify}

2. The ABA baby-led attachment visual guide and video. https://www.breastfeeding.asn.au/resources/baby-led-attachment

3. *Happy Mama Movement* #231. The Real Truth about How your Brain Changes with Parenthood – with Chelsea Conaboy ^{Apple} 🎙 ^{Spotify}

4. *The Midwives' Cauldron* S2 E7. 18.4.21 Breastfeeding: the early days ^{Apple}🎙^{Spotify}

5. *The Midwives' Cauldron* S4 #3. Infant sleep. An interview with Lyndsey Hookway. ^{Apple}🎙^{Spotify}

6. YouTube video, School of Health & Social Care, Swansea University: 'Why you might want to put the baby books down'. https://www.youtube.com/watch?v=DagfgMeMSXI&list=PLoflLgxNjBdyr7i2Zx-Arw-TEU2PwXWgf4&index=4

7. *The Midwives' Cauldron* S4 #7. An interview with Professor Helen Ball – SIDS, bed-sharing and an anthropological look at motherhood and infancy. ^{Apple Spotify}

Chapter 7

Early Mothering and the
Fourth Trimester with Clémentine

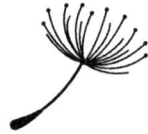

Meeting Clémentine

Clémentine and I met when she was pregnant with Charlie; she was attending pregnancy yoga classes that I had the privilege of teaching. I could listen to Clémentine talk all day. Her beautiful French accent, so melodic, came from an obviously strong woman. (Her name is pronounced in the French way: 'Clé-mon-teen', rather than Cle-men-tyne.)

It was a joy for me to watch her baby bump grow and know that the yoga was bringing her some relief from her nausea. Already a practitioner of yoga, Clémentine fully embraced her practice as a pregnant woman.

When she and Charlie returned for postpartum yoga, it was wonderful to see them. Clémentine's experiences are deeply distressing to read at times, but her raw honesty and her deep wish for you powers through her words: find your voice and speak up.

Have your favourite cuppa and nibbles ready. Underline, draw happy or sad faces, whatever flows for you as you read her words. Also, please sit with the feelings they evoke, make notes about what you wish to be clarified and chat about with your care provider. Share the emotions that have come up for you with someone you trust, and take care of yourself. Be. Breathe.

Mama of Charlie and Alizée, here is Clémentine's letter to you

"Have a voice!"

Dear Mama,

Here is my letter, explaining the birth of my first daughter, Charlie. I apologise in advance to the mamas-to-be, as it is not what we would like to hear and certainly not what society, medical staff, people around us, books and especially movies will show us. I'm hoping that my experience might help some of you not feel alone anymore.

For those who are not yet pregnant, those who are and will soon be expecting, and those who experienced trauma like mine, remember that it is your body, your soul, your sanity, and your absolute whole that you are about to give or have given. Never let anyone diminish you in your rights, and make you feel like nothing more than an oven.

Have a voice!

And if you can't have it on that special day, make sure you have someone with you who will be your voice when you can't be. It is not just about the baby; it is and should be about you first.

Giving birth and raising your children in a foreign country is extremely challenging. I was born in France and emigrated to Australia in my late twenties. Becoming a mother is already a crazy experience; even more so when you don't have any family support close to you. Being lucky to give birth in a developed country makes you feel that you don't have the right to complain. And then you let them discard your body and dehumanise you as a woman, thinking that they are the professionals.

While I was in excruciating pain at the maternity ward, I remember the difficulty of having to think and express myself in English. Even though I'm fluent and perfectly understand everything, my head was screaming from the pain and confusion. Everything was so blurry and distressing. I felt that it was asking me for extra effort on top of going through so much pain. In this state, your brain can't function normally; having to produce this extra effort to listen to and speak your second language is extremely difficult. I remember wishing that the staff and my husband could speak and understand French to relieve me of that strong emotionally and physically draining life experience.

The only great part of it was when I couldn't contain my pain and emotions after 20+ hours of labour. Finally, I yelled and screamed to insanity in my mother tongue – after having been so silent and trying to hold it in, because we shouldn't display any moment of distress or unforgettable pain. Having to push in front of an army of midwives, doctors, nurses and, of course, my husband was distressing, but the pain would be so strong that you would not care anymore if one more person would enter the room and violate your intimacy by watching you like an object, so vulnerable and exposed. At last, I could open the tap and let loose all the insults and bad thoughts, while thinking: *This is it. I am dying. All this pain is killing me.*

I don't really know how to bring the right words to my experiences. This is the fourth time that I have attempted this letter. Every time, I find it way too personal and can't stop thinking that I'm complaining; when reading it again, I can't stop seeing the word 'I' written everywhere and feeling that it is really self-centred and narcissistic.

I have given birth twice and both experiences haven't been the best. The second time might have been a bit easier because I knew what to expect from the hospital. Still, it couldn't prepare me for the coldness, inhumanity and disregard towards me from certain staff members.

Before Charlie was born in 2018, I read a lot of books and information regarding pregnancy, birthing and maternity. My best friend, who had a child before I did, gave me some great advice and I can never thank her enough. Advice, such as trying to wait at home as long as you can when contractions start, otherwise they will send you back there. She also sent me a book and a special oil to massage my perineum, as nobody ever told me that massaging that area (another kind of small torture) would help prevent tearing yourself up to the anus.

After 7 hours of strong and painful contractions at home, I arrive to be 'welcomed' by an overwhelmed maternity. It was on bypass because 2 maternity wards in my area had recently been shut down. That means my small maternity had to take the burden of all those patients. After waiting on a chair in the hallway for a while, I was told – without being checked – that I would have to go to another hospital.

I refused!

Being in so much pain, I couldn't see myself moving and having to jump in a car for another 25 minutes of driving. The midwife decided to examine me and told me that I would stay there as I was already 5 cm dilated. I was then lucky to have on my side 2 beautiful angels, 2 midwives who clearly practised their job the way it should be. Because they wanted to be there, to help the mamas feel as secure as possible, and empowering them the best they could. I will always be thankful to them, for they held me under their loving care.

After doing my best to bring Charlie into this world drug-free, I couldn't anymore. I asked to get the epidural. This was a bit late as I was already opened to 7 cm, but I was insistent and the midwife said yes.

When the anaesthetist arrived 2 or 3 hours later, I was lying on the bed. Before having to lie on that bed, I was constantly moving around the room, trying to have some warm water on my aching back, rolling on the ball, trying to do some yoga postures (thank you, Wendy) that I practised while being pregnant. This helped a lot at that time.

The first thing the anaesthetist said on entering the bedroom was: "Oh okay, great. I didn't even touch her and she is already complaining and crying." I can't even describe what I felt at that time, but I had to try really hard not to burst into tears. He created such emotional distress, when I was clearly at one of the most vulnerable moments of my life and in so much pain. At this point, I'd been having contractions for 15 hours, but I didn't say as much. I hid the fact that I wanted to scream from the pain I was feeling.

I felt unempowered and didn't have the strength to reply. At first, I wasn't sure if I heard right. And secondly, he retained all the power! (Would you contradict someone that was going to insert a 10 cm needle into your spine?) I remember the more experienced midwife telling him off gently. You could tell she didn't have much power either. His attitude was then disgusting. He was extremely diminishing in his way of talking to me, pushing on my back, squeezing my huge belly, and accusing me of moving when I was trying to hold still while having extremely strong contractions. It was horribly painful and resulted in me feeling humiliated again.

Of course, the epidural stopped my contractions, which means that I went back to 4 cm and I had lower left leg numbness, but with the rest of my body awake. As a first-time mother-to-be, I didn't have the knowledge of what I could express or not, if it was normal or not. My mistake was certainly to shut up and not complain about anything. After releasing some of my emotions, while the anaesthetist was there, I felt like I was wrong. That I wasn't strong enough to fulfil my duty of becoming a good mother. The epidural hadn't worked. I felt absolutely everything.

It did stop my contractions, however. This resulted in an injection of hormones to start labour again! Now I went from 4 cm to 10 cm in no time. It was extremely violent and painful. Trying to hold your breath and push – while being so big and in so much pain – was the biggest effort I have had to make in my whole life. The pain I felt is just not possible to describe, so excruciating that you believe you will never get there.

When Charlie was stuck in the pelvic bone for a little while was the worst moment. At that point, I couldn't endure it, not anymore. I believe that my mind protected itself, that it left my body to cope with the experience. I remember seeing myself on the bed, watching myself from above. Some people would refer to this as sort of a near-death experience.

Charlie was finally born after my obstetrician (who followed me for the births of my 2 children and whom I regard highly) had to do an episiotomy with my consent, when he was starting to get worried because Charlie's head wouldn't go through. My husband told me later that we could see her crown, but I wasn't large enough to deliver her. I believe that he had to cut me twice to have her. The sensation of torture and relief at the same time was very weird. It almost felt that I was losing my guts instead of giving birth.

I didn't hold my daughter (that *thing* I had just expulsed from my body) straight away, as the midwives had to take her for their necessary routine. Something was wrong; she wasn't crying and her lips were blue! She wasn't breathing! I found this out later, because at that stage, I was so exhausted from the labour that I was barely conscious. Still, I was trying to understand what was happening. Why couldn't I have my baby? They brought her to me after I heard her crying for the first time. Things were starting to get real.

When they put her on my chest, I could finally identify her as a baby – not necessarily my baby, but it was definitely a little baby – and that it was already trying to find my breast.

At that moment, you think: *That is it. It's finished!* But you still have to make an extra effort of pushing the placenta out and need to be stitched up. I couldn't really care anymore as the pain stopped and all these people in the room were chatting about their weekend, like I wasn't there. My obstetrician was assisting a nurse doing my stitches. I remember being slightly worried at this point, because a few months earlier one of my friends told me how they stitched her up tighter (an old practice that used to be done to satisfy the husband).

Charlie was on my breast for about 2 hours after a long labour. I just wanted one thing, to not be hurt anymore, for my body to be left alone, and to go to sleep! It was already midnight.

Unfortunately, I was one of those who suffer in breastfeeding as well. This was so unbearable that I was screaming in my head. I couldn't really tell which pain was the more excruciating. Between your vagina being destroyed, your perineum being stitched up, your breast being pulled, bitten, pinched and sore, or your uterus starting to contract itself back to its normal size every time you breast feed – who could tell?

I did breastfeed for about 4 months and the fourth month was a real torture. The pain never left me and I would end up in tears every single time. I was extremely thankful when one kind midwife visiting me at home told me about the nipple shield. It really helped me to reduce the pain.

After the first breastfeeding session, my husband didn't have the right to stay with me in the hospital. I tried to stay composed, while inside I was slowly decomposing and crumbling. It was very scary for me. Coming from a country where the fathers have the right to stay and often do stay and help, with his own bed next to his partner and the baby, it was a shock that he could not spend the night.

I recall not really knowing what to do when Charlie was crying in her crib and I was so exhausted. I was singing lullabies and trying to rock her crib while slowly dying of pain and tiredness. I was doing my best for her to be quiet, as I was sharing the room with another lady. It took me a while to understand that what the baby needed was to be on my breast again. It might feel unrealistic, but I can assure you that I was in another world and it didn't occur to me that, after staying on the breast for 2 hours, the little thing needed to be on it again!

The night of torture continued as the staff were constantly coming in the room to care for my neighbour who had had a c-section and therefore needed constant care. I couldn't rest. I had the terrible experience of midwives coming to wake me up every hour and a half to force me to wake up Charlie to breastfeed her. My gut told me that this wasn't right, but you just think the staff know better and again your voice is muzzled. We were in winter, but because Charlie wanted to sleep, they forced me to undress her to wake her up so she could take the breast. I thought it would never end. When I did ask if they could take the baby for a little while and give her a bottle of formula, they laughed and were extremely rude and diminishing, stating that I had to feed her.

The next morning, I remember asking one of the midwives when I would start my perineal education (rehab) and if she would give me a referral to see a physio. She looked at me in a condescending way and abruptly asked me why I needed to see a physio; my birth was normal, she said, and I didn't need it. Another fall from my chair. Again perineal re-education in France is a right that every woman has after giving birth. It is provided and paid for by the Medicare equivalent and you have as many sessions as you need (generally about 10). Now I could understand why I met so many women who told me they were suffering from prolapses, weak pelvic floor etc.

A few days after coming home, I started having visits from 2 different midwives. When the first one asked me how I was coping with breastfeeding, I told her honestly that we had given her a bottle of formula the night before, as I didn't have any more milk and Charlie was still hungry. That woman started lecturing me and told me that I had made a big mistake; I shouldn't have given my child a bottle of formula. I felt like I'd killed my baby and that I was a horrible mother. I did hold my tears back very hard, but as soon as she left, I cried out everything I had. I still recall the guilt I felt. Fortunately, the second midwife, who checked on me few days later, was wonderful and extremely gentle. She told me a few words that gave me a bit of strength back and was just so caring.

Here we are, almost 6 years later and I can still remember everything. I really hope that reading my experience will prevent you some of the suffering, anguish, uncertainty and humiliation that I went through. I hope you never feel the guilt I felt and still feel to this day that I should have done better for myself and my child.

Always remember to use your voice. You have rights. We are not just the vessel that has to bring this child into this world. We are not unimportant. We chose to do this willingly and should be respected for this commitment.

I wish you all the best.

Avec tout mon amour,

(With all my love,)

Clémentine

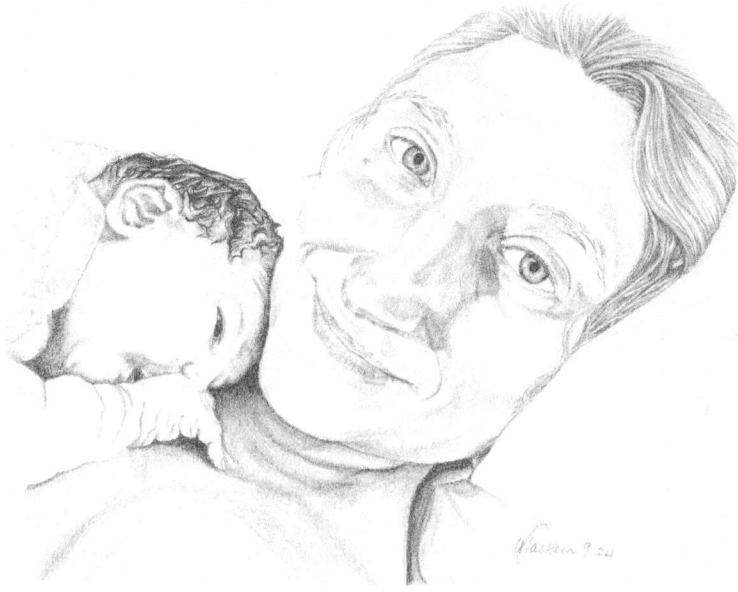

Clémentine with Charlie after her harrowing birthing experience. The depthless love and relief expressed through tired eyes, all while smiling, are testament to the boundless power of a birthing mother.

🌼 Dear Mother Becoming,

Okay, that was hard to read and absorb. Feel the feelings. Incredulity, sadness and rage. Many women can relate to the experiences and emotions Clémentine felt during her labour, birth and early postpartum. Clémentine still does. Big breaths, mama. Tea, chocolate, whatever you need to comfort yourself right now. This is why we are here – to prevent this happening. We want mothers to arrive in their postpartum physically and emotionally well.

Here we are in your fourth trimester with Clémentine. You have arrived at the most important, powerful, transformative evolution of yourself. You are a mother. Forever.

The invisible umbilical cord wound through your entire being transforms 'me to we'. However many times you experience birth, every thought and action automatically considers the 'other', your baby, your child. No matter how old your children are, that cord is with you, grown within you, birthed by you, nourished by you in your heart, mind, body and spirit. There is no return to the woman you were. No 'bouncing back'.

And why would we want to? Through all you have learned of your physiological changes, hormonal influences, your brain, your behaviours, thoughts and feelings, you are altered to the core. We don't need to go back because we have evolved into *something more*. More. That needs to be celebrated, acknowledged, appreciated, valued, treasured and nurtured. I'm so infinitely proud of you, dear mother.

Here, the much-lamented phrase, "Nobody told me what it would be like!" is going to be discussed and put to rest. Because all the letters you have read have told you that mothering is challenging. It is not what society portrays. We'll be discussing the darker side of mothering that no one talks about, because it is perceived as shameful. But it isn't.

Here, we put all we have created together into practice. The foundational elements of self-love, rest, warmth, sleep, nourishing food and support will hold you. Time isn't important. Schedules don't rule. This is a blur where expectations hold no sway. You are the most important being in your world right now. When you are steady, your child will thrive.

Oh, and we can't put a baby back when mothering becomes tough. There's a no returns policy! Yes, occasionally, the "what-the-hell-have-I-done" will surface. You may find yourself saying, "This isn't what I signed up for!" These thoughts, in the haze of fatigue and change, will cross your mind. That's okay and completely normal. This book is about understanding that becoming a mother is an extraordinary life-altering experience. The aim is to arrive at the end of your fourth trimester emotionally, psychologically and physically well, or on the way to being so.

Here are more wise words from Vanessa Olorenshaw: "You thought there were only three trimesters? Well, that's what they want you to think. A couple of days' lie-in if you're lucky. Then get on with it. Back to work with you. Don't be lazy. Share that baby, like a good girl. In fact, many cultures have variations on the fourth trimester theme. The first three months after the birth when the mother is cared for, as she in turn cares for her helpless babe. Yup. Our babies are in need of direct physical contact and sensitive care. Dare I say maternal care? Dare I?"[1] Maternal care is not a concept to be reduced, ignored or shunned, because it is the very foundation of our society.

Feminism left the fourth trimester behind, yet 61% of women in Australia give birth.[2] As Andrea O'Reilly states in her book *Matricentric Feminism, Theory, Activism, Practice*, "Indeed, a mother-centred feminism is needed because mothers – arguably more so than women in general – remain disempowered despite forty years of feminism. [O'Reilly's book] does not rationalise or defend the need for a mother-centred feminism, as it takes it as a given."[3]

Matricentrism values and supports mothers, and understands all the intricacies of matrescence in pregnancy, birthing and the fourth trimester. It is required in this space. *Mother Becoming* is gentle matricentric feminism in action, because it changes the narrative around becoming a mother. Changing the narrative in our own minds from 'less' to 'more', from fear, anxiety, self-silencing and subservience to self-trust, empowerment and confidence in thought and action.

Matricentrism alters how we see and value ourselves, how we hold autonomy and sovereignty over our bodies. It ensures we accept nothing less than respectful language and fully informed care. It also fills us with confidence to make our own consented choices and have those choices respected. It moves us to demand best practice based on the overwhelming evidence for continuity of midwifery carer. Research that benefits pregnant and birthing women, reduces intervention, birth trauma and primary caesarean section needs to be put into action in a timely manner, not up to 20 years later! It advocates for a system of maternity care that values women over the dollar.

In your fourth trimester, rest needs to come from a place of strength, rather than a place of shame or laziness. Asking for support is a normal thing to do. Value your recovery from birth with the integrity and respect it deserves, no longer coming from a place of 'failing' because you can't do and be it all. In our culture, unattainable expectations are placed on new mothers. This chapter highlights how your village flies into action to support you! That is the way we evolved – to be nurtured and supported in this unique, vulnerable time of recovery. It's when you learn the cues of your baby and fall deeply in love.

You matter, precious mother. Your evolutionary matrescence journey is in full, magnificent, frustrating, bewildering upheaval right now. And that's okay. It's normal.

Our culture of 'you win' if you recover from childbirth, get back to normal and back to the workplace the fastest is damaging. This attitude needs to be overturned. What do you win in this race exactly? Whose approval are you seeking? What ideal might you be trying to live up to? Is it real or an illusion?

A lot of this change will come from you, dear mother, and we will continue to explore empowering you – in your identity, autonomy, agency, and in finding authentic ways to mother that work for you.

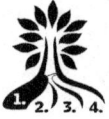

The Physical, Hormonal and Emotional Influences on the Fourth Trimester

This is a time to nurture the mother, who in turn will be stronger to nurture the baby, providing an environment of closeness, safety and bonding outside of the womb. It's when we recognise and support the mother as she undergoes significant hormonal, physical, emotional and neuroplastic changes; it is a time of recovery and transition. If we began to recognise the fourth trimester as a necessary, normal and honoured time to support the new mother in our culture, who knows what benefits would arise?

While reading and researching for this chapter, I found remarkable similarities in the care of new mothers from differing cultures worldwide. There are 5 core elements that are all interlinked and complement each other. They honour the sacredness of this time, and boost oxytocin as a bonus.

Five core elements to honour in the fourth trimester

Retreat from the world with a wise investment in rest: A gentle landing into this altered way of life means sleep, doze, get deep rest on your bed when your baby sleeps, without the temptation to be busy. Day and night melt together in these early months, the babymoon. Please don't rush. Take time and soften into slow living. Respect and acknowledge your body and its needs. Take time to learn your baby's cues and find the rhythm of feeding, comfort, alert times and sleep for both of you. Try to be in bed and around the bed, pottering for the first 2 to 3 weeks or so. Don't lift anything heavier than your baby. Ask other children to climb on the bed to cuddle, rather than lifting them.

Warmth and cosiness: Minimise cold draughts, bright light and media stimulation. Channel all your energy into recovering from birth, healing and promoting breastfeeding. It takes time to heal from birthing, heavy blood loss, a perineal injury or wound or from surgery. Take regular pain relief if you need it, as your comfort is so important for resting, replenishing and restoring. Be comfortable with a belly-bind to support your body.

Nourishing and comforting foods: Eat nourishing foods, snack and drink plenty of fluids, preferably prepared by someone else! Consume snacks during the night too, boosting energy for feeding. Have the freezer well stocked beforehand, even filling the neighbour's or a friend's freezer if possible! Have the pantry well stocked too. The meal train from your village is on the go. If you don't have much family support, employing someone to provide postpartum food is a worthy investment. Someone else does your food shopping, or shop online, having prepared your regular list of items before giving birth.

Touch that is loving: Loving touch is not only for baby, with skin-to-skin, gentle baby massage and kangaroo or carrying care, but also for the mother. Hugs with your partner and other children, gentle head massage and temple rub, neck and shoulders worked out, foot rubs, leg massages or full body. All this shows you love and fills you with a sense of wellbeing. It is a passive form of exercise until physical activity directed at abdominal and pelvic recovery begins. A postpartum doula would do this for you.

Support and companionship: Get support from people who listen, and who hold all those big emotions without judgement or unsolicited advice. This is where we embrace tears, leaky boobs, big pants, hairy legs, mess, baby sick and exhaustion. Receive help from the village with grace. Use that brand-new tool of asking for assistance without fear of being judged. A supported and nourished mum has more capacity to care for her baby as well as herself. Be strong in your boundaries with visitors (helpers) in these early weeks; minimise visiting time unless they are cooking, cleaning, caring for other children, bringing you drinks and snacks, or doing the washing!

We will be exploring more of the above, and how they are practised in other cultures later in this chapter, to help us form new rituals of care. Our westernised medical model of postpartum care is a Cinderella service (the poor relation of maternity care) and provides so little for new mothers. It's time to make changes that honour the importance of postpartum recovery.

Remember, your brain is changing, learning new skills and forming new ways of thinking, seeing the world differently, exchanging priorities, behaving differently. The amazing rewiring process – initiated by hormones and very receptive to oxytocin – happens for your own wellbeing during this time. Your brain does not fall out with the placenta. Your 'mum brain' is a marvel, not to dismissed as 'baby brain' in a derogatory manner by anyone, including yourself. If you put the car keys in the fridge and the milk in the pantry, so what? Your brain is focusing on what is important and doing so in a haze of fatigue.

- **Wishlist** 🌱 *Newborn Mothers* #25. 'Caring for the World's Mothers after Childbirth' ᴬᵖᵖˡᵉ🎙Spotify Talking to Jenny Allison, author of *Golden Month: Caring for the World's Mothers*, is a must-listen episode. Smiley face, gentle nag, please enjoy.
- *Australian Birth Stories* #386. With neuroscientist Dr Sarah McKay ᴬᵖᵖˡᵉ🎙Spotify To help understand the normality of intrusive thoughts and baby blues. It has insight into postpartum depression and the rare occurrence of postpartum psychosis.

Breastfeeding is a full-time job

Prolactin and oxytocin continue to be the major musicians playing through the mind and body, remaining with the mother as long as her breastmilk is suckled from her. Colostrum (first milk) nourishes the baby until transitional milk is produced. This process is often referred to as 'the milk coming in', which happens at 36 to 96 hours after birth. Breasts become very full and tight, also known as becoming engorged, and can be very uncomfortable. Hand expressing some milk to soften the nipple and areola so the baby can latch will help.

Breastmilk becomes mature by about 9 to 30 days postpartum, which is why mum needs to eat and rest in this first month; the energy required to lactate is considerable. She is also learning the skills of feeding, latching, and understanding and responding to baby's cues, while recovering and healing from birth.[4]

Remember, baby's stomach is the size of a cherry in the first few days and feeding every 2 to 3 hours is normal. By day 3, their stomach has grown to the size of walnut, the same time mum is producing more milk (22–27 ml). By the age of one week, the stomach is the size of an apricot at 45–60 ml. By one month, it's an egg with room for 80–150 ml each feed.[5]

Babies are born different sizes, unique in their own little characters. Their suckling is telling mum, "More milk please." Be it 2-, 3- or 4-hourly, they will tell you. Feeding is baby-led. They don't know about clocks or the concept of time. Removing expectations is important, especially if breastfeeding is what you want to do. You have no idea what you are going to experience. A trustworthy and consistent source of support and advice during this time is invaluable. The Australian Breastfeeding Association has a virtual village. Having a doula or a lactation consultant to call or come to the home are further options. The financial cost for these services needs to be considered before birthing, if breastfeeding is something you value deeply.

Typically, mothers' emotions around breastfeeding are not considered enough. Breastfeeding is hard work. How a woman feels about breastfeeding is important and there is no right way to feel. There isn't much honest antenatal education or knowledge among family and friends to support this. Mothers are discharged from hospital with a few visits from the midwife, then a 10-day visit from the child health nurse as a means of support. It's as if they have been left to take a step off a cliff into the unknown without anyone to catch them.

In her book, *Why Breastfeeding Grief and Trauma Matter*, Amy Brown states: "Breastfeeding is more than latching a baby on. It's about understanding normal baby behaviour: how much they feed (lots), how much they sleep (little) and how much they like being put down (basically never) and then how building milk supply and responsive frequent feeding build into all of that to make breastfeeding work."[6] Instead, mothers are often waved off with, "Good luck with that, breast is best, get on with it and succeed, otherwise you have failed." They become isolated with their deep wish to feed, but are advised by well-meaning others to give the baby a bottle and have a bit of a rest, because they come from a generation where bottle-feeding was common. This is why chores like cleaning, laundry, cooking and having support with the care of other children is necessary.

Again, there is no room for judgement for decisions about feeding because each mother's situation and experience is unique. Breastfeeding doesn't flow smoothly for every mother. There may be delay in transition milk production due to a difficult birth. Challenges with the latch of the baby to the breast or tongue tie may make drawing milk from the breast difficult, which leads to reduced milk supply. Then there's sore nipples, different advice, frustration, tears and disappointment. Women so often struggle alone with feelings of grief and failure. They can be angry at being told breastfeeding is natural and instinctive, while having their expectations crushed through lack of informed and compassionate support.

Emotional stress inhibits the flow of oxytocin due to the rise in cortisol from the fight-or-flight response, just like in labour. A mother's emotional wellbeing is extremely important to the flow and production of breastmilk.

There is also a rare condition called dysphoric milk ejection reflex (DMER), where negative emotions are felt with the letdown reflex. This may be a deep hollowness in the stomach, anxiety, hopelessness and dread. Such extreme emotions with breastfeeding make this journey so hard. If this is you, dear mother, please reach out for support and tune in to *The Midwives' Cauldron* episode shared in the resources.

When a mum is struggling, she needs to be seen, acknowledged for her hard work and for doing the best she can with what she has. Language like 'failure to breastfeed' and mum 'gave up' is so damaging. It is important to have a strategy in place before birth: where to go and who to call for support.

- **BA virtual village.** After registration, there are free resources.
  Helpline: 1800 mum2mum or 1800 686 268

- **ABA #11.** 'Supporting the new mother' Apple 🎙 Spotify

- **ABA #E8.** 'Where is my village?' Apple 🎙 Spotify

- **Wishlist** 🌿 **YouTube. Illustrates the flow of water and fat in breastmilk during a feed.** Foremilk, near the nipple, is watery. Hindmilk, back of the breast, is full of fat.
  https://www.youtube.com/watch?v=_Kxr5rzB4ck

- *The Midwives' Cauldron* S4 #13. 'Breastfeeding aversion, agitation and dysphoric milk ejection reflex' Apple 🎙 Spotify

- *Happy Mama Movement* #197. 'Finding Peace with Breastfeeding' Apple 🎙 Spotify

Your and your baby's sleep

In all of this, sleeepppp and rest are significant for establishing breastfeeding. Instead of looking at the clock, listen in to the rhythms of your baby and your body. No expectations or time restrictions. No places to be, other than at home. Soften into the moments. The rock and sway and pat, pat, pat to settle your baby. The long inhalations and long exhalations. Slow down. Pop a 'do not disturb' on the door. Put your phone on silent, with just one friend and family group communicating with you and for you.

This is such a short breadth of time in the whole of your life. Embrace the timeless, the messy, the slow, the help and the support. This is your purpose right now. Mum. Solace. Comfort. Food. Warmth. Security. Touch. Love … For both of you. All the elements to coax and keep oxytocin flowing.

Red light keeps a baby sleepy during the night; white and blue light from TVs, iPads and smartphones stimulates wakefulness. At bath time, usually a few hours before a (flexible) bedtime, the bathroom ceiling lights are like a sun shining in their eyes. That, with toys, is stimulation, not winding down.

When using sound to help baby go off to sleep, it needs to stay on repeat the entire nap or sleep time. Otherwise, when it stops, it stimulates alertness, because the comfort is no longer there. Awareness of being alone in the cot kicks in. Babies' sleep cycle is 50–60 minutes. They surface a bit then. If anything in their environment is different, they wake more fully.

Alpha music is more of a sound and has a 60 bpm rhythm. Leave a single track on repeat. This is similar to the comforting noises of being inside mum, listening to her heartbeat, gurgling intestines and rhythm of her breath. It is nice and familiar and boring. Have a listen to 'Gentle sleep music for babies', available on Spotify, iTunes and other services, to get an idea.

It is important to be in the same room while they sleep, day and night. The first 3 months or so, a baby carrying sling is perfect for warmth, security and breathing in your natural smell. These little beans have been enveloped in a continuous, warm hug inside mum. It's quite a shock to be exposed to bright light, cold air and loud noise. We are a mammalian carrying species. A sling simulates this, while keeping our hands free. We are sold so many devices that encourage separation. Cuddling or sleeping on mum, dad or partner is completely normal.

Smell is useful too. Beyond 3 months, wear a dab of a gentle aromatherapy oil like mandarin, lavender, petitgrain or chamomile. When they sleep in a basket, car seat or cot, a drop nearby will be comforting for the baby.

· **Wishlist** 🌿 *Birth-Ed* S1 #7. 'Understanding Infant Sleep' with Sarah Ockwell-Smith, author of *Why Your Baby's Sleep Matters* ^{Apple} 🎙 ^{Spotify}

Supporting mums worldwide and what we can learn

The most similar westernised society to Australia that provides dedicated postpartum care is the Netherlands. There, it is covered by social insurance and is a legal right. The *kraamzorg*, a registered maternity care provider, who is qualified in postnatal care and breastfeeding support, also helps with light home chores, cooking and fending off too many visitors. They do 3 to 8 hours of work per day in the home. This subsidised postnatal care has an out-of-pocket cost of approximately $8 per hour and is available for an average of 49 hours over 8 days.

The Netherlands has the highest homebirth rate in Europe of between 13 and 14% and takes perinatal care seriously. Some comments from Dutch mothers about the early days were: "We were totally unprepared," and "If you're a new mum or dad, you have no idea." One mother said, "I'm a doctor, so you would expect that I'd know something, and I knew some things, but you really don't have a clue."[7] These mothers treasured having a kraamzorg to be there purely for them, with all the knowledge and support they brought with them.

In Australia, our equivalent is a postnatal doula. We have no subsidy or private insurance provision for this type of care. However, it could be worth considering and saving for a doula to be there for you.

Jenny Allison's book *Golden Month: Caring for the World's Mothers after Childbirth* describes the wisdom of lost practices of postpartum care. Her knowledge of Chinese medicine and collection of lived oral stories from multiple cultures around the world provides the foundation we need to relearn.[8]

The Asian recognition of 6 weeks or 40 days as a time of rest and recovery coincides with the length of time it takes for the placental site inside the uterus to heal, and for blood loss known as *lochia* to settle. Heavy blood loss (*lochia rubra*) usually lasts from 3 to 5 days. *Lochia serosa*, which is thinner and browner, lasts until about the tenth day after birthing. Settling to a yellow to white, *lochia alba* may last up to 6 weeks. If lochia remains heavily red beyond 5 days, it may indicate that some placental or membrane tissue is still in the uterus; if it has a green tinge to it and is smelly, this indicates infection. Both need further investigation and care.[9]

The 40 days is often honoured as 10 days in bed, 10 days around bed, 10 days around the home and then 10 days in the neighbourhood. Indian Ayurvedic wisdom and that of other Asian cultures, such as the Chinese golden month of 4 to 6 weeks, adopt a holistic approach to nurturing the mother. The 40 days is practised in many African and Arabian countries, Russia and Greece. The 6 weeks of *cuarentena* in Latin America also features the 5 elements mentioned on page 259. This time is for retreating from the world, with rest and sleep, warmth, nourishment, loving touch, support and companionship.[10] Sleep, doze and be with your baby to establish breastfeeding. Rest is precious.

Warmth is a key feature, right back to a time when hot water wasn't plentiful and there was no central heating or hair dryers. The essence of the practice is the mother using all her energy to rest, heal and feed, rather than trying to keep warm. So, if you hear about Asian women not washing their hair for 40 days, this is cultural heritage, not being unclean.[11]

And fooooooddddd is a big thing too – nourishing, easy to digest and consumed warm. Four main purposes for the food you eat at this time are: replacing blood loss, replenishing nutrients, repairing damaged tissue and supporting breastfeeding. Bone broth-based soups are frequently promoted as a source of protein and nutrients in Asian cultures. You need foods full of protein, carbohydrates and fats. This may mean easy-to-digest, slow-cooked meals, like soups and porridges. And make sure they're calorific.[12] This isn't a time to think of slimming down, as your body needs energy to recover and fuel to feed your baby.

Allison talks about daily massage, especially the lower legs, to prevent any blood clots, because blood remains *hypercoagulable*, which means it clots more quickly. This is part of the pregnant body preventing too much blood loss at birth. Lack of movement may lead to what is called a *deep vein thrombosis*, a clot in the lower leg, which can cause other medical complications that require immediate medical care.[13] This is why midwives nag mothers about moving the lower legs after having recently given birth. You might point and flex the feet regularly when in bed, or when pottering to the loo. Or do some calf raise exercises.

The use of massage is a passive form of exercise, which encourages good circulation in the legs. Some practices massage the mother with a warm compress and warmed oils filled with warming herbs and spices. The whole body is massaged, including gentle massage of the abdomen in a clockwise rotation, imitating the movement of food through the small and large intestines. This is thought to assist with resettling the abdominal organs, toning the muscles and easing the sense of emptiness after having given birth.[14] Self-massage is soothing too. Postnatal doula Julia Jones demonstrates how to do this in her video in the goody box. It is so nurturing and can be done with your baby too. How good would it be to receive a massage every day? Mmmmm yummy.

Modern women may find some of the older customs of 10 days, 10 days, 10 days and 10 days too restricting. However, we can take elements of these practices and experience a postpartum period that supports and nourishes us as much as possible. We must truly believe we are worthy and in need of this, because it prevents postnatal depletion, which is sadly a common experience in our society.

Preventing postnatal depletion

Prevention of postnatal depletion is better than having to cure it, let alone suffer it. As Dr Oscar Serrallach, the author of *The Postnatal Depletion Cure* describes: "In my clinic, I do not see mothers who have failed or who are not trying hard enough. What I do see every day are mothers who are physically and emotionally depleted, exhausted, and stressed. They are at the end of their tether with no relief in sight."[15] He explains that this is caused by "the time and resource demands of motherhood [being] higher than ever, and unfortunately, it's becoming increasingly difficult for parents to easily access the non-hired help of a family and community to assist in looking after children. This mismatch between expectation and support, stacked on top of nutrient depletion, leads directly to mothers feeling overwhelmed. A new mother's biology is not designed and shouldn't be expected to have to deal with this level of ongoing and constant demands."[16]

Dr Serrallach has a lovely way of talking about postpartum as a 'feminine upgrade' with all the changes of matrescence. He has a holistic representation of the physiological, emotional and psychological perspective. Seeing this as a 'superpower' of mothers is a beautiful narrative for reframing the challenges mothering can bring. His definition of postpartum is 7 years after a birth, not 6 weeks for physical recovery, not 6 months for a check-in on mum's psychological wellbeing. He states: "Postnatal depletion is a constellation of symptoms affecting all spheres of a mother's life after she gives birth. These symptoms arise from physiological issues, hormonal changes, and interruptions of the circadian day/night rhythm of her sleep cycle, layered with psychological, mental, and emotional components."[17]

So, it isn't just one thing. It's everything. Invest in yourself. Invest in rest, recuperation and restoring your long-term emotional wellbeing too. If you are already a mum and are feeling deeply fatigued, you could see a holistic or integrative GP practitioner. They investigate all the essential micronutrients, minerals and vitamins, and hormonal and cortisol levels, alongside physical and emotional wellbeing and lifestyle.

One of the main aims of this book is to provide ways of approaching your pregnancy, birthing and postpartum experience to prevent postpartum depletion. Living a slow postpartum is key. Many families in Australia are immigrants, so extended family assistance may not be possible. Among Asian cultures, mothers, mothers-in-law or grandmothers come to stay for 3 to 6 months to support the new mother by taking over household chores and cooking.

By creating a village, a virtual village of support and information, and by harnessing friends, family, neighbours and surrounding community, maybe having saved for a postpartum doula or lactation consultant, we can create a different kind of family and postpartum experience. In one Australian state, an aunties community of mature women provides meals for isolated mums. We need more aunties.

- Self-Massage with Julia Jones. YouTube
  https://newbornmothers.com/blog/the-newborn-mothers-ultimate-guide-to-self-massage
- Wishlist 🎙 *Happy Mama Movement* #111. 'Postnatal Depletion with Dr Serrallach' Apple 🎙 Spotify
- 'Village aunties supporting new mums in action' YouTube.
  https://www.youtube.com/watch?v=S8CDfosvK0Q

Practical recovery information and tips

As we chatted about with Alysia, comfort is really important, so regular pain relief, hygiene, rest and good nutrition all promote healing.

Spritz your bits

As a nurturing and comforting practice, try the following spritz from *For Modern Mothers*. Keep a spray bottle (glass if possible) in the fridge handy. Lightly use on your vulva and perineum after a wash or after having a wee or poo.

For each 100 ml:

50 ml witch hazel (from any chemist)

50 ml cooled boiled water

5 drops lavender essential oil

5 drops tea tree essential oil (or 10 drops lavender if tea tree is too expensive)

Shake the ingredients together and spritz your bits for comfort.

Another fabulous hack for a cool pack is to lightly smooth some aloe gel (with nothing else added) on a pad, then lightly spray on the above spritz (not soaking the pad). Fold and freeze plenty in a ziplocked bag or box. When you need to change your pad, take one out of the freezer. After a few minutes, it is soft enough to pop in your pants. Bliss. Prepare some before birth, then have one of your dream team continue to prepare them for you.

Leaking wee, fanny farts, farts, and poop accidents!

Nothing is off limits in our discussion in this physical element. We will explore leaking wee, fanny farts, farts, heaviness or bulge in the vagina, and poop accidents. So often, mothers are embarrassed by these symptoms and suffer in silence. This needs to stop. I don't want to scare you out of becoming a mother, but pelvic recovery is an issue that doesn't have enough air time or resources to prevent possible issues in the first place. We don't want you to wonder: *Why did no one tell me?* This is why we started the pelvic floor connection with Samantha in the middle months of pregnancy in Chapter 2.

I introduced the video, *A simple way to find your pelvic floor muscles*, from the Continence Foundation of Australia. The 'Pelvic floor health for expectant and new mums' PDF by the Pregnancy Centre and Continence Foundation of Australia is on Samantha's **wishlist** .

No matter what kind of birth, even caesarean, there is no need to put up with a urine leak, fanny farts, farts, or a slight poop when lifting a toddler, jumping, exercising or sneezing after giving birth. Pelvic floor exercises are really important and rectify most of these symptoms.

If this is happening, after doing your exercises or even if you haven't, please don't suffer in silence. Currently, if severe pelvic floor injury is recognised as a chronic health condition lasting over 6 months, Medicare offers 5 appointments in a calendar year via a plan that has 3 health professionals on the team. These are: your GP, who you need to see to arrange this; a physiotherapist; sometimes an obstetrician or psychiatrist.

The lack of postpartum pelvic recovery support in Australia really isn't good enough. As Clémentine mentioned in her letter, in France every new mother is offered 10 free sessions with a pelvic health physiotherapist, no matter how they have birthed. We need this too. Please talk to someone. You are not alone. Gentle nag.

We chatted with Katie about Dr Thompson's work, where she says: "Women are suffering birth injuries and are left feeling unprepared, unheard, disbelieved and dismissed. This needs to change."[18] We don't go around with an outward sign of injury and weakness of the pelvic floor, but we do get lots of adverts for pads to cover 'oops' moments. That's not okay. It's not okay to let us just put up with it. I think every pad should come with a peel-off sticker that says, 'Have you seen a pelvic health physiotherapist?' Then we need to provide pelvic health recovery for every mother as part of postpartum care.

The tummy gap

Now on to the tummy gap, called *diastasis rectus abdominis* (DRA), where the muscles of the abdomen part as the body makes room for the expanding uterus. This is why, after birthing, there is a feeling of 'jelly belly' as the muscles take time to come back together. It can feel as if the organs of the body are wobbling all over the place, unsupported. Belly-binding or a belt can be source of support and comfort after birth. They are not a substitute for the gentle exercises though!

In her book, *Why Did No One Tell Me? How to Protect, Heal and Nurture Your Body Through Motherhood*, Emma Brockwell tells us that the abdominal muscles draw together again in the weeks after birth. However, for about one-third of mothers, a gap between the muscles remains. It's not clear why, but the risk factors of many babies, genetics, heavy and poor lifting technique, straining for a poo, coughing, sneezing, straining and excessive load in exercise early after birth have been identified as coinciding with increased intra-abdominal pressure, which in turn doesn't help DRA.[19] Vicious cycle.

Having DRA doesn't mean you are broken, but it can affect your self-esteem and mental health. With proper rehabilitation advice, abdominal wall function can heal. However, as Brockwell notes, "...

fear and lack of understanding of DRA are some of the most limiting factors for anyone living with it".[20] Working with a physiotherapist and or a good personal trainer helps, as does avoiding constipation. So, plenty of fluids and nourishing foods that get poop going. Take your time with exercise. Be mindful of posture and careful of how much weight you're lifting. As always, sleep and rest when you can.[21] Nag, nag.

In the resources there is a video on how to feel for diastasis recti. There are also exercises to help repair, tone, strengthen and restore the abdominal muscle function. If DRA is significant, the same Medicare rebate as for pelvic floor complications is available.

Can you see the theme running through this element? Rest, food, time for you, care for your body. You matter.

- Reminder: *Beyond the Bump* S1 #35. 'All things pelvic floor (and why we shouldn't put up with pissing ourselves)' Apple 🎙 Spotify

- Reminder: *Great Birth Rebellion* #21. 'Perineal suturing' Apple 🎙 Spotify

- Reminder: *Great Birth Rebellion* #19. 'Perineal bundle' Apple 🎙 Spotify

- 'Spritz your bits' recipe from For Modern Mothers. https://www.formodernmothers.com/blog/soothing-spray-pads-for-your-post-baby-perineum

- Reminder: A simple way to find your pelvic floor muscles'. YouTube 'https://www.youtube.com/watch?v=q0_JAoaM6pU&t=4s

- Reminder: Pelvic floor health for expectant and new mums PDF https://continence.my.salesforce.com/sfc/p/#A0000000KUc9/a/5K0000003lek/nEDoZ3oU8.RlEab2f0E7RQ_RYNAeSA1rtAjEgDcSf0g

- 'Diastasis Recti' Physiotherapist Michelle Kenway. YouTube. https://www.pelvicexercises.com.au/diastasis-recti-exercises/

- Reminder: Active Pregnancy Foundation website. 'Find Your Active' downloadable guides https://www.activepregnancyfoundation.org/findyouractive

---

Healing after caesarean birth

Healing from a caesarean includes everything we have talked about so far – and healing from major abdominal surgery. So, with a few bells and whistles added on. Please remember, deep in your bones that you, dear mother, have achieved the extraordinary. Anyone having this surgery would normally be off work for 6 weeks, which isn't a luxury you have. Not only are you recovering from major surgery, but you are also healing from being pregnant, with the added request of your body to make milk on broken sleep. You are amazing.

The milk coming in may be a little delayed due to recovering from surgery, but that doesn't mean it won't happen. Lots of support with skin to skin, suckling time and love bombing your baby helps immensely. The ability to lift, hold, carry and position your baby to feeding in comfort helps oxytocin to flow. Here, being in the present, hour by hour, day by day, slow, gentle, kind, patient, and with gracious acceptance of support, is needed. Having a village of support will be incredibly comforting if caesarean birthing is your experience.

The average hospital stay is 3 to 4 days and you may be sent home with Clexane injections (blood thinning medication) because they are usually prescribed for about a week.[22] Your midwife will show you how to give yourself these injections or show your partner. You'll also get a disposable sharps box to take back to the pharmacy when finished.

Recovery from caesarean birth will take longer than vaginal birth, and there is an 8% chance of a wound infection. It's difficult to see over your belly, so look at the wound in the mirror or have your partner do so. If there is any redness or swelling, discharge or opening of the wound, please call your GP. Adequate pain relief to support mobility is incredibly important, because being able to get in and out of the bed or chair, as well as go to the toilet in comfort, helps healing.[23]

· Australian Birth Stories website. 'Mothers stories of caesarean birth' https://australianbirthstories.com/

Resuming your sex life after birth. No longer a taboo subject

Here we have another minefield of a topic that is rarely properly or openly discussed with common sense and sensitivity. The spontaneity of romantic sex rarely happens in the first few years after birth. The reality of little people's needs interrupts the mojo. A bit of planning is required.

The main thing is to not feel pressured that you 'should' be resuming intercourse, because libido is deeply affected after birth. The same hormone that promotes milk production (prolactin) decreases the sex hormones oestrogen and testosterone, so libido is suppressed. So, breastfeeding is a bit of a libido dampener. Quite often, women feel sensual with the surge in oestrogen around ovulation, which makes sense from a biological perspective, because that's when conception occurs. However, with oestrogen dampened down during exclusive breastfeeding, ovulation is supressed. (This is not a completely fail-safe option for contraception though.)

The new mother is also getting plenty of oxytocin hits from breastfeeding and skin-to-skin cuddles, so there isn't as much need to get it from her partner. In Dr Serrallach's words: "If your body has to choose between the needs of a breastfeeding baby and those of an eager-beaver partner, whom do you think is going to get chosen? Your baby of course!"[24] If both partners know what is happening on a biological and family needs level, it takes the pressure off. Broken sleep for both parents isn't sensuality-inducing either.

Emma Brockwell's book acknowledges women's worries about having sex after childbirth. Worries include feeling decidedly unsexy, unsure of their changed body, and fearful that penetrative sex will be painful or pull apart any scar (which it won't). Women need to feel desirable, to feel desire, and to have time to become aroused and uninhibited enough to fall into sensuality. This is lot to ask when tired, when sex hormones are suppressed, and when possibly feeling touched-out after having children permanently attached.[25]

For the first few times of intercourse, being on top with plenty of lube and controlling the depth of penetration and motion may make you feel more confident. It's also normal with orgasm to let down breastmilk, because lots of oxytocin has just been produced. For 20% of mothers, urine leaks during orgasm too, which can be due to a weak pelvic floor or overactive bladder. Please try not to be embarrassed. You are not alone. It would be a shame if it put you off having sex. Having a wee before intercourse helps, as well as doing pelvic floor exercises. If leaking persists, or if intercourse is painful, please see your GP and get a referral to see a pelvic health physiotherapist.

With a drier vagina when breastfeeding, a tight pelvic floor or scarring, painful sex called *dyspareunia* may occur, which is why I mentioned lube.[26] Putting up with pain is simply not okay. Something can be done to help you. Your sex life matters.

> · **Wishlist** 🌿 *Beyond the Bump* #232. 'Will I ever feel like having sex again? with sexologist Juliet Allen' Apple 🎙 Spotify
>
> In this conversation, nothing is off the table. They cover feelings of uncertainty around when to resume sex after birth, readiness, discomfort, communication with your partner around resuming intimacy, loss of libido, lube, time needed to get the mojo going and ways of sensual expression other than penetrative sex.

Contraception for spacing pregnancy

So, having talked about sex after birth, a chat about contraception might be useful here! Better Health Channel is a good go-to website, with advice on when to begin contraception after birth. You will need to choose what suits your body and lifestyle from the types of contraception available.

If breastfeeding exclusively night and day for 6 months, ovulation will be suppressed. This is because prolactin inhibits the ovaries' response to the **follicular stimulation hormone** and a few other hormones that would be involved in getting an egg ready for release. With exclusive breastfeeding, menstruation usually returns at 4 to 5 months, but can take as long as 2 years. However, ovulation can still be happening, so contraception is advisable from 3 months. Choice of contraception is limited while breastfeeding because some contraceptives will suppress lactation.

If not breastfeeding, contraception should begin 3 weeks after giving birth, which is a big must-know. Commonly, mothers are guided to wait for the 6-week check-up with the GP and talk about contraception before resuming their sex life then. This is unrealistic as not every mother wants to wait that long, so contraception with a barrier method is a must.

> · Contraception. Better Health Channel website.
>
>   https://www.betterhealth.vic.gov.au/health/healthyliving/contraception-after-giving-birth

Talking about postpartum depression and anxiety

New mothers' emotional and psychological wellbeing is of paramount importance. This chapter holds the deep wish to prevent or rapidly identify postpartum depression, birth trauma and PTSD. This is why there have been many resources, ideas and practices, scattered throughout – we want to reduce the risk. We don't always have family and friends for emotional or practical support, particularly as we are a country of many immigrants. Building a village may be hard, especially if the mother is experiencing social anxiety and depression in pregnancy and postpartum. Even in the best of circumstances, new parenting can be extremely challenging.

Postpartum depression and anxiety **do not discriminate.** Pregnancy and birth could have been smooth, glowing, with a lovely supported physiological birth, and plenty of help through a village. Or full of vomiting, a rough time being pregnant, disliking every moment, with a long unsupported labour and traumatic birth, and no village whatsoever. It can hit any new mother. No matter her circumstances.

No matter her pregnancy or birth experience. No matter how wanted the baby is.

As mentioned previously, one in 5 mothers experiences postpartum anxiety and depression. These are just the mothers we know about. Because of the associated stigma, shame and feelings of failure, there are mothers out there suffering alone. Society and the system have failed these mothers. Opportunities to care for mothers are being missed, and these gaps in points-of-contact with mothers need to be filled. Mothers also need to feel unjudged and able to reach out for support.

Intrusive, horrible thoughts are common. Mums rarely share these thoughts because they feel appalled and ashamed of themselves for thinking them, but thoughts such as *I don't want to do this anymore* are not unusual. Listen to 'Intrusive Thoughts? You're not alone' with Dr Caroline Boyd.

Important note: We use 000 for emergencies in Australia. Ask for the Emergency Department, not Accident and Emergency.

None of this is meant to scare you or take away from the want, excitement and joyfulness of becoming a mother. However, the hard facts are that the occurrence of postpartum depression in Australia is significant. This book has journeyed towards identifying it, reducing it, and removing the shame, stigma and failure in our internal and external narrative. So, what else can we do? In her book *Why Postnatal Depression Matters*, Mia Scotland writes that we don't have time for culture to change; we can acknowledge mothers' and fathers' support needs now. She offers DIY steps if you think you may have depression.[27]

Drawing from and expanding on Mia's steps:

- **Tell people:** Lift the silence and suffering. You have not failed in any way. This is a huge step, but please take it. Listen to those who love you if they say they think you might have depression. It may be confronting, but please take notice of them and try not to be angry or feel judged on your mothering skills. Sometimes it's difficult to find clarity when you're treading water with your nose barely above to take a breath.

Speak to your midwife or child health nurse. PANDA has a great PDF form called 'I need help', which is an extra **wishlist** 🖋 item in this section. It will help you see how you are travelling and has tickbox answers and space to write what else you want to say. It can then be used to show someone what is happening with you, if you do not have the words.

Make an appointment with your GP. Give the 'I need help' form to your GP, because it highlights the significance of your feelings. The "all mums are tired and get a bit down" answer given by GPs isn't enough. Don't be fobbed off. Ask your GP to refer you to the Gidget Foundation for free telehealth counselling, and give them a call, especially if you are a rural or remote mum.

- **Accept offers of help:** If your GP offers to refer you to a counsellor, psychologist or psychiatrist as part of a mental healthcare plan, please take it. Medicare subsidises 10 sessions with a mental healthcare plan. If you need treatment in the form of medication for a while, it's okay. Dearest mother, you are stronger for acknowledging you need help and softening enough to accept it with grace. Allow practical help. Stay strong in emotional boundaries, and tend to your emotional needs, rather than others'. It's okay not to love being a mum. It's not okay to be lost in feelings of confusion, overwhelm, grief, shame and utter despair, while not sleeping, being wired all the time and exhausted beyond hope.

- **Ask for help:** Reach out. Ask to be held, told you are loved and are doing the best you can. Ask for space … Some time to yourself, even for an hour. Get a cleaner, go to a yoga class alone, take a walk in a park with nothing to hold but a bottle of water. Begin to find yourself again.

Amy Taylor-Kabbaz, in her book, *Mama Rising: Discovering The New You Through Motherhood*, gently points out: "We have lost the ability to listen to our own wisdom and treat ourselves like we would our best friend. We have completely disconnected from our true self, so we go searching for anything that feels a little like connection in the form of our phones. But what we are really aching for is a connection to ourselves."[28]

Through the breathing practices, meditations and yoga, the intention to reconnect mind, body and spirit has been held throughout this book. To acknowledge that mind, body and spirit are intricately linked has been an essential part of finding ways to reconnect to your own extraordinary abilities. Use these practices to self-soothe and soften into in times of distress and bewilderment, with the intention of kindness and self-compassion. At this point, listen to *Happy Mama Movement's* 'Why we struggle receiving help' to help clarify your thoughts and know you are worth being supported. You don't have to do it all alone.

Another resource to draw from if experiencing anxiety and depression is the online video courses for new and expecting parents on the PANDA website. They are free, with email registration to join the learning hub. Your COPE app and partner emails will be continuing to support you too. Why not pop onto their websites to find what you need? Having contact numbers and resources ready is part of supporting your fourth trimester. That way, in the fog of fatigue, if you need to reach out, the useful information is easily accessible. Remember, emotional and psychological vulnerability is not a failing; it just is.

The 6-week postnatal check with the GP looks at physical recovery and wellbeing, touches on mental health and explores contraception. Baby is examined too. There is a time constraint though. Although we now see greater awareness of maternal mental health assessment at 6 weeks, I would encourage you to make an appointment just for you too. This tends to be the last point of contact for maternity care that has any focus on you. The focus of health care from here on is now primarily on your baby.

As a touchstone, please complete the PANDA 'I need help' form, mentioned just before. Be honest with yourself as you do. Remember, your physical and emotional health come first. When you are being cared for, you are more able to care for your baby.

We talked a lot about birth trauma with Katie. Reading the letters from Katie, Alysia and Clémentine has made this very real. We have seen how birth trauma leads to physical and psychological pain, bewilderment, feelings of failure and isolation. We know that one in 10 mothers who experience birth trauma develop PTSD. Offered with Katie, here is a gentle reminder to have another look at the Make Birth Better 'Am I Traumatised?' PDF questionnaire. If you tick any of those boxes, print it out and take to your GP at any time. PTSD doesn't fit a timeline of 6 weeks. It can be many months or even years before symptoms happen. That is the same with PND.

Partners matter too. If they are struggling, please encourage them to complete the PANDA 'How to find help for partners' PDF and see their GP. Recommendation 5 of the NSW inquiry into birth trauma proposes to "improve mental health support for women and families affected by birth trauma by including psychological support in public postnatal care, ensuring that parents have access to psychological support beyond the immediate post-partum period, reviewing the funding needs … to increase Medicare-rebatable psychological support for new parents to reduce gap fees and enable access to the number of sessions clinically required".[29] Bring it on.

- **Wishlist** 🪶 Pregnancy Uncut S1 #4. 'The Silent Sea: Postnatal depression and anxiety' ^Apple 🎙 Spotify
  In this episode, Dr Kara Thompson chats with Jo, a mother who shares her story of her silent suffering. She speaks of how opportunities to care for her were missed. When crisis finally hit Jo and she just couldn't get out of bed, this became the turning point in her journey of recovery. Hannah Jenson, a clinical psychologist, identifies gaps in care, where things can be missed, and the points-of-contact to reach out to for support.

- *Birth-Ed* S2 #4. 'Intrusive Thoughts? You're not alone' with Dr Caroline Boyd ^Apple 🎙 Spotify

- **The Gidget Foundation website.** Provides a free 'Start Talking' telehealth service and is full of useful supportive information for partners and families too.
  https://www.gidgetfoundation.org.au/support/start-talking-telehealth
  Phone: 1300 851 758
  Email: Self-referral contact@gidgethouse.org.au

- *Happy Mama Movement* #165. 'Why we struggle receiving help' ^Apple 🎙 Spotify

- **Hub on the PANDA website.** https://learning.panda.org.au/external/catalogue?tenancyId=2
  Reminder: PANDA PDF 'I need help' https://pandasfoundation.org.uk/wp-content/uploads/2024/02/I-need-help-womenbirthing-people.pdf

- **Reminder: MBB 'Am I Traumatised?'** https://www.makebirthbetter.org/pdf-downloads-parents

- PANDA 'How to find help for partners' PDF https://pandasfoundation.org.uk/wp-content/uploads/2024/01/How-to-find-help-partners.pdf

Strong posture as a foundation for recovery

The foundation for recovery is good posture: standing in a way that engages the legs, pelvis, abdomen, head and spine in good alignment. The tone and strength of this foundation allows for postpartum recovery, as you engage the core, protect the lower back and draw the abdomen inwards. This assists in engaging the pelvic muscles too. Good posture also prevents and eases backache. Strong posture when baby-wearing will be a wonderful exercise in itself. In the moments like waiting for the kettle to boil or cleaning your teeth, use them as a reminder to stand there and practise pelvic floor exercises.

Find a postnatal yoga or Pilates mums and baby class, not only for the physical, but also to connect or reconnect with other mums for that all-important community to nourish the spirit too. You could even form a walking group together.

Practice offering: Ishwara Pranidhana and shower meditation

Ishwara Pranidhana is from the Yoga Sutras of Patanjali. It is often interpreted as surrender, devotion, and love of the Divine or a higher power.[30] We begin the practice of ishwara pranidhana with recognising the Divine within ourselves as a beautiful part of life in the context of our vast universe.

Here, it may be surrendering into this new evolution of yourself as a mother. Now that 'me' has become 'we', you may need some softening of the ego, no longer holding on to 'I' during this early time of transition. This will allow the space for evolution to take place, reducing conflicting emotions and identities. You are still you. Yet now more. You may be lost for a little while in the blur of newborn care. Here's a gentle reminder to surrender to the hours of feeding, pacing, patting and calmly shushing. Allow yourself time to just be. You are Divine.

This time-out shower meditation allows the breath and senses – in mindful, present awareness – to do the talking for you. Time slows as a minute expands, feeling so much longer than usual. This is peaceful yet attentive rest just for you.

- See water streaming in droplets as a spray, ready to welcome you. Begin to breathe deeply, fully, expanding for a long, slow, steady count in until full to brimming with moisture-laden air. Allow the breath to fall away in a sigh, fully emptying on a looonnnggg outward breath, shoulders releasing.

- Step into the fall of water slowly, noticing the feel of thousands of drops of water landing on your skin. Just stand, facing the spray, and continue your breathing pattern. Feel, see, smell and listen without doing anything for a long, delicious minute.

- When busy thoughts come in, without judgement, come back to the breath and senses.

- Pop your face under the fall of water, allowing it to kiss your skin in a position that feels comfortable for you. Breathe in. Just stand there. No expectation, no demands, just be. Notice what feels nice. Feel the warmth, the gentle massage of thousands of water drops, the warmed moist air travelling through your nose.

- Another minute passes by, but feels longer somehow.

- Take your time to reach for the soap. Purposefully, gently massage your body as though you had all the time in the world. Note the changes in sensation and smell. Wrap your arms around yourself in a gentle hug or place your hand on your heart. Just stand as the soap rinses away.

- Step out, wrap yourself in a towel and breathe again. Notice the differing quality of sensation on your skin. It may be a tingle, warmth, the soft touch of the towel. Slowly dry your face, neck and body.

- Once again, just stand and take a few long breaths.

- With no sense of hurry, reach for your moisturiser or some oil. Gently massage it into your skin. Long sweeping strokes of the limbs with a clockwise swirl over your belly. Allow it to sink in, brushing your hair or cleaning your teeth, as it absorbs.

- Aaaahhhhhhh … fresh, clean, tingly, ready for the rest of the day or night.

Practice offering: Neck and upper body stretch

This lovely neck and upper body stretch is another soothing practice to release from the bent over, forward-folding position adopted during seated feeding. Being aware of posture and doing some gentle movement while breastfeeding may be a perfect way to decompress.

- Scan through your body, noting where you may be holding any tension.

- Wiggle a little, your baby having a wiggle with you.

- Begin with lengthening from the base of the spine to the top of the head on the in-breath, then releasing and softening on the out-breath.

- Use a gentle seated Cat–Cow stretch, inhale wide and deep with a long count of 5.

- Open the chest outwards and roll back the shoulders.

- Allow your head to feel heavy as it drops back, lengthening the chin upwards.

- As you exhale, curl over your baby, shoulders roll in, chin to chest, head heavy, expelling the breath on a long count of 6.

- Feel into the lengthening of the entire spine and neck.

- Take a shallow breath here and send it to your neck, upper back and shoulders, seeing them opening and lengthening, softening.

- Sigh it out.

- On the next inhalation, come back to sitting upright.

- With the out-breath, allow your head to fall towards one shoulder, releasing and lengthening the opposite side of the neck.

- Take another breath here and see it opening the vertebra in the neck with soft white light.

- Inhale, coming back to upright.

- Exhale, taking the head to the other shoulder, repeating the neck-opening breath.

- Repeat as many times as you like, becoming present in the moment with yourself and baby.

- Calm any racing thoughts and let go of the temptation to be distracted by social media or the buzzing of notifications.

- Listen to music or an audiobook instead.

- Your baby will sense you settling into a calm energy. They pick up on everything.

We began exploring ahimsa with Liesja in Chapter 1, particularly in how we speak to ourselves. When thinking about returning to exercise, do so with those qualities in mind: gentleness and compassion extended to your body without haste or judgement. Take your time when you begin to exercise again and really listen to your body. Bring patient awareness to the contraction and release of muscles as you exercise. Tone, strength and stability will return with time.

- Posture and Alignment Pilates with Lucy Filce YouTube. https://www.youtube.com/watch?v=an96ARErOkE

- 'Heal abdominal separation and rest' YouTube. Shows how the essence of ahimsa is embodied in this yoga practice, which is gentle, slow and restorative. https://www.youtube.com/watch?v=8YH9Crd5pWA

- 'Mum and bub yoga playtime' YouTube. Gentle practice with graduated change with your baby present. https://www.youtube.com/watch?v=FcZUiQl7N4w

- 'Build core strength 1' YouTube. If you have had a caesarean, start after 6 to 8 weeks. Remember, we can only see the outside scar, the layers of muscle, tissue and the wound on the uterus are healing too. With this in mind, have patience before engaging in stronger exercise. https://www.youtube.com/watch?v=r26RqJrmOOM

Fourth trimester yoga flow: Restore and bond

Welcome back! Yoga with your baby is an entirely different experience. Be prepared for plenty of interruptions the first few times you practise together. Your baby will gradually learn that yoga with you is a fun interaction, and will feel calm with you at the end of the practice. This flow works on strong posture, bringing the rectus abdominus muscles together and strengthening the pelvic floor and lower back. Skip standing sequence 14–19 if you are too tired today. Be kind to yourself. It's not a competition to 'bounce back'. No such thing. The changes that pregnancy and birth have made to your body are unique to you. Postpartum yoga needs to be practised with the qualities of ahimsa. Gentleness, compassion and patience towards your body and mind.

When attending a class, please don't feel frustrated if you only do half it, or none of it, due to feeding or if your baby is unsettled. You will still learn the postures to do at home by listening and observing other mums. Yoga is also about community and connection. Feed and change your baby whenever they need it. Have a mat and toys for your baby and be ready to move them as you move postures. It's fun when babies begin to crawl and investigate each other!

1. Begin in a reclined or side-lying position, baby beside you. Use props if you wish. Scan through your body and notice any tension or discomfort and send your breath with a thought to soften that area. Practise 3-part breath for 5 rounds. Begin to find a sense of stillness within your mind and body.

2. Move to a comfortable seated position, baby in front of you or in your lap. Sit tall. Soften the pelvic floor then practise 5 rounds of pelvic floor lifting. Begin by isolation of the urethra only. It may just be

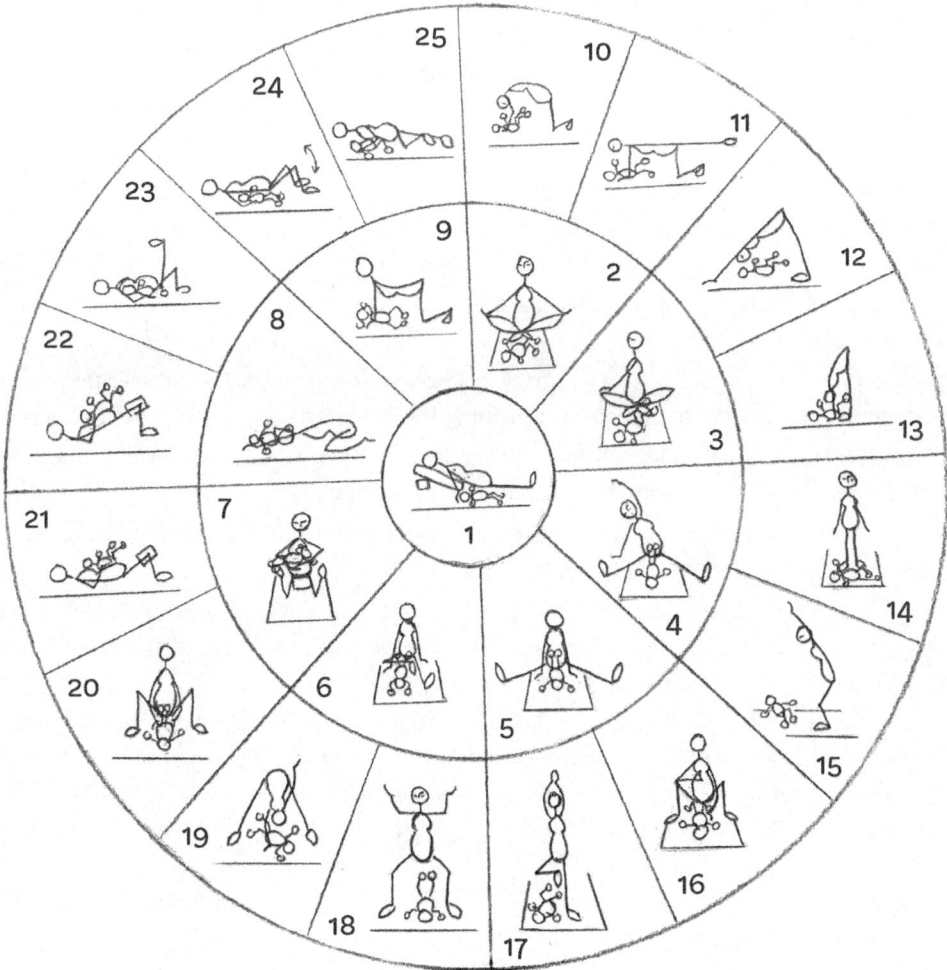

a thought to that area; imagine it lifting to begin with. That's okay. Reconnection comes with time. Lift, lift a bit more, hold for one breath cycle. Lower a little then full release. Repeat with the vagina, then the anus. Then all 3 together. Fully soften the pelvic floor between postures.

3. Place the left hand on the right knee, right hand on the floor behind you. If baby is in your lap, just the right hand behind you. Inhale, sit tall. Imagine a line between the hip bones drawing them together and engage your abdominal muscles. Again, this may feel very slight to begin. It's okay. Exhale, turn to the right, look over your right shoulder. Inhale to upper chest, exhale into the twist a little more, then release. Repeat on the other side, then both sides twice more. Keep your abdomen engaged.

4. Wide-legged sideways bend, one arm overhead and one hand on the floor or your baby. Look up to the raised elbow. Keep your abdomen engaged, particularly on the lift to sit upright. Both sides 3 times.

5. Wide-legged forwards fold. Sit tall, fold forwards at the hips, hands either side of your baby. Blow kisses to them. Tickle them as you sink a bit more with each exhalation onto your forearms. Engage your pelvic floor as laughter in this pose might leak wee. That's okay too!

6. Seated forwards bend with bent left knee, the sole of your left foot to the inner right thigh. Engage the pelvic floor and bend forwards, with right toes to ceiling. Baby is on the inside of your right leg. More tickles as you gaze at your baby. Repeat for the left side.

7. Move to upright kneeling with a bolster or cushion between your legs, toes tucked under. Hold your baby close to your body if needed. Notice the bolster against your groin, lift the pelvic floor, draw your abdomen in. Inhale and press into the toes and knees to come to upright kneeling, arms extended overhead. Exhale and sink back slowly. Then release the pelvic floor and abdominal muscles. Rest through one breath cycle. Repeat twice.

8. Move to Child's pose. Baby is between your extended arms to touch and reassure them. Soften and release your body. Rest here awhile.

9. Inhale to all fours. Baby's face is directly under yours. Cow pose.

10. Cat pose. With Cat pose, bend your elbows and kiss your baby or blow raspberries on them. Cow to Cat pose 3 times.

11. All fours with a neutral spine, look at your baby, engage your abdomen. Inhale and extend the right leg behind you, pelvis parallel to the floor. Two breath cycles. Exhale to all fours. Repeat on the left side.

12. In all fours, look at your baby and inhale. Exhale and lift to Downward Facing Dog. Pelvic floor soft. Three breath cycles. Walk the hands either side of your baby towards your feet.

13. Step your feet either side of your baby, your arms crossed or hands soft on their belly. Head hangs. Loll a while. Skip 14–19 if you are too tired today. Be kind to yourself.

14. Inhale, with a slight bend in your knees press into feet, uncurl one vertebra at a time and move to Mountain pose. Baby can still be between your hip-width feet. Body fully engaged. Three breath cycles. During your day, remind yourself to return to this posture.

15. Inhale, engage abdomen and pelvic floor and raise the arms over your head. Exhale, bend the knees as if about to sit on a chair. Chair pose. Remain here. Inhale. Exhale, arms straight as they move down past the body to open out like wings behind the hips. Inhale, lift arms up while still in chair pose. Three cycles of breath with the arm movements. Inhale to stand and soften the body. Hold your baby close while in chair pose if needed.

16. Move to a squat, baby in front of you. Do Cow Cat 3 times while in the squat. Lift pelvic floor in Cow, fully release in Cat. Rock from side to side.

17. Press through the feet and come to Mountain pose. Transition to Tree pose. Three breath cycles both sides.

18. Turn to face the long edge of the mat with your baby between your feet. Mountain pose, body engaged. Inhale and widen your stance, arms up in the air into a star shape. Exhale, sink to Goddess pose. Three cycles of breath.

19. Inhale, straighten the legs. Exhale, bend forwards, hands to floor, with a slight bend in the knees if needed. Straight arms. Inhale, reach the right arm up and look to the ceiling. Exhale, hand back down. Tickle your baby. Repeat on the other side. Repeat twice.

20. Move to a squat, baby in front of you. Do Cow Cat 3 times while in the squat. Lift pelvic floor in Cow, fully release in Cat. Rock from side to side.

21. Lie on your back, knees bent with a block held between them, feet on the floor. You may want to put your baby on your chest and belly, their head towards or away from you. Imagine the line between the hip bones and draw it tight. Lift your pelvic floor and tuck your pelvis under, pressing your mid back beneath your belly button into the floor. Keep pressing the block with your knees. Three cycles of breath. With an exhalation, release the press into your back, untuck the pelvis, fully soften the pelvic floor. Take a breath. Repeat twice.

22. Repeat the sequence of 21, press into the feet and lift the pelvis up into Bridge. Press the knees a little more to hold the block more firmly. Lift a little higher with an inhalation. Exhale and slowly uncurl the spine, pelvis and fully soften. Take a breath. Repeat twice.

23. Place your baby beside you so you can concentrate on this abdominal exercise. Repeat the sequence of 21 to support your abdominal muscles and lower back as you extend your right leg. Inhale and slowly lift your right leg up, toes to the face. Exhale and slowly lower it down with a slight pause just before the heel touches the floor. Repeat on the left side. Repeat full sequence twice.

24. Windscreen wipers to wind down.

25. Sávāsana. Meditative rest. Lie on your back, bolster under your knees, baby tucked close. Or lie on your side and breastfeed or cuddle. Wiggle in. Long, slow breaths in and longer breaths out as you scan through your body. Return to natural breath rhythm. Practise the "Oceans embrace a continent" visualisation and meditation at the end of Clémentine's chapter, page 288. Embrace yourself generously. Attend the birth of a new you. You are the One who embraces All that you are. An amazing woman and mother.

Cultural, Herstorical and Political Influences on the Fourth Trimester

Still with me? Great! How many dints are there in the wall from the times you have thrown this book at it? We have had enough herstory, don't you think? So, here we are exploring the cultural and societal expectations of mothering and motherhood that exist right now. The aim is to make some much-needed changes in the way mothers are seen, valued and supported.

"Why didn't anyone tell us this stuff?"

Why did we not know about the monotony, misery, boredom and repetition, about the complexity of mothering? Why is everyone pretending everything is okay, putting a mask on it? When Susan Maushart, journalist and author, had her 3 young children, she was part of an informal mothers group that gathered weekly and asked these questions. She wrote a book about it: *The Mask of Motherhood: How Becoming A Mother Changes Our Lives and Why We Never Talk About It.* In the book, she questions the conspiracy of silence that stops women from speaking about the darker side of their mothering experiences and from acknowledging their fears and feelings. Maushart states: "For most contemporary women, then, the transition to motherhood is like some arcane initiation rite to a secret society to which the price of admission is (as with the birthing process that preceded it) an oath of silence."[31]

Silence has been a theme running through these pages. Let's blow the lid off. Here we are having some real conversations.

Maushart writes: "In order to gain life in new motherhood, she must lose life. To mask the magnitude of this sacrifice with silence, guilt, and denial is to trivialise a genuinely heroic journey into selfhood."[32] What might this mean?

That to become a mother, a woman's life changes permanently. Yes, it certainly does.

That our society belittles her new identity as somehow lesser than she was before. Yes, it does.

That she is denied the recognition and transition of her mother becoming rite of passage and the pride and confidence due her. Yes, she is.

That the reality of her self-sacrifice and hard mother-work is shrouded with invisibility and silence. Yes, it is.

That reducing a mother's self-worth after the extraordinary changes she has experienced is cruel. Yes, it is.

That this leads to feelings of shame, self-denial and guilt that isolates mothers in our society, denying them the recognition they deserve, and the environment and the opportunity to thrive in their matrescence. Yes, it does.

And this is why we are here – to change it. As Maushart says: "To mask the magnitude of this sacrifice with silence, guilt and denial is to trivialise a genuinely heroic journey into selfhood."[33]

Intensive mothering isn't healthy

We live in a culture of *intensive mothering*. First coined by sociologist Sharon Hays, it describes how societal and cultural expectations are placed on mothers, particularly in westernised cultures with unrealistic ideals. These norms put demands on mothers, which cause anxiety, guilt and a sense of inadequacy. The pressure to be present for their child is 24/7. The expectation is to provide constant emotional support, encouragement, affection, reassurance and investment. And to provide educational enrichment via activities that enhance the child's intellect. Sacrificing their own time, hobbies, relaxation, career and passions. Holding themselves to impossibly high standards in their role as mother, home maker, social secretary, nutritionist and more …

An excessively child-centred mania has taken over, putting busyness and the child's wellbeing ahead of all else, while the mother is expected to be nurturing and unselfish. Mothering has never been so intensive, time-consuming or as costly as it now.[34] This leads to burnout.

In addition, with Samantha in the middle months of pregnancy in Chapter 2, we touched on the nasty phenomenon of mum-shaming in our culture. We are going to explore that a bit more here and how to tackle it.

It is a huge responsibility to look after a vulnerable human child, being responsible for their health and safety, and nurturing their growth. There is no one-size-fits-all way of caring for and raising them. Each family is unique and no baby behaves the same as another. There is too much judgement and criticism for the way we feed, co-sleep and bed-share. Then there are the dreaded 'sleep training' conversations and questions like, "Is your baby good?" There is judgement about whether you work or stay at home. Judgement about child development milestones, and competition between mothers over the best 'stuff' for the baby. Judgement about the cleanest house, for being back in pre-pregnancy jeans, for parenting styles.

All this judgement undermines a mother's sense of ability, worth and identity, and brings insecurity, anxiety, loneliness and can deeply affect her mental health. Being held to unrealistic expectations sets mums up to feel they have failed. The perfect superficial world of Facebook and Instagram leads to that insidious feeling of 'comparisonitis'. Who posts the truth without filters?

The words of Amy Taylor-Kabbaz in *Mama Rising* ring true here: "If we work, we are judged. If we stay at home, we are judged. We were pitied, no matter what we chose: 'poor working mum missing out on so much' or 'poor stay-at-home mum, stuck in the kitchen tied to the sink.'"[35]

With over-expectations and mum-shaming, confidence is ground down. This causes further spiralling, can lead a mother to withdraw and become filled with 'mum guilt', which at its worst leads her to stop taking care of herself. In isolation, frustration, guilt and unhappiness, sadly this can come out as maternal rage and anger.

Maternal rage is real

This book speaks out about what is silenced, to prepare you for the raw reality that may be your experience sometime. Maternal rage is a real experience.

Sometimes motherhood makes us feel such deep anger that we are shocked by it. We are sold a bliss myth that mothering brings untold joy and fulfillment, without the truth that it also wears mothers down. There is a lack of preparation that mothering is hard. Who posts the truth about being fed up and bored with the daily repetition? The mess, heap of laundry, cereal for dinner, tears, frustration, resentment, no time to catch your breath and of being 'touched-out'?

Mothers are held to unrealistic ideals of the 'super mum', who not only manages it all, but does it with grace and serenity. Added to this is the injustice that partners' lives seem so unaffected! The sensory overload of constant criticism from media and society as a whole, and the fatigue and overwhelm are expressed as maternal anger, which is hard to calm.

Dr Caroline Boyd's website and blog explain maternal anger and give voice to mothers who tell their stories with anonymity, all held in a non-judgemental space. Anger is so often an expression of unmet needs. Have a look at the 'stories of maternal anger' on Caroline's blog and know you not alone. Also listen to *Beyond the Bump*'s 'Am I the only one with mum rage?' at this point.

There is no perfect way to mother. Each mother is doing her best and mistakes are okay. Something good that came from the 1950s is the term, the 'good enough mother', which was first described by the British paediatrician and psychoanalyst Donald Winnicott in 1953. This was when women's place was firmly in the home after giving birth. He noticed that babies and children benefitted when their mothers failed them in manageable ways.[36] Babies and children are resilient. They do not need us to be perfect, sacrificing everything of ourselves for them, being their constant source of care and entertainment. There are a million ways to get it right. So often, we don't focus on them; we focus on the little failings instead. It's enough to be enough.

Empowered mothering

A way to change the beliefs and behaviours of intensive mothering and to relieve the pressure cooker of pent-up maternal rage is what Andrea O'Reilly describes as 'empowered mothering'. We met O'Reilly in the introduction when defining matricentric feminism. This is an evolving concept, where mothers don't think childcare is their sole responsibility or that 24/7 mothering is necessary for children. They co-opt partners, friends, family and an involved community to assist with childcare as 'co-mothers' or 'other mothers'. These are not gender-specific roles. This philosophy of empowered mothering allows room to combine work, being a mum and having time for yourself. There is no place for maternal guilt and shame, or the concept of failing. It fully embraces being 'a good enough' mother.[37]

To help your empowered mothering journey, minimise 'what I wish I knew beforehand', read the article, 'The hidden load: How thinking of everything holds mums back'. This describes what so many mothers experience today: how, when it comes to household responsibilities, women perform far more cognitive and emotional labour than men. Have the discussion with your partner to prepare for what your roles are going to be as parents. The age of praising a man for changing a nappy or 'babysitting' their own child is over. Also, agree on which of the people in your village will have a part in caring for and raising your child.

- *Survive and Thrive* #15. 'How our ideas of parenthood make us feel like we are failing'. Apple 🎙 Spotify This resource provides insight into what parenthood is like and helps lower expectations of yourself.

- Dr Caroline Boyd website. 'Maternal Anger explained' https://drcarolineboyd.com/blog/maternal-anger-what-happens-physiologically-plus-the-distinction-between-anger-and-rage

- Dr Caroline Boyd Blog. 'Stories of maternal anger'
  https://drcarolineboyd.com/blog/stories-of-maternal-anger

- *Beyond the Bump* #112. 'Am I the only one with mum rage?' with Yara from Life After Birth Psychology Apple 🎙 Spotify

- 'The hidden load: How thinking of everything holds mums back' https://www.bbc.com/worklife/article/20210518-the-hidden-load-how-thinking-of-everything-holds-mums-back

---

Matricentric feminism and early mothering

Motherhood is a social ideal that refers to the set of cultural, societal and historical expectations, roles and norms that shape how mothering is understood and practised. It defines what it means to be a "good mother" based on societal values, rather than the biological act of birthing and mothering a child. That ideal has to change. Mothering needs matricentric feminism because motherhood is the structure in which a mother does her mothering.

As I wrote in the introduction about matricentric feminism, "It values emotional, nurturing and caregiving labour as skills, and a source of strength and knowledge. It argues that these skills and experiences are valuable and should be recognised and respected in all aspects of life." Matricentric feminism provides a foundation for activism that challenges policies and practices to support, empower and liberate mothers and their families. This is exactly what we need in the pregnancy, birth and early mothering space.

Mothering needs to be supported and respected with realistic expectations, so a mother can thrive in her experiences of mothering. Mothers need to be well in body, mind and spirit, knowing they are worthy of recognition and support. This is such a vulnerable time in a mother's life. As we have journeyed together, we have discovered values and strengths and looked at setting boundaries, to instil self-trust and autonomy, not only in pregnancy and birthing but here in the fourth trimester too. This is your personal matricentric feminism in action.

The words of Amy Taylor-Kabbaz describe how feminism has left mothering behind, leading to busy, busy, busy intensive mothering and the fallout that comes from that. "Feminism has brought amazing benefits to millions of women, but an unintentional side effect has been the supreme undervaluing of 'just' being a mother and wife. Stay-at-home mums feel like they are always having to justify their worth or explain why they are not working. And they often find themselves filling their lives up to look busy, because that's success, right?"[38]

Returning again to the wisdom of Vanessa Olorenshaw, her words resonate deeply here when we think of empowering ourselves as mothers. She writes: "Maternal feminism. Matricentric feminism. Mother-centric feminism. Justice and fairness for mothers. We are women and we are mothers. How can we tolerate our culture, feminism and socio-economic policy continuing to deny and neglect a core part of our identity, a huge range of our needs and the importance of what we do?"[39] Yes! Huge cheer!

So, attitudes and support towards mothering need to change. A huge part of the shift is the language we use to describe our evolution of becoming a mother. That means adopting and using 'matrescence'. In this word, where a world of understanding takes place, we have a voice to describe the psychological, spiritual, social, economic, cultural and physical influences that take place as we transform into our mothering identity. Our entire journey together has been a discovery into this world and word.

Dear Mother, all you have learned is now ready to be practised, to protect yourself and your family from a culture that doesn't value mothering. You are a light to show the way towards healing the intergenerational damage our westernised culture has caused to mothering. You are a beacon to other women, friends, community and your children, towards bringing back a matricentric focus.

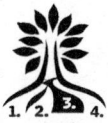

Social, Economic and Media Influences on the Fourth Trimester

Babymoon and boundaries

Your newborn bubble of time is precious and must be treated respectfully. In your 'support the new family' chat, establish boundaries and express your expectation that visitors become helpers. If you need help wording these boundaries, here are some examples.

- Please don't visit if you are sick.
- Wash your hands on arrival.
- Leave your stresses and worries at the door.
- Be the host for us instead of expecting to be hosted.
- Provide lots of tea and water.
- Bring a meal, snacks, some shopping, tidy up a bit, pop some laundry on.
- Please don't give parenting advice unless asked for.
- Please don't expect to hold the baby on your visit. It may not be the right time.
- Please help with other children, walk the dog, offer school pick-up/drop-off.
- Please don't overstay or make us feel guilty if we cancel.

Finding your people is so valuable. Seek out your mum village that aligns with your values and philosophy, and is real, non-judgemental and supportive. Look for those who have compassion for each other, respect each other's choices and provide an environment to flourish in. Share stories with each other, build companionship.

Find a place where laughter, tears, raw emotions and real struggles can be held with safety, and where people celebrate your small successes. "Yay, you managed a shower today!" is a real boost from those in the know. Go where mistakes can be talked about, because mistakes are okay. We are not primed with the ability to mother perfectly. There is no such thing. This parenting experience is new and you are learning. How often did we get 100% at school? We are not perfect and do not have to be. Remember, it's enough to be good enough, not perfect.

Do shop around for this support. There are some groups where the 'who has the best baby buggy' and 'who got back into their jeans soonest' competitive edge can make a mum feel terrible. I hope this attitude changes over time, because those mothers are often feeling lost and alone, and too frightened to be truthful about their feelings. Mum and baby yoga or other exercise classes that you started in pregnancy may thrive here for social connection and a village.

Social media, with its parenting advice that floods the senses and sells something that 'fixes you' or 'fixes your baby's sleep', can be daunting, overwhelming and confusing. Avoid being drowned by too much information, especially when time is precious and your brain is tired, by having some trusted sources available. They might be:

- the ABA, your doula or a lactation consultant
- BASIC for sleep
- Active Pregnancy Foundation
- COPE
- your favourite podcasts
- other sources you might have found helpful and reliable throughout this book
- your own.

Building a boundaries shield

Build an imaginary, shimmering, translucent wall around yourself that only lets in what nourishes and supports you. No need for comparisons, because how can you compare one unique situation – baby, mother or family dynamic – to another?

- Other people's opinions, goals, parenting styles, feeding and sleep methods are theirs.
- Other people's comments, judgements and 'helpful advice' don't matter.
- Other people's false illusions on Facebook and Instagram are irrelevant.
- Turn them off.
- Let them all ping off your shield.
- Maintain your boundaries to support yourself and your family.

Tips for managing tough days

We have chatted about the village and partner support, but there will be days when your baby, infant or toddler just wants you. There will be days and nights when you are alone. Loneliness, and the feeling of isolation, can have profound effects on a new mother. The sheer overload of fatigue and emotions swirl in the body and mind with no comfort or outlet. The distress of new mothers in seclusion is very real. There will be days when nothing you hoped to achieve gets done at all. The mess doesn't matter. Your state of mind and physical wellbeing does. To get you started:

- Have you eaten and had a drink? Made the time to brush your teeth? That's a great beginning to feel a bit better. Pyjama days, comfy clothes and messy hair are the new trend. Practise the mindful sensory shower meditation. Clean knickers feel good too.

- Whenever you begin to feel rattled, unsure, cross or sad, come back to your practice of deep breaths. Long inhalation through the nose, even longer exhalation … Calming the nervous system, slowing your heart, lowering your blood pressure. Your breath is your anchor, always with you, ready to help.

- Listen to a podcast, music or have the radio on when you are alone.

- What is it you really have to do today? If you don't do it, is it life-threatening? No? Okay, that email and call back can wait. Reschedule. Reduce your expectations and don't give a fig about anyone else's.

- Surrender … Yes, as if it's so easy! We have been conditioned to believe that only control and the success of achievement are worth anything. Let go of 'I should' be doing this, this, this and this. Let it become 'I could' or simply surrender into just being today.

- Go outside, barefoot. Breathe, feel, smell, see, listen. Feel the earth or grass underfoot.

- Acknowledge your emotions. They are yours after all. Write them down. As you do so, the emotions no longer have such a tight hold over you, because they are outside of you now.

Tough days are just that. In the *Tips for Managing Tough Days* podcast, host Nikki McCahon talks about renaming them 'cuddle days'. Brilliant. Cuddles bring out the oxytocin, so they are a great activity. As long as you feed yourself and are drinking plenty of water too, cuddle days are in. Oh, and it's totally okay to rock up to school in pyjamas with a three-month-old covered in baby sick while dropping off older children. How awesome are you to get any other children fed, dressed and ready for kindy or school! You rock! Do a happy dance at any disapproving stares.

- *Birth-Ed* S2 #5. 'Consciously Preparing for Parenthood' with Dr Maryhan, a psychologist and parenting adviser. Apple 🎙 Spotify

- **COPE website** 'Loneliness' https://www.cope.org.au/new-parents/emotional-health-new-parents/loneliness-in-early-parenthood/

- *Seasons of Matrescence* S3 #4. 'Tips for Managing Tough Days' Apple 🎙 Spotify

- **Raising Children Network. Newborns** https://raisingchildren.net.au/newborns

---

The economic effects of becoming a family

Remember the economic effects of becoming a family that we discussed with Samantha in the middle months of pregnancy? That was a while ago now and a lot has happened since, so pop back and have quick squiz to refresh your memory.

In her 2004 article, 'Hitting the Maternal Wall', Joan Williams, a professor of law, discusses workplace assumptions that women's commitment, competence and dedication to their work lessens when they become pregnant and return as mothers. She writes about barriers and bias that halt professional advancement. We need cultural change in attitudes towards flexible, at-home, family-friendly work arrangements with parental leave policies for both parents. We need to break through that maternal wall. We need to create more equity and support for mothers.[40]

With the new feeling of becoming a mother, we have what we call competing devotions. This is the conflict that arises with the multiple roles and responsibilities and the unending dollops of maternal guilt that go with it.[41] Hmmm, what to choose? Career or family? Hmmm, care for myself or care for others? Hmmm, hang on to individual identity or embrace maternal identity? Hmmm, time for children, time for partner or time for me? Hmmm, cultural expectations of me as a mother or personal boundaries?

Navigating all of this is a minefield.

Add to the mix the need for supported lactation breaks in a comfortable place other than the toilets and adequate storage facilities for breastmilk if you return to work. Pop onto the ABA website for their easy information about expressed breastmilk storage. Our culture and society needs to support and value mothers who work.

Each mother's journey will be unique. Find a balance and cultivate self-trust by returning to your values, strengths and needs in your new role and identity as a mother. This will help ease the transition during this matrescence challenge. Do this with pride, ignoring that nasty inner voice and throwing maternal guilt out the window. This is a tall order and it won't be easy. You are bucking an ingrained system of belief that you must sacrifice yourself. Attain a balance, with awareness of your wellbeing, and, self-worth. Your little one is learning from your behaviours.

The 4 podcasts offered in the goody box cover a wide range of financial considerations after becoming a family, including healthcare costs, staying home choices, returning to work, and finding your value on your return to work. The information will help you with your choices.

In *Australian Birth Stories*, Sophie Walker chats with Dr Eliza Hannam about Medicare rebates and the cost of allied health services. No rebate is available for lactation consultants unless they are an endorsed midwife. Dr Hannam also talks about mental health plans. Dr Hannam now offers the gold standard of postpartum care after having children herself and witnessing the lack of options for new mothers. She trains other GPs to provide this service too. Bring it on nationally.

In *Beyond the Bump*, 'How can we be smarter with our money once we start a family?', financial journalist Frances Cook provides guidance on preparing for maternity leave and planning for your future financial security. Remember the ATO contributions splitting to keep your superannuation growing that we mentioned with Samantha in Chapter 2? The podcast chats through practical, everyday savings tips, mortgages, efficient ways of investing for your children, and more, in the context of the current economic climate. Have a listen if financial security is causing some anxious moments.

Beyond the Bump's 'How does one return back to work after baby?' talks about the emotions and practicalities of when and how to go back to work. Having a baby has turned your life upside-down. Before the invisible umbilical cord began yanking, you had decided you would go back to work full-time after 6 months or a year. Now you want to work part-time, negotiate some flexibility and wonder if your employer is obliged to accept this or not.

The podcast also discusses how to avoid being passed over for promotion when someone with less experience is also applying for the job, returning to part-time work, setting and maintaining boundaries of actual part-time hours and more. Then, there's the competing devotions, maternal guilt, mental load and breastmilk pumping at work. After all that, we wonder if it is all worth it because of childcare fees. If this is you, listen in as it also comes with tips on how to leave the house in the morning.

Lastly, in the *Beyond the Bump* episode 'How to know our worth and ask for more $$$ (as woman and postpartum mama)', businesswoman Meggie Palmer chats about the gender pay gap, strategies for returning to work with confidence, talking about money more openly, and approaching increases in pay strategically. With tips for changing from full- to part-time work and setting realistic expectations instead of being and doing it all, Palmer certainly boosts the confidence for return-to-work mums, particularly singing their praises as they are more efficient.

Oh, here is another snark from me. Returning to a work culture sucks when we have to show no emotion about our private lives or the stresses of sick children, because that would be 'unprofessional'. To work as if we don't mother and mother as if we don't work – pffftttt. Workplace over-expectation and lack of empathy and understanding of what is truly involved in becoming a mother has to change. Going back to work or starting work as a mother isn't easy, especially with pesky competing devotions, maternal guilt and the maternal wall to navigate. Be kind to yourself, precious mother.

- ABA website. 'Expressed milk storage' https://www.breastfeeding.asn.au/resources/storing-ebm
- *Australian Birth Stories* #399. 'Postpartum care Options + Costs' Apple 🎙 Spotify
- *Beyond the Bump* #194. 'How can we be smarter with our money once we start a family?' Apple 🎙 Spotify
- Wishlist 🌿 *Beyond the Bump* #172. 'How does one return back to work after baby? with Naomi, writer, and postpartum doula' Apple 🎙 Spotify
- *Beyond the Bump* #113. 'How to know our worth and ask for more $$$ (as woman and postpartum mama)' Apple 🎙 Spotify

---

Back to media for the last snark

Our current culture of hard marketing and consumerism affects mothers deeply. Mothers are exploited in every way possible to buy products and services to make them feel they are a 'good' mother. Tatjana Takševa, Professor of English and Women and Gender Studies, in her article, 'The Commercialisation of Motherhood and Mothering in the Context of Globalisation', highlights: "… the commercialisation of motherhood and mothering has appropriated, exploited and depends for its success on the perpetuation of many of the deeply embedded cultural types of mothering, such as intensive mothering, as well as New Momism".[42]

New mumism is intensive mothering with all the stuff that makes her the ideal mother. A mother has to devote her entire physical, emotional, and intellectual being 24/7 to her children and enjoy every minute of it.

How can we turn this around and know that our self-worth is not found in having more stuff? Our self-worth is not in being switched on 24/7 with a fake face of happiness. It is not in being and doing everything, when our brains and behaviour didn't evolve the way modern intensive mothering or new mumism demands.

Takševa proposes: "Empowered mothering in the present context may mean finding innovative ways of avoiding the commercialization that seeks to define the relationship between mothers and their children, and that capitalizes and exploits the desire of mothers to nurture their children."[43]

So, how might you avoid commercialisation? Purchasing second-hand items, forming a village, ensuring items are passed on and shared? For birthday parties, pass on a book that has been treasured and outgrown. Perhaps offer experiences such as 'baking together at our house'. Maybe it's a drawing and painting day, a visit to a farm, museum or library, a picnic day, play date or film day. Offer a dads/

partners activity day, which is a win-win as the men take the children on an adventure and spend time with their child. There are so many possibilities. Do what feels good for you. Children just want to spend some time with friends, family, mum and dad. Offer an experience instead of adding to a mountain of stuff.

Postpartum body image

Body image is a hot topic running through these chapters. In 'Postpartum Body Image with Kyla Blacksmith', body image is explored with honesty and with sensitivity. Kyla is a dancer and openly expresses that she struggled with an eating disorder when younger due to the pressure of body image. She talks about:

- sadness at the competition between women to get back to pre-pregnant weight and body shape and how unreal that expectation is
- honesty about body changes and what women wished they had been told about before giving birth
- the realities of the first few months of physical changes
- how painful afterpains can be, how heavy blood loss can be and how sore it was to move around after stitches in the first days
- having what feels like rocks on the chest as milk comes in, which affects sleep positions due to tender boobs
- the difficulties with breastfeeding and feelings of guilt and shame at using formula
- shock about hair loss and how it affected her confidence (It does grow back!)
- owning all these changes and emotions, both temporarily and permanently
- comfort and practicality in clothing, wearing husbands' clothes and jocks, saving a fortune on in-between clothes, and husbands who complain about milk stains.

Bodies change after their incredible feat of growing, birthing and feeding a baby. It is important to acknowledge and own the feelings this evokes. You are beautiful just as you are.

- *Beyond the Bump* S1, #50. 'Postpartum Body Image with Kyla Blacksmith' Apple 🎙 Spotify

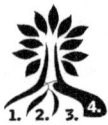

Self-identity, Beliefs and Values, and Spiritual Influences on the Fourth Trimester

Here you are, mum. What a journey we have been on together

We expand in our sense of self, becoming immersed in the responsibility and nurturing of this new life, and prioritising the care of our child. We have this maternal identity. We navigate and adapt to new roles in our relationship, family, community, society and work. Identity shifts from 'me to we', with the invisible umbilical cord entwined into every part of our lives.

Acknowledge the physical, hormonal and emotional adaptations that have forever changed our body, ways of thinking and emotional bonds. We may lose our sense of self for a while in this melting pot of new demands and roles. Yet, at the same time, with a sense of purpose, returning to the anchors of our values, strengths and cultivation of self-trust, we acknowledge that this period of transition takes time.

It is challenging and realising our self-worth in this brings a deep sense of achievement and enrichment too. You are still you. You have also become more, while claiming the identity of mother as respected, strong and powerful.

We began with Aurélie Athan's definition of matrescence, and how it encompasses all the aspects of our lives. Combined with matricentric feminism, it inspired the mother becoming tree of matrescence as a framework to help you journey through this book. Here we return to Athan in the final spiritual part.

In Athan and Miller's article, 'Spiritual Awakening Through the Motherhood Journey', the authors interviewed first-time mothers and found similar themes of 're-awakening' to realities of life not experienced before becoming a mother. Their use of intensely spiritual language to describe their experiences aligned with the language of compassion, surrender, patience and Divine love.

Athan and Miller suggest: "Motherhood is an opportunity for creative spiritual growth and transformation in women. This potential lies latent in the intense emotional experiences inherent in mothering which are designed to be and to accelerate spiritual development."[44]

They also suggested that the mothers' stories constantly reminded them of the basis of our universal hero/heroine myths, where "in deciding to mother a child, women are in fact spiritual heroines called to the daunting adventure of motherhood, where through a series of trials they are brought forth into a richer, more mature condition".[45] They conclude that our culture does not recognise, honour or value this extraordinary mothering experience. Their suggestion to recognise mothers' spirituality as a way of enriching themselves and their children towards a rebirth of society is a beautiful intention.

Through the letters and words in these pages, maybe you have a sense of becoming connected to something greater. Connection to a matricentric village and rediscovering the wonder of the Divine within. Connection to heart, mind and body with the capacity for unconditional love and compassion for yourself. It is all part of the transformation and evolution of becoming a mother, while navigating the challenges and achievements along the way. I hope to have moved mothering towards being revered again. You are extraordinary.

Closing the bones ceremony

Our journey comes to an end for now, as we explore a *closing the bones* ceremony. This is a ritual and spiritual practice of acknowledging and celebrating the woman and mother you have become. Closing the bones recognises the transition from the fourth trimester to the rest of your mothering life. Practised in many cultures, but particularly in South America, this ceremony is usually performed around 40 days, or 6 weeks, after birth but can be performed at any time as a ritual way of finding closure.

It involves massage of the abdomen with warmed and possibly fragrant oil, then the use of long scarves, traditionally the Mexican rebozo scarf. In Mayan culture the mother's spirit travels through the universe when in labour to find and gather her baby's soul so they can be birthed together. When the bones are closed, the mother's spirit is fully recalled and closes energetically.[46]

Scarves are placed under the mother's lower back, pelvis and upper thighs, then crossed over above her to gently rock her side to side as though encouraging the 'bones to close' by realigning muscles, ligaments and joints. The scarves are tied closed, binding the bones, particularly the pelvis, together again. It is a nurturing and comforting practice thought to encourage the mother's organs to settle into place. It encourages the pelvis to close again once the effect of the hormone **relaxin** has settled.

Getting creative, you can borrow scarves, raid op shops, or use old sheets to make it an inexpensive experience. We can bring this ritual into every new mother's life to celebrate her, as we did in pregnancy in a mother blessing.

This postpartum ritual isn't just a physical realignment, but an opportunity for the mother to explore her emotions around birthing and becoming a mother. The ritual creates an environment that provides support, connection, and acknowledgment of the mother's transition, feelings and identity. She explores her story, beginning to regain a sense of equilibrium, peace, closure and strength. We mentioned how powerful this would be for a mother experiencing stillbirth. It would be deeply emotional for all involved, but would benefit the mother by acknowledging her. Although her arms are empty, her body, spirit and soul still need support in recovery, healing and emotional release. Through ritual, we acknowledge she is always a mother for her lost baby.

- 'Closing the Bones' YouTube. Ceremony with Sophie Messager
  https://www.youtube.com/watch?v=vi_2WP3cEt0

Practice offering: Embrace yourself generously meditation and *Santosha*

Another of the niyamas of the Yoga Sutras of Patanjali is *Santosha*. Its literal meaning is contentment. It is about finding joy in the little things, with acceptance and appreciation of what we are and where we are. We can move through the flow of mothering with this attitude. It doesn't mean putting up with anxiety, pain, poor care, poor relationships, silencing the self, or resigning ourselves to those things. It is finding contentment in the strength to do something about what troubles us.

We don't live in a perpetual state of the mothering bliss myth. It's challenging. Yet within that, there are beautiful moments of achievement, love, wonder and joy. Breath by breath, moment by moment, step by step, hour by hour, day by day ... Your evolution in matrescence and mother becoming never ends. It's a journey of constant change and adaptation, tears and laughter, fright and joy, and overwhelming emotions. And of course, there are the times when you think: *If had I known it would be like this, I would never have thought myself capable of it!* This is you now, changed to the very core of your being and utterly incredible.

As a final offering, verse 56 of the Yuki Practices by Lorin Roche in his Radiance Sutras is the source of our last mindful, breathing and visualisation meditation.[47] The words have been a balm for me over happy and troubled times. I hope they are for you too. Each interpretation is unique, personalised to our needs, and this is just one way I visualise you, dear mother becoming.

Verse 56
Oceans embrace a continent.
Space welcomes the sun.
Embrace yourself this generously.
Form your arms into a circle
And cherish the rising of serenity.
Attend the birth of something new.
Thoughts dissolve into peace,
As you become the One who embraces All. [26]

- Wiggle into your comfortable spot, gently scanning through the body as you have practised so many times already.

- Choose your favourite breathing method and melt a little more into comfort.

- Your breath is your anchor, vitality in the energy of your lifeforce.

- Visualise yourself as a continent, a wide place of earth, kissed by the sun, wind and rain, all held in an enfolding hug by the salty tang of the ocean.

- Embraced with life, land, air and sea, held in this vast space, warm and nourished by the sun.

- With each breath in, feel, see, touch, smell and listen ... expand ...

- With each breath out, soften and gently release tension, worries, any frustration or anger.

- Flow with the breath, as many times as you need to, until you can begin to embrace yourself as generously as an ocean kissing the shore.

- Now you become the sun, the centre of our solar system. The centre of your family. Radiate your warmth, compassion and love.

- See your arms forming a circle, holding yourself, your baby, your partner, family, friends and community, the earth and spill outwards ... One by one by one. Held with love and cherished.

- Each breath in, begin with you ... Cherish yourself.

- Next breath, go to your baby ... Cherish them.

- Each breath out, melt into an arising serenity of cherishing yourself, your baby ...

- You are attending the birth of something new, the birth of you. Each breath, each moment, each hour, each new day, attend to you first. Embrace yourself with honour and gratitude.

- Allow peace to settle, in the acknowledgment that you are doing the best you can and that you are enough.

- Your breaths now allow for a window of gracious knowledge that you, dear mother, are the centre of the universe. You are The One, worthy, embracing The All that this journey of mother becoming has entailed.

Mother Becoming Inspired Actions in the Fourth Trimester

Here, we arrive at the end of our long journey together. It has been quite a trek, with challenging country to navigate as well as beautiful views. Shrug off the pack and boots. Take a rest. Have a cuppa and your favourite snacks, imagining Liesja, Samantha, Ashleigh, Ally, Katie, Alysia and Clémentine joining you for company. What questions might you ask them as you gather together?

I hope you have scribbled, underlined, agreed, disagreed, and doodled love hearts, happy, sad, and angry faces, and exclamation marks all over the pages. Feel free to journal again now, making a list of all you have discovered and what you might want to explore more.

Talk to your partner, dear friends, support network and colleagues about what you have discovered after taking the time to reflect on whatever has resonated with you. How have these words landed?

Please practise a slow postpartum. It's over to you now, dear mother.

With so much love,

Wendy x

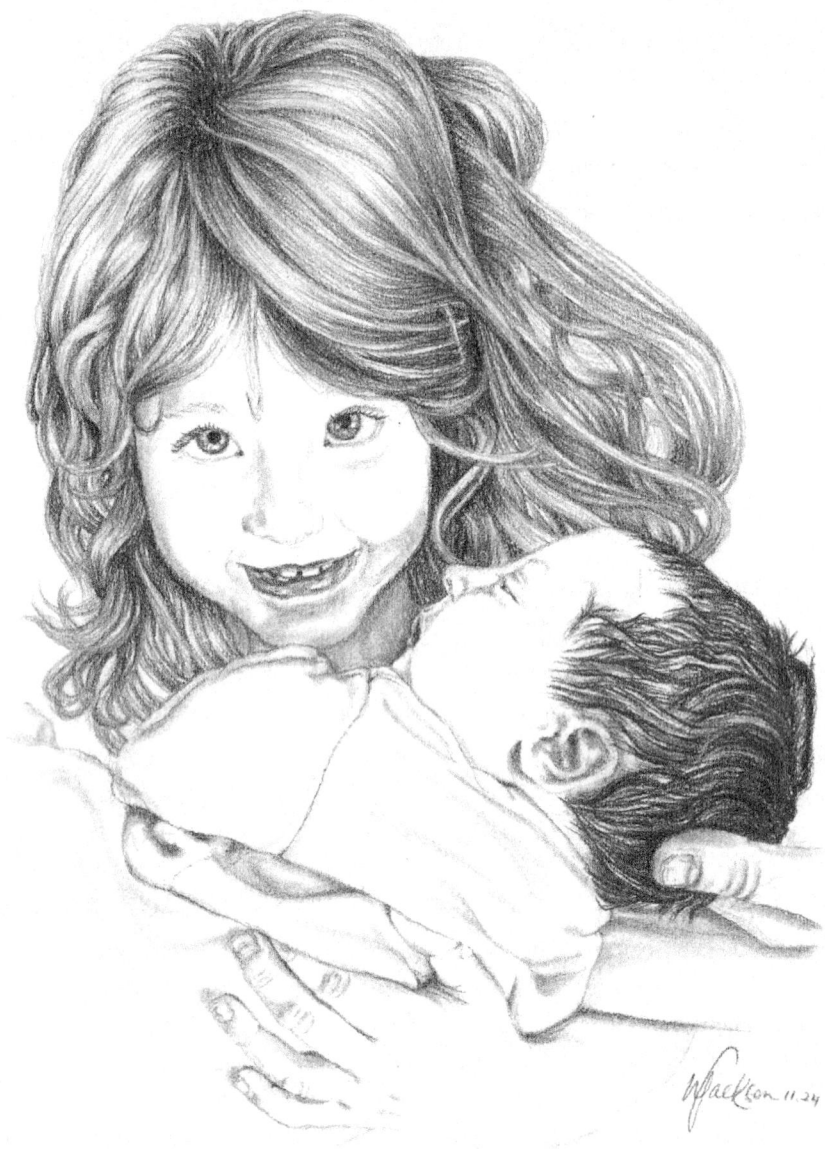

Charlie holding her baby sister, Alizée, for the first time with the support of the loving hands of Clémentine. Oh my goodness! Look at the radiant joy on Charlie's dear little face. Such a proud moment for her; it captures her delight.

How might it be for you ...

- If, in our culture, the fourth trimester were acknowledged as normal and as an honoured time to support new mothers?

- If you were given time to apply all the elements of support, nourishment, rest and sleep, massage, respect, and assistance from visitors?

- If the village, networks, community and authentic connections in mothers groups were judgement-free?

- If mum-shaming had no place and the mother were cherished?

- If you continued to choose you first, knowing you are worth nourishing, normalising rest, embracing it?

- If you asked for help?

- If you knew you were good enough just as you are?

- If our current Cinderella service for postpartum care were made matricentric and lasted much longer?

- If midwifery COC were available up to 6 weeks postpartum, minimum?

- If breastfeeding were far more supported and normalised in public, not undermined?

- If pelvic health physiotherapy appointments for every mother were provided as part of postpartum care?

- If you had conversations before birthing with partners about the reality of sharing care, home duties, finances, each other's emotions, returning to intimacy, and experiencing this new family life?

- If these conversations continued with respect for each other because this evolution affects both of you?

- If there were less silencing about returning to sexual intimacy, because your sex life matters?

- If silence, self-blame, shame and stigma associated with postpartum depression were erased, with more input into emotional wellbeing and support services?

- If we lived in a culture where maternal depletion didn't exist because it was prevented in the first place?

- If the bliss myth around mothering were debunked, and no longer exploited for commercial gain?

- If feelings of maternal guilt no longer held sway?

- If the spirituality of mothering were recognised as enriching, an experience to be held with respect and valued as a foundation of mother becoming?

- If we took the time to practise the offerings for health in mind, body and spirit for postpartum recovery?

- If you had a ritual of your own, like the closing the bones ceremony, to celebrate birthing, and becoming a mother the way you celebrated your mother blessing in pregnancy?

- If our focus were matricentric rather than baby-centric?

- If matrescence were known, understood, respected and supported in our westernised culture?

- If family needs were part of return-to-work policy, planning and support?

- If you had a place to go, a place of advocacy to make change for yourself and women of the future, a place to make changes you feel passionate about?

- If you found your advocacy feet?

A place for you to go to make change

To make change for yourself, your daughters and the women of the future. To make changes you feel passionate about. Here are some places of advocacy.

- **Maternity Choices Australia.** A reliable source of information on all things pregnancy and birth. MCA provides a PDF template for positive change in maternity care for each state. For example:

  - For an increase in midwifery COC from 8% to 75%; this will save $127 million annually in WA

  - For publicly funded homebirth and Birthing on Country models to be expanded nationwide

  - For a Chief Midwifery Officer to be appointed to every state, because the current Chief Nursing and Midwifery Officers come from a nursing, not midwifery background. Which means midwifery interests and therefore yours are not sufficiently represented.

  Attach the PDF for your state, and email your state and federal MPs and senators with a brief explanation about why these aspects of pregnancy care are important to you.

  Choose your state. https://www.maternitychoices.org/advocacy

- **Maternity Consumer Network (MCN)** https://www.maternityconsumernetwork.org.au/about

  For powerful advocacy in the political arena to improve maternity care for all women in Australia

  For their maternity campaigns: For more midwifery group practice pre-written letter templates https://www.maternityconsumernetwork.org.au/team-1

- **ICM Bill of Rights for Women and Midwives.** https://internationalmidwives.org/resources/

  Click on Human Rights, then click on Download Resource for the PDF

  Attach the PDF to an email, as above, explaining which part is important to you.

Fourth Trimester References and Wishlist

1   V Olorenshaw, *Liberating Motherhood: birthing the Purple Stocking Movement.* Womancraft Publishing, 2016, p59. ISBN 978-910559-192

2   Australian Institute of Health and Welfare. Women and Babies. https://www.aihw.gov.au/reports/mothers-babies/australias-mothers-babies/contents/overview-and-demographics/state-and-territory

3   A O'Reilly, *Matricentric Feminism, Theory, Activism, Practice.* Demeter Press, 202, p42. ISBN 9781772583762

4   Breastfeeding Protocols. 'How the breast works'. Ontario. Canada. https://breastfeedingresourcesontario.ca/sites/default/files/PDF/BFI_How_the_Breast_Works_web.PDF

5   M Harris. *Men, Love and Birth.* Pinter and Martin, 2017, p144. ISBN 9781870662251

6   A Brown, *Why Breastfeeding Grief and Trauma Matter.* Pinter and Martin, 2019.,p110. ISBN 9781780666150

7   E Beddington, Guardian Article. 'A home help for eight days after giving birth. Why the Dutch maternity care is the envy of the world'. https://www.theguardian.com/lifeandstyle/2023/oct/25/a-home-help-for-eight-days-after-giving-birth-why-dutch-maternity-care-is-the-envy-of-the-world

8   J Allison, *Golden Month. Caring for the world's mothers after childbirth.* Beatnik Publishing, 2016. ISBN 9780992264840

9   G Chauhan, P Tadi, 'Physiology, Postpartum Changes'. In: StatPearls [Internet]. Treasure Island (FL): StatPearls Publishing; 2024 Jan-. Available from: https://www.ncbi.nlm.nih.gov/books/NBK555904/

10   Allison, *Golden Month*, p14.

11   Allison, *Golden Month* ,p55-7.

12   Allison, *Golden Month*, p58.

13   Allison, *Golden Month*, p51.

14   Allison, *Golden Month*, p54.

15   O Serrallach, *The Postnatal Depletion Cure. A Complete Guide to Rebuilding Your Health & Reclaiming Your Energy. For Mothers of Newborns, Toddlers and Young Children.* Hachette Australia, 2018, p7. ISBN 9780733640322

16   Serrallach, *The Postnatal Depletion Cure*, p7.

17   Serrallach, *The Postnatal Depletion Cure*, p4.

18   K Thompson, 'Birth injuries are a feminist issue. An obstetrician explains why'. https://womensagenda. com.au/latest/birth-injuries-are-a-feminist-issue-an-obstetrician-explains-why/#:~:text=An%20ob-stetrician%20explains%20why,-by%20Kara%20Thompson&text=%22We%20need%20to%20lift%20 the,been%20ignored%20for%20too%20long.%22

19   E Brockwell, *Why Did No One Tell Me? How to Protect. Heal and Nurture Your Body through Motherhood.* Vermillion, Penguin Rando House, 2021, p194-202. ISBN 978178504336

20   Brockwell, *Why Did No One Tell Me?* p199.

21   Brockwell, *Why Did No One Tell Me?* p200.

22   C Goggin, *Why Caesarean Matters*, Pinter and Martin, 2018, p123. ISBN 9781780665405

23   Goggin, *Why Caesarean Matters*, p123.

24   Serrallach, *The Postnatal Depletion Cure*, p257.

25   Brockwell, *Why Did No One Tell Me?* p203-9.

26   Brockwell, *Why Did No One Tell Me?* p209.

27   M Scotland, *Why Postnatal Depression Matters*, Pinter and Martin, 2019. p136-9. ISBN 9871780665603

28   A Taylor-Kabbaz, *Mama Rising: Discovering The New You Through Motherhood*, Hay House, 2019, p41. ISBN 9781401958985

29   New South Wales Parliament Legislative Council Select Committee on Birth Trauma, Report. 2024; p xv ISBN: 978-1-922960-38-2 https://www.parliament.nsw.gov.au/lcdocs/inquiries/2965/FINAL%20 Birth%20Trauma%20Report%20-%2029%20April%202024.PDF

30   Easy explanation of the Yamas and Niyamas in the Patanjalis Yoga Sutras, https://www.ekhartyoga.com/ articles/philosophy/the-yamas-and-niyamas

31   S Maushart, *The Mask of Motherhood: How Becoming a Mother Changes Our Lives and Why We Never Talk About It*, Penguin Books, 2000, p107. ISBN 0140291784

32   Maushart. *The Mask of Motherhood*. p114.

33   Maushart. *The Mask of Motherhood*. p114.

34   S Hays, *The Cultural Contraindications of Motherhood.* Yale University Press; 1996. ISBN 978030076523

35   Taylor-Kabbaz, *Mama Rising*, p24.

36   M Wedge, Psychology Today. 'What is a "Good enough Mother'? https://www.psychologytoday.com/au/ blog/suffer-the-children/201605/what-is-good-enough-mother

37   O'Reilly, *Matricentric Feminism*, p173.

38   Taylor-Kabbaz, *Mama Rising*, p23.

39   Olorenshaw, *Liberating Motherhood*, p23.

40   J Williams, 'Hitting the Maternal Wall'. Academie; 2004 (90) 6 doi:10.2307/40252700. https://www.researchgate.net/publication/246380119_Hitting_the_Maternal_Wall

41   S Goodwin, K Huppatz, *The good mother in theory and research*. Sydney University Press; 2010 p 1-23. ISBN: 9781920899530. https://www.researchgate.net/publication/305851753_The_Good_Mother

42   T Takševa, (2012). The Commercialization of Motherhood and Mothering in the Context of Globalization: Anglo-American Perspectives. *Journal of the Motherhood Initiative for Research and Community Involvement*, 3(1).p 134-148. p136. Retrieved from https://jarm.journals.yorku.ca/index.php/jarm/article/view/35343. https://jarm.journals.yorku.ca/index.php/jarm/article/view/35343/32068

43   Takševa, The Commercialization of Motherhood and Mothering, p146.

44   A Athan, L Miller, (2005). 'Spiritual Awakening Through the Motherhood Journey'. *Journal of the Motherhood Initiative for Research and Community Involvement*, 7(1).p17-31. P17. Retrieved from https://jarm.journals.yorku.ca/index.php/jarm/article/view/4951. https://www.researchgate.net/publication/288827864_Spiritual_awakening_through_the_motherhood_journey

45   Athan, Miller, Spiritual Awakening Through the Motherhood Journey, p17.

46   K Lina. Bone closing ceremony. 'What it is and where is comes from.' The Educated Birth. https://www.theeducatedbirth.com/articles/bone-closing-ceremony-what-it-is-and-where-it-comes-from#:~:text=It%20helps%20a%20parent%20find,with%20the%20birth%20and%20motherhood

47   L Roche, *The Radiance Sutra*, Verse 109, Yuki Practice, Sounds True, 2014, p91. ISBN 978-1-60407-659-2

Wishlist

1. *Newborn Mothers* #25 'Caring for the World's Mother's after Childbirth.' Apple 🎙 Spotify

2. YouTube. Illustrates flow of water and fat in breastmilk during a feed. https://www.youtube.com/watch?v=_Kxr5rzB4ck

3. *Birth-Ed* S1 #7 'Understanding Infant Sleep' with Sarah Ockwell-Smith. Author of 'Why Your Baby's Sleep Matters.' Apple 🎙 Spotify

4. *Happy Mama Movement* #111 'Postnatal Depletion with Dr Serrallach' Apple 🎙 Spotify

5. *Beyond the Bump* #232 'Will I ever feel like having sex again? With sexologist Juliet Allen' Apple 🎙 Spotify

6. *Pregnancy Uncut* S1 #4 'The Silent Sea: Postnatal depression and anxiety.' Apple 🎙 Spotify

7. *Beyond the Bump* #172 'How does one return back to work after baby? with Naomi, writer, and postpartum doula.' Apple 🎙 Spotify

Glossary of Anatomical and Medical Terms

Acidaemia	If there is too much acid in the blood it can affect how organs work.
Amniocentesis	A small sample of amniotic fluid (the fluid surrounding the baby) is taken to test chromosomal disorders like Down syndrome and genetic diseases.
Anaemia	Low iron in the blood and reduced oxygen carrying capacity
Alveoli	Milk sac in the breast
Amniotic sac	The sac that holds amniotic fluid that surrounds the fetus
Amygdala	Small, almond-shaped part of the brain that plays a major role in processing emotions, especially fear, stress and pleasure. Triggers the "fight-or-flight" response
Augmentation	Speeding up labour by medical means
Birth injury	Damage to the pelvic organs, muscles, nerves
Caesarean	Surgical birth by incision through the lower abdomen and uterus
Cerebellum	Part of the brain that helps with balance, movement and coordination. Located at the back of the brain, just above the spinal cord
Cervix	Lower, narrow part of the uterus that connects to the vagina
Circadian rhythm	Your body's natural 24-hour clock that controls when you feel awake and when you feel sleepy. Also helps regulate sleep, hunger and body temperature
Clitoris	The small and highly sensitive visible part of the clitoral organ
Colostrum	The very first fluid a baby drinks from the breast
Chorionic villus sampling	Taking a small sample of tissue from the placenta to test for chromosomal disorders and genetic diseases
Corpus luteum	What is left over after ovulation on the ovary
Crura	Internal, erectile tissues that extend from the visible part of the clitoris to line the pelvic arch
Decidua	The lining of the uterus during pregnancy. It forms when the uterine lining (endometrium) thickens and changes to support the growing baby.
Dystocia	When labour slows down or stops
Episiotomy	A surgical cut to the perineum
Eustress	Positive stress that motivates and helps you perform better
External cephalic version	A hands-on technique used by doctors to turn a baby from a breech position (bottom first) to a head-down position before birth
Ferguson reflex	A reflexive urge to push triggered by the stretching of the cervix
Fetus	What a baby is called while still inside the mother
Fistula	A hole between the vagina and either the bladder or the rectum as a result of prolonged, obstructed labour
Friedman's curve	A graph to measure progress in labour
Forceps	A pair of surgical instruments. Two spoon-shaped blades are inserted into the vagina and placed around the baby's head near the ears.
Fundus	Top of the uterus
Haemorrhage	Significant blood loss before or after birth

Hypercoagulable	Blood clots too easily or too much
Instrumental birth	Use of medical instruments during delivery to assist in the birth of a baby. Usually by forceps delivery and vacuum extraction
Immunoglobulin	A protein in the blood that helps the body fight infections. Also called antibody
Lactation	Production of breastmilk
Letdown	A reflex that pushes milk to the baby when breastfeeding
Levator ani	Muscles in the female pelvis that form part of the pelvic floor. They support the bladder, uterus and rectum, and play a role in childbirth, urination and bowel control
Limbic system	Part of the brain that controls emotions, memory and motivation
Lithotomy	A position for birth with the mother on her back. Hips and knees bent, and supported in stirrups. Used for access for instrumental birth
Macrosomia	A larger than average baby
Menarche	The first occurrence of menstruation in a female. The onset of puberty
Microbiome	The microorganisms (bacteria, fungi, viruses and other microbes) that live in and on the human body
Morbidity	Injury, disease, illness or poor health
Mortality	The frequency of death in a given population over a defined period. Also called the mortality rate
Multiparous	Has given birth to one or more babies
Neocortex	The outer layer of the brain responsible for thinking, problem-solving, language and decision-making
Neonatal encephalitis	This is brain swelling (inflammation) in a newborn baby.
Neuroendocrine	The way the nervous system and hormones work together to control body functions
Neuroplasticity	The brain's ability to change by forming new neural connections
Nulliparous	Not given birth before
Nutation	The top of the sacrum tilts forward, and the tailbone moves backward.
Obstetric dilemma	Evolutionary biology that proposes why human childbirth is difficult
Occipito-posterior	Position of baby's head at or in the pelvis. Baby's back to mum's back
Oligosaccharides	A type of carbohydrate (sugar) made up of a few simple sugar molecules linked together. Found in foods like vegetables, beans and human breast milk
Os	The opening of the cervix to the uterus
Pathological	Description of disease or abnormal conditions, ill-health
Partogram	A graphical tool used in labour to monitor the progress of childbirth and the wellbeing of both the mother and baby
Perineum	The area between the vagina and anus
Placenta praevia	The placenta covers the cervix (the opening of the uterus)
Pheromones	Natural chemical signals that living things release to communicate with others of the same species
Physiological	Refers to how the body and its systems normally function

Piriformis	Small, yet important muscle in the lower back, deep in the buttocks
Puerperal sepsis	Severe bacterial infection of the uterus and surrounding tissues after childbirth, and can spread throughout the body
Sacrum	A triangular-shaped bone at the base of the spine. Part of the pelvis
Sacroiliac joint	Connects the sacrum to the iliac bones of the pelvis
Symphysis pubis	The joint at the front of the pelvis where the 2 pubic bones meet
Syntocinon	Syntocinon is a brand name for a synthetic form of oxytocin
Suturing	The process of stitching a wound or surgical cut to help it heal
Tocophobia	An intense fear of childbirth
Uterus	The womb between the bladder and rectum. The organ of female fertility and childbirth
Vacuum	The use of a suction cup (vacuum) is applied to the baby's head to help guide it through the birth canal
Vagal nerve	A major part of the parasympathetic nervous system, which counterbalances the "fight or flight" response
Vertebra	Bone of the spine
Vestibula bulbs	Part of the clitoris, a pair of erectile tissues located on either side of the vaginal opening

Acknowledgments and Thanks

To all those who agreed to review the book:

Professor Sara Bayes, Vice Chancellor's Professorial Research Fellow Edith Cowan University, WA. Thank you for telling me I needed endorsement and offering advice on who to approach, and giving me the confidence to do so when I felt like a little fish in a very big pond;

Obstetrician Liza Fowler for her insight from a medical perspective and writing such beautiful words in her foreword;

Dr Marina Weckend for detailed feedback on Ally's chapter and Katie's chapter;

Christine Parry, Senior Aboriginal Liaison Officer for Boodjari Yorgas MGP, for reviewing my writing on Birthing on Country;

Amy Taylor-Kabbaz, author and matrescence pioneer, who offered these wise words. "Just hold the intention of this book. May it be in every mother's hands and may my fears step aside so that this book can do what it is meant to do.";

Emma Snelgar, who offers birth trauma debriefing, for reviewing Katie's chapter.

Ashleigh Farquhar, grammar fiend, (from Chapter 3) for helping me proofread the book!

For the words of praise for this book:

Vicki Hobbs, Back to Basics Birthing educator and doula, and doula trainer with Doula Training Academy Australia;

Dr Catherine Bell, author, doula, birth cartographer and director of Maternity Choices Australia;

Mandy Becker-Knox, creator of the Hatha Yoga Method and director of Kookaburra Yoga.

Professor Sara Bayes, Vice Chancellor's Professorial Research Fellow, Edith Cowan University, WA

Your words have given me confidence that this book is needed.

To all the researchers and authors who gave me permission to quote and cite their work.

To the women who got me to the finish line:

Kris Emery for telling me that I was on track with a developmental edit of Liesja's chapter, then taking on the developmental edit of the whole book and beginning the editing process;

Julie Taylor, proofreader and editor extraordinaire, who took over from Kris. For doing the final editing, teaching me the technical stuff that gives me hives and then formatting the book. Your patience and endless encouragement made completing the book a far easier experience than it could have been;

Megan Hele for designing the book cover and bringing my vision and art of *Mother Becoming* to life;

Ruth McCann, website and socials creator. For taking the fear out of tech for me and creating a digital piece of art together.

Heartfelt thanks to Liesja, Samantha, Ashleigh, Ally, Katie, Alysia and Clémentine, for making this book real. For giving me a purpose and way to express my passions. For joining me in this conversation to empower women and mothers in their pregnancy, birthing and early mothering. You fill my soul cup always.

To my husband, Ant, for constantly saying "book first".

To my children, Robert and Rebecca, for telling me how proud they are of me.

To Mum and Dad for cheerleading all the way with daily FaceTime catch-ups from the UK.

To my faithful fur baby Lorien, giver of unconditional love. Passed 17.10.24

To the sisters of my heart, thank you for your total faith in me and this book, supporting me over the challenging years of its evolution. Especially my bestie, Nancy, for telling me as it is when I might not want to hear it, telling me the hard stuff, and laughing when I tell her, "I don't like you right now!"

To the circles of friendship in my life, the Mother Becoming mums, yoga group Jo, Bek, Amanda and Bec. You are infinitely precious to me.

To family and friends far and wide in this world for cheering me on over the miles.

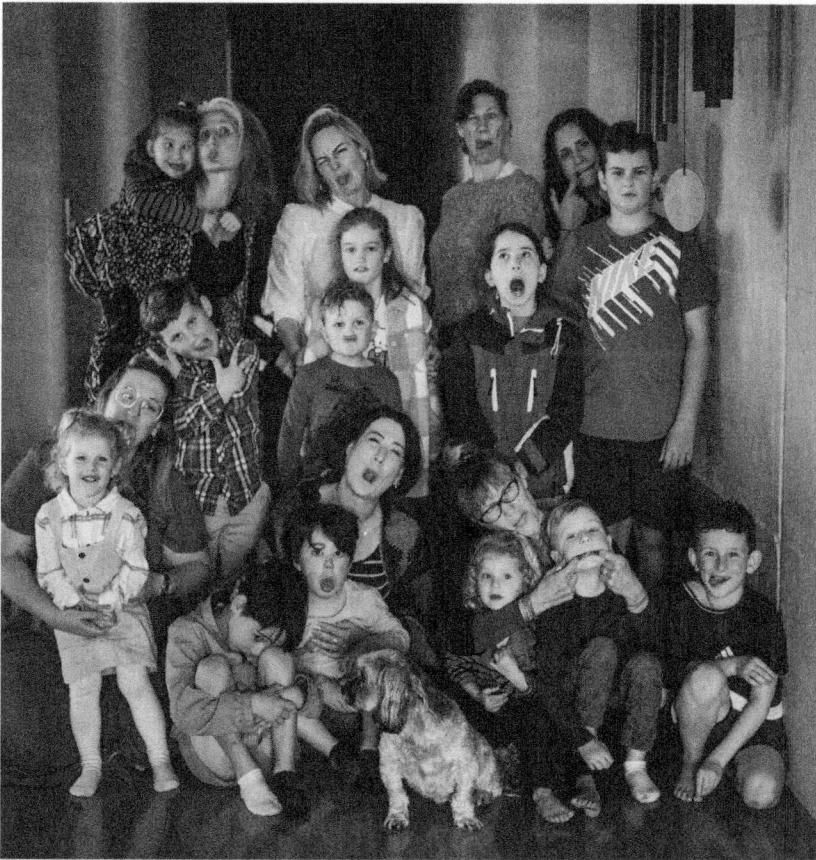

Love from all of us

Further Information

Bulk orders

If you would like to place a bulk order for this book, please email: wendy@motherbecoming.com.au

If there is a profit made from this book, 50% will go to the Stillbirth and Neonatal Death Society, the Gidget Foundation and Maternity Choices Australia.

Previous publication

Wendy Jackson. Breastfeeding and Type 1 diabetes mellitus. March 2004. British Journal of Midwifery. 12(3):158-165 DOI:10.12968/bjom.2004.12.3.15361

Meet me on the *Happy Mama Movement* podcast #232 'Healing without a timeline with Wendy Jackson' Apple Spotify YouTube https://www.youtube.com/watch?v=OEudeilZojM

Please join me in a matricentric village of support and nourishment at **www.motherbcoming.com.au**

Free resources on the website

Mother Blessing Ceremony Guidance PDF
Birth Space Privacy and Respect Poster PDF
Village and Fourth Trimester Support and Information PDF
Directory of Support and Information PDF

The **Wishlist** will be updated as change happens.

Join the Mother Becoming village on Facebook and Instagram

https://www.facebook.com/MotherBecoming/

https://www.instagram.com/mother_becoming_book/

Printed in Dunstable, United Kingdom